Clinical Cases in
Gastroenterology

Clinical Cases in Gastroenterology

Editor

Rajesh Upadhyay
MRCP (UK) FRCP (Glasgow) FICP FIAMS FACP (USA) FISG
Senior Director and Head
Department of Gastroenterology and Hepatology
Max Super Specialty Hospital
New Delhi, India

Foreword
D Nageshwar Reddy

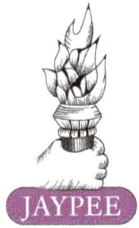

JAYPEE BROTHERS MEDICAL PUBLISHERS
The Health Sciences Publisher
New Delhi | London

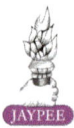 **Jaypee Brothers Medical Publishers (P) Ltd.**

Headquarters
Jaypee Brothers Medical Publishers (P) Ltd
EMCA House, 23/23-B
Ansari Road, Daryaganj
New Delhi 110 002, India
Landline: +91-11-23272143, +91-11-23272703
+91-11-23282021, +91-11-23245672
Email: jaypee@jaypeebrothers.com

Corporate Office
Jaypee Brothers Medical Publishers (P) Ltd
4838/24, Ansari Road, Daryaganj
New Delhi 110 002, India
Phone: +91-11-43574357
Fax: +91-11-43574314
Email: jaypee@jaypeebrothers.com

Overseas Office
JP Medical Ltd.
83, Victoria Street, London
SW1H 0HW (UK)
Phone: +44 20 3170 8910
Fax: +44 (0)20 3008 6180
Email: info@jpmedpub.com

Website: www.jaypeebrothers.com
Website: www.jaypeedigital.com

© 2024, Jaypee Brothers Medical Publishers

The views and opinions expressed in this book are solely those of the original contributor(s)/author(s) and do not necessarily represent those of editor(s) or publisher of the book.

All rights reserved. No part of this publication may be reproduced, stored or transmitted in any form or by any means, electronic, mechanical, photocopying, recording or otherwise, without the prior permission in writing of the publishers.

All brand names and product names used in this book are trade names, service marks, trademarks or registered trademarks of their respective owners. The publisher is not associated with any product or vendor mentioned in this book.

Medical knowledge and practice change constantly. This book is designed to provide accurate, authoritative information about the subject matter in question. However, readers are advised to check the most current information available on procedures included and check information from the manufacturer of each product to be administered, to verify the recommended dose, formula, method and duration of administration, adverse effects and contraindications. It is the responsibility of the practitioner to take all appropriate safety precautions. Neither the publisher nor the author(s)/editor(s) assume any liability for any injury and/or damage to persons or property arising from or related to use of material in this book.

This book is sold on the understanding that the publisher is not engaged in providing professional medical services. If such advice or services are required, the services of a competent medical professional should be sought.

Every effort has been made where necessary to contact holders of copyright to obtain permission to reproduce copyright material. If any have been inadvertently overlooked, the publisher will be pleased to make the necessary arrangements at the first opportunity.

Inquiries for bulk sales may be solicited at: jaypee@jaypeebrothers.com

Clinical Cases in Gastroenterology

First Edition: **2024**

ISBN: 978-93-5696-394-8

Dedication

I would like to dedicate this book to my parents without whose support and guidance I would not be who I am today. I am grateful to them for imparting good values, encouraging me to pursue the path of learning and knowledge, and persevering despite difficulties.

To my wife, Veena, whose love, unwavering support, and encouragement have been the pillars through which this book has come to fruition.

To my esteemed teachers, the guiding lights who imparted not only medical knowledge but also the art of compassionate care. Their wisdom echoes in this book, and it stands as a tribute to the lessons learned from them.

Contributors

AC Anand
MD (Medicine) DM (Gastroenterology) FICP FSGEI
FRCP (London) FRCP (Edinburgh) FACP FACG FAMS
Professor and Head
Department of Gastroenterology and Hepatology
Kalinga Institute of Medical Sciences
Bhubaneswar, Odisha, India

Ajay Duseja
MD DM FAMS FAASLD FACG FSGEI FISG FINASL
Professor and Head
Department of Hepatology
Postgraduate Institute of Medical Education
and Research
Chandigarh, India

Ajay Kumar MD DM MAMS FRCP
Chairman
BLK-Max Hospital—Institute for Digestive
and Liver Diseases
New Delhi, India

Akash Roy MD DM
Consultant
Institute of Gastrosciences and Liver Transplantation
Apollo Multispecialty Hospitals
Kolkata, West Bengal, India

Anant Gupta DNB DrNB
Consultant Gastroenterologist
SR Kalla Memorial Gastro and General Hospital
Jaipur, Rajasthan, India

Anupam Prakash MD
Director Professor of Medicine and Head
Department of Accident and Emergency
Lady Hardinge Medical College
New Delhi, India

Arka De MD DM
Assistant Professor
Department of Hepatology
Postgraduate Institute of Medical Education
and Research
Chandigarh, India

Ashish Chauhan MD DM
Assistant Professor
Department of Gastroenterology
Indira Gandhi Medical College and Hospital
Shimla, Himachal Pradesh, India

Ashish Kumar
MD DM FRCP (Edinburgh) FACP FISG MISG FINASL
Professor and Senior Consultant
Department of Gastroenterology and Hepatology
Institute of Liver, Pancreatico-Biliary Sciences
Sir Ganga Ram Hospital
New Delhi, India

Avesh MD
Consultant
Department of Gastroenterology
and Hepatology
Max Super Specialty Hospital
New Delhi, India

Bhabadev Goswami MD PhD
Former Professor and Head
Department of Gastroenterology
Gauhati Medical College and Hospital
Guwahati, Assam, India

Bipadabhanjan Mallick MD DM
Associate Professor
Department of Gastroenterology
and Hepatology
Kalinga Institute of Medical Sciences
Bhubaneswar, Odisha, India

BJ Gokul MD DM MACG FAGIE
Consultant Gastroenterologist
Department of Gastroenterology
MedIndia Hospitals
Chennai, Tamil Nadu, India

D Nageshwar Reddy
MD DM DSc FAMS FRCP FASGE FACG MWGO FAGA FJGES
Chairman
AIG Hospitals
Hyderabad, Telangana, India

Daya Krishna Jha MD DM
Consultant Gastroenterologist
Department of Gastroenterology
Army Hospital (Research and Referral)
New Delhi, India

Deepak Lahoti MD DM
Senior Director
Department of Gastroenterology
and Hepatology
Max Super Specialty Hospital
New Delhi, India

Deepanshu Khanna MD DNB DrNB
Senior Resident
Department of Gastroenterology
Max Super Specialty Hospital
Ghaziabad, Uttar Pradesh, India

Dibyalochan Praharaj MD DM
Assistant Professor
Department of Gastroenterology
and Hepatology
Kalinga Institute of Medical Sciences
Bhubaneswar, Odisha, India

Goutham Reddy Katukuri MD DM
Consultant Gastroenterologist
Asian Institute of Gastroenterology
Hyderabad, Telangana, India

Govind Makharia MD DM DNB
Professor
Department of Gastroenterology
and Human Nutrition
All India Institute of Medical Sciences
New Delhi, India

Harshil Trivedi MD
Consultant
Max Centre for Gastroenterology, Hepatology
and Endoscopy
Max Hospitals
New Delhi, India

Jayanthi Venkataraman MD DM
Senior Consultant and Gastroenterologist
Gleneagles Global Health City
Chennai, Tamil Nadu, India

K Raja Yogesh MD DM MRCP FAGIE
Consultant Gastroenterologist
Department of Gastroenterology
MedIndia Hospitals
Chennai, Tamil Nadu, India

Kaushal Madan MD DNB DM
Principal Director and Head
Department of Clinical Hepatology
Max Hospitals
New Delhi, India

Kunal Das MD DM FRCP
Director and Head
Department of Gastroenterology
Yashoda Super Specialty Hospital
Ghaziabad, Uttar Pradesh, India

Madhura Prasad MD MRCP FTE DNB
Consultant Gastroenterologist
VGM Hospital
Coimbatore, Tamil Nadu, India

Mahesh Kumar Goenka
MD DM MNAMS AGAF FACG FASGE
Director
Department of Gastroenterology
Institute of Gastrosciences and Liver
Transplantation
Apollo Multispecialty Hospitals
Kolkata, West Bengal, India

Mahiboob Sayyed MD DNB
Consultant Gastroenterologist
Asian Institute of Gastroenterology
Hyderabad, Telangana, India

Manav Wadhawan MD DM
Senior Director
Institute of Liver and Digestive Diseases
Head, Hepatology and Liver Transplant
(Medicine)
BLK-Max Hospital
New Delhi, India

Manu Tandan MD DM
Senior Consultant
Department of Gastroenterology
Asian Institute of Gastroenterology
Hyderabad, Telangana, India

Contributors ix

Mayank Bhusan Pateria MD
Senior Resident
Department of Gastroenterology
Institute of Medical Sciences
Banaras Hindu University
Varanasi, Uttar Pradesh, India

Mayank Jain MD DNB
Senior Consultant
Department of Gastroenterology
and Hepatology
Arihant Hospital and Research Centre
Indore, Madhya Pradesh, India

Meenakshi Jain
MD PG Diploma in Diabetes Management
Director
Department of Internal Medicine
Max Super Specialty Hospital
New Delhi, India

Mithra Prasad MD DM
Consultant Hepatologist
VGM Hospital
Coimbatore, Tamil Nadu, India

MS Prasad MS
Consultant Surgeon
Department of Gastroenterology
MedIndia Hospitals
Chennai, Tamil Nadu, India

Naveen Bhagat MD DM
Resident
Department of Hepatology
Postgraduate Institute of Medical Education
and Research
Chandigarh, India

Neha Berry MD DM
Consultant
BLK-Max Hospital—Institute for Digestive
and Liver Diseases
New Delhi, India

Nitin Bhople DNB DrNB
Consultant
Department of Gastroenterology
and Hepatology
Max Super Specialty Hospital
New Delhi, India

Nitin Gupta MD DM
Senior Consultant
Department of Gastroenterology
Rajiv Gandhi Cancer Institute
New Delhi, India

Nitin Jagtap MD DNB
Consultant Gastroenterologist
Asian Institute of Gastroenterology
Hyderabad, Telangana, India

Omesh Goyal DM FISG FINASL FIACM MNAMS
Professor
Department of Gastroenterology
Dayanand Medical College and Hospital
Ludhiana, Punjab, India

Pavan Dhoble MD DNB
Junior Consultant
Department of Gastroenterology
PD Hinduja Hospital
Mumbai, Maharashtra, India

Philip Abraham MD FCPS DNB
Consultant
Department of Gastroenterology
PD Hinduja Hospital
Mumbai, Maharashtra, India

Preetam Nath MD DM
Associate Professor
Department of Gastroenterology and Hepatology
Kalinga Institute of Medical Sciences
Bhubaneswar, Odisha, India

Preeti Sarma MD
Registrar
Department of Gastroenterology
Gauhati Medical College and Hospital
Guwahati, Assam, India

Premashis Kar MD DM PhD
Senior Director and Head
Department of Gastroenterology
Max Super Specialty Hospital
Ghaziabad, Uttar Pradesh, India

Prerna Goyal MD FIACM
Assistant Professor
Department of Medicine
BJSD College and Hospital
Ludhiana, Punjab, India

Contributors

Priyanka Ojha MD
Senior Resident
Department of Gastroenterology and Hepatology
Max Super Specialty Hospital
New Delhi, India

Rajesh Upadhyay
MRCP (UK) FRCP (Glasgow) FICP FIAMS FACP (USA) FISG
Senior Director and Head
Department of Gastroenterology and Hepatology
Max Super Specialty Hospital
New Delhi, India

Reethesh SR MD DrNB
Consultant
Hepatology and Liver Transplant (Medicine)
BLK Super Specialty Hospital
New Delhi, India

Rupjyoti Talukdar MD FICP AGAF
Director (Pancreatology)
Asian Institute of Gastroenterology
Head
Pancreas Research Group and Division of Gut Microbiome Research Institute of Translational Research, Asian Healthcare Foundation
Hyderabad, Telangana, India

S Sathiamoorthy MD DM FAGIE
Consultant
Department of Gastroenterology
MedIndia Hospitals
Chennai, Tamil Nadu, India

Sagar Tyagi MD
Associate Consultant
Department of Vascular and Interventional Radiology
Max Super Specialty Hospital
New Delhi, India

Sandeep Nijhawan MD DM
Senior Professor
Department of Gastroenterology
SMS Medical College
Jaipur, Rajasthan, India

Sanjay Banerjee MD DNB DM MNAMS FRCP
Head
Department of Gastroenterology
ILS Hospitals
Kolkata, West Bengal, India

Sanjeev Sachdeva MD DM
Director–Professor
Faculty, In-charge (GI Physiology) and Head
Department of Gastroenterology
GB Pant Hospital
New Delhi, India

Sarat Chandra Panigrahi MD DM DNB
Associate Professor
Department of Gastroenterology and Hepatology
Kalinga Institute of Medical Sciences
Bhubaneswar, Odisha, India

Saroj Kant Sahu MD DM
Assistant Professor
Department of Gastroenterology and Hepatology
Kalinga Institute of Medical Sciences
Bhubaneswar, Odisha, India

Sethubabu DNB DM
Senior Consultant
Department of Gastroenterology and Hepatology
Krishna Institute of Medical Sciences
Hyderabad, Telangana, India

Shami Kumar DNB DrNB
Gastroenterologist
Department of Gastroenterology and Hepatology
Max Super Specialty Hospital
New Delhi, India

Shishirendu Parihar MD
Assistant Professor
Department of Gastroenterology
Institute of Medical Sciences
Banaras Hindu University
Varanasi, Uttar Pradesh, India

Shivam Kalia MD DM
Senior Resident
Department of Gastroenterology and Hepatology
Kalinga Institute of Medical Sciences
Bhubaneswar, Odisha, India

Soumya Jagannath MD DM
Assistant Professor
Department of Gastroenterology
Indira Gandhi Medical College and Hospital
Shimla, Himachal Pradesh, India

Contributors xi

TC Viveksandeep MD AB (Med) AB (Gastro) MACG
Director of Endoscopy
Department of Gastroenterology
Augusta University Medical Center
Medical College of Georgia
Augusta, Georgia, USA

Teja J MD
Consultant
Department of Gastroenterology
and Hepatology
Krishna Institute of Medical Sciences
Hyderabad, Telangana, India

TS Chandrasekar
MD DM DSc FRCP FASGE FACG AGAF FAMS FICP FIMSA MWGO
Founder, Chairman and Chief Interventional Gastroenterologist
Department of Gastroenterology
MedIndia Hospitals
Chennai, Tamil Nadu, India

Uday C Ghoshal MD DNB DM FACG RFF FAMS FRCP (Edin) MISG
Professor and Head
Department of Gastroenterology
Sanjay Gandhi Postgraduate Institute
of Medical Sciences
Lucknow, Uttar Pradesh, India

Ujjwal Sonika MD DM
Associate Professor
Department of Gastroenterology
GB Pant Hospital
New Delhi, India

Uzma Mustafa MD DNB
Assistant Professor
Department of Gastroenterology
Sanjay Gandhi Postgraduate Institute
of Medical Sciences
Lucknow, Uttar Pradesh, India

Vamsi Murthy K MD DM FAGIE
Consultant
Gastroenterologist, Hepatologist
and Therapeutic Endoscopist
VGM Hospital
Coimbatore, Tamil Nadu, India

VG Mohan Prasad
MD DM (Gastro) FRCP(E) FCCP FSGEI FICP FASGE
Senior Consultant
Department of Gastroenterology, Hepatology
and Therapeutic Endoscopy
VGM Hospital
Coimbatore, Tamil Nadu, India

Vinod Arora MD DM
Assistant Professor
Department of Hepatology
Institute of Liver and Biliary Sciences
New Delhi, India

Vinod Kumar MD
Assistant Professor
Department of Gastroenterology
Institute of Medical Sciences
Banaras Hindu University
Varanasi, Uttar Pradesh, India

Vishal Sharma MD DM
Associate Professor
Department of Gastroenterology
Postgraduate Institute of Medical Education
and Research
Chandigarh, India

VK Dixit MD DM FRCP FAMS FICP FINASL FSGEI FISG
Professor and Head
Department of Gastroenterology
Institute of Medical Sciences
Banaras Hindu University
Varanasi, Uttar Pradesh, India

VK Gupta MD DM
Director
Department of Gastroenterology and Hepatology
Max Super Specialty Hospital
New Delhi, India

VS Gaurav Narayan MD
Senior Resident
Department of Gastroenterology and Hepatology
Max Super Specialty Hospital
New Delhi, India

Yogesh K Chhabra MD DM
Principal Consultant
Department of Nephrology
Max Hospitals
New Delhi, India

Foreword

I congratulate Dr Rajesh Upadhyay, a well-known and very much respected and appreciated Senior Medical Teacher and Academician in Gastroenterology for coming up with this book, *Clinical Cases in Gastroenterology* that will have positive impact on students and also young practitioners.

Dr Upadhyay is presently working as the Senior Director and Head, Department of Gastroenterology and Hepatology, Max Super Specialty Hospital, New Delhi, India. He has held several academic and administrative posts in several associations and has been the Dean of Indian College of Physicians. He has been a Postgraduate Examiner and is a Member of Special Advisory Board, and National Board of Examination (NBE).

Even though there are many excellent books on clinical aspects in gastroenterology, a paucity of concise book on practical aspects of gastroenterology, written in simple, easy-to-understand language is felt by students, young teachers and practicing physicians and medical gastroenterologists. In this book, he has provided in-depth clinical case discussions for postgraduate students in gastroenterology along with brief note on approach to common gastroenterology and liver symptoms and various conditions under gastrointestinal tract, liver, hepatobiliary and pancreatic systems, which can be applied in day-to-day life. This book has all the essentials to make postgraduate students, competent gastroenterologists, and also benefit teachers to refresh their knowledge and skills of bedside clinical examination. The topics are covered in lucid, clear, and easy-to-understand language. Most recent advances have been incorporated.

I am sure this book will be read not only by all the postgraduates but also by practicing physicians and gastroenterologists to update their knowledge and also improve their clinical skills. I wish Dr Rajesh Upadhyay all the best for the success of this book and future endeavors.

Best Regards

D Nageshwar Reddy
MD DM DSc FAMS FRCP FASGE FACG MWGO FAGA FJGES
Chairman, AIG Hospitals
Hyderabad, Telangana, India
Padma Shri (2002) and Padma Bhushan (2016) Awardee
Past President of World Endoscopy Organization
Recipient of Rudolf Schindler Award

Preface

Welcome to the dynamic and intricate world of Gastroenterology, a field that continually evolves with groundbreaking discoveries, technological advancements and a profound commitment to understanding the complexities of the digestive system.

It is interesting the way this book was conceptualized. During one of our regular postgraduate classes, I witnessed a case presentation by the 1st Year DNB student in our unit. During our conversation about the case, I conveyed my dissatisfaction with his presentation approach and inquired about the availability of books on clinical case presentations. To my astonishment, I discovered that there were scarce resources in terms of books specifically catering to postgraduates in gastroenterology for clinical case presentations. It was then that the need for 'filling the gap' in medical literature unfurled a cascade of ideas that eventually became the foundation for my book.

This book is an attempt to incorporate clinical cases seen in day-to-day practice, with an exhaustive discussion aimed to sharpen and enhance the thinking ability of the reader. As a postgraduate, embarking on a journey of specialization in Gastroenterology, you are entering a realm that not only demands a comprehensive grasp of fundamental principles but also necessitates adaptability to the ever-expanding landscape of knowledge. The most effective method for acquiring practical knowledge in disease management and consequently preparing students for examinations and clinical practice, is through case presentations and discussions.

This textbook is meticulously crafted to serve as your trusted companion throughout your academic pursuit, offering a thorough exploration of the multi-faceted aspects of gastroenterology and hepatology. It is designed to provide a solid foundation in the core principles, diagnostic techniques, therapeutic interventions, and recent advancements that define this rapidly evolving discipline. The book caters to the diverse needs of both postgraduate students and clinical practitioners, fostering a deeper understanding of the subject matter and its practical applications. As you navigate through the pages of this book, you will find an emphasis on evidence-based medicine, critical thinking, and a patient-centered approach. We encourage you to actively engage with the material, incorporating clinical reasoning and problem-solving skills that will be crucial in your future practice.

In this book, distinguished authors have delved into a diverse array of pertinent cases. The objective is to instruct on the presentation of clinical problems and the formulation of strategies for diagnosis and management. In these pages, you will encounter a diverse array of cases carefully selected to encapsulate the breadth and depth of gastroenterological conditions. From common ailments to rare presentations, each case has been chosen to challenge and expand your clinical reasoning, encouraging you to navigate the intricate web of signs, symptoms, and investigative findings that define gastroenterology.

I would like to extend my gratitude to the contributors—experts in the field who have generously shared their knowledge and experiences. Their insights serve as valuable signposts, guiding you through the twists and turns of clinical decision-making.

May this collection of clinical case presentations inspire you to approach each patient encounter with intellectual rigor, empathy, and a dedication to unravelling the mysteries of gastroenterology. I wish you success in your academic endeavors and fulfilment in your pursuit of excellence in patient care.

Rajesh Upadhyay

Acknowledgments

I would like to express my sincere gratitude to all those who played a crucial role in the creation and publication of this book. Their support and contributions have been invaluable, and I am truly thankful for their dedication.

First and foremost, I extend my deepest appreciation to the talented authors, medical professionals, researchers, and educators whose work has paved the way for advancements in gastroenterology. Each one's contribution of their expertise, creativity and passion is reflected in the pages of this book. Your commitment to excellence has made this project a reality and I am honored to have collaborated with such a remarkable team. Your collective efforts have laid the foundation for the insights presented in this book.

Next, I would like to thank the publishers, M/s Jaypee Brothers Medical Publishers (P) Ltd, New Delhi, India, for their unwavering support. Their guidance, professionalism, and commitment to quality have been instrumental in bringing this project to fruition. A special mention of Mr Priyansh Saxena for his coordination in shaping this book.

A special note of thanks goes to my Secretary, Ms Indu Sharma, for providing continuous support.

To everyone who played a part, big or small, in the journey of bringing this book to life—thank you. Your support has made this endeavor a rewarding and fulfilling experience.

This book is a result of collaborative efforts and shared passion for advancing knowledge in gastroenterology. I am truly grateful for the support and contributions of everyone involved.

Last but not least, I would like to thank my wife and my children for their love, and unwavering support throughout this journey.

Contents

Section 1
Approach to Common Gastrointestinal and Liver Symptoms

1. Returning to Basics Always Helps 3
   Vinod Kumar, Shishirendu Parihar, VK Dixit

2. Fever, Pain Abdomen, and Altered Liver Tests 6
   Sandeep Nijhawan, Anant Gupta

3. Fever with Jaundice 13
   Vinod Arora, Anupam Prakash

4. Approach to Dysphagia 18
   Pavan Dhoble, Philip Abraham

5. Approach to Renal Dysfunction in Chronic Liver Disease 26
   Yogesh K Chhabra

Section 2
Diseases of the Esophagus

6. Perplexing Cases of *Candida* Esophagitis 33
   Sanjay Banerjee

7. Refractory Gastroesophageal Reflux Disease 40
   VG Mohan Prasad, Vamsi Murthy K, Madhura Prasad, Mithra Prasad

8. Management of Dysphagia 47
   Ashish Chauhan, Soumya Jagannath, Govind Makharia

Section 3
Gastrointestinal Bleed

9. Nonvariceal Upper Gastrointestinal Bleed 57
   Kunal Das

10. Obscure Gastrointestinal Bleed 64
    Neha Berry, Ajay Kumar

11. Gastric Variceal Bleed 72
    Rajesh Upadhyay, Sagar Tyagi, VS Gaurav Narayan

Section 4
Diseases of the Liver

12. **Nonalcoholic Fatty Liver Disease** 81
    Ashish Kumar

13. **Alcoholic Hepatitis** 92
    Rajesh Upadhyay, VS Gaurav Narayan, Priyanka Ojha

14. **IgM Anti-HEV Positivity in a Patient with Suspected Severe Alcoholic Hepatitis: Cause or a Red Herring?** 99
    Harshil Trivedi, Kaushal Madan

15. **Acute on Chronic Liver Failure** 105
    Akash Roy, Mahesh Kumar Goenka

16. **Intrahepatic Cholestasis** 112
    Rajesh Upadhyay, VS Gaurav Narayan

17. **Herb-induced Liver Injury** 121
    Bhabadev Goswami, Preeti Sarma

18. **Autoimmune Hepatitis** 125
    Reethesh SR, Manav Wadhawan

19. **Recompensation and Reversal of Cirrhosis: Myth or Reality?** 130
    Naveen Bhagat, Arka De, Ajay Duseja

20. **Sickle Hepatopathy** 134
    AC Anand, Shivam Kalia, Dibyalochan Praharaj, Preetam Nath, Sarat Chandra Panigrahi, Bipadabhanjan Mallick, Saroj Kant Sahu

Section 5
Diseases of the Gallbladder and Biliary Tract

21. **Choledocholithiasis** 141
    Nitin Jagtap, D Nageshwar Reddy

22. **Obstructive Jaundice** 146
    Deepanshu Khanna, Premashis Kar

23. **Spontaneous Rupture of Cystic Artery Pseudoaneurysm Presented as Hemobilia** 150
    VK Dixit, Mayank Bhusan Pateria, Vinod Kumar

24. **Immunoglobulin G4-related Gastrointestinal Diseases** 153
    TS Chandrasekar, BJ Gokul, S Sathiamoorthy, K Raja Yogesh, MS Prasad, TC Viveksandeep

Section 6
Diseases of the Pancreas

25. **Management of Acute Pancreatitis** 165
    Goutham Reddy Katukuri, Rupjyoti Talukdar

26. **Autoimmune Pancreatitis** 172
    Nitin Gupta

27. **Pancreatic Mass Lesion—A Diagnostic Dilemma** 175
    VK Gupta

Section 7
Diseases of the Intestines (Luminal Disorders)

28. **Chronic Constipation** 181
    Omesh Goyal, Prerna Goyal

29. **Chronic Diarrhea** 194
    Daya Krishna Jha, Vishal Sharma

30. **Chronic Constipation: Frequently Asked Questions** 202
    Mayank Jain, Jayanthi Venkataraman

31. **Gallstone Ileus Presenting as Subacute Small Bowel Obstruction** 209
    Sethubabu, Teja J

32. **Small Bowel Neuroendocrine Tumors** 213
    Mahiboob Sayyed, Manu Tandan

33. **An Interesting Case of SIBO/Dysbiosis** 219
    Sanjeev Sachdeva, Ujjwal Sonika

34. **Amoeboma Masquerading as Carcinoma Colon** 228
    Deepak Lahoti, Shami Kumar, Nitin Bhople, Avesh, Meenakshi Jain

35. **Constipation–Functional Dyspepsia Overlap** 232
    Uday C Ghoshal, Uzma Mustafa

Index *239*

Section 1: Approach to Common Gastrointestinal and Liver Symptoms

1. **Returning to Basics Always Helps**
   Vinod Kumar, Shishirendu Parihar, VK Dixit

2. **Fever, Pain Abdomen, and Altered Liver Tests**
   Sandeep Nijhawan, Anant Gupta

3. **Fever with Jaundice**
   Vinod Arora, Anupam Prakash

4. **Approach to Dysphagia**
   Pavan Dhoble, Philip Abraham

5. **Approach to Renal Dysfunction in Chronic Liver Disease**
   Yogesh K Chhabra

Returning to Basics Always Helps

Vinod Kumar, Shishirendu Parihar, VK Dixit

INTRODUCTION

A 45-year-old lady presented to us with fever × 15 days which was high-grade and associated with chills and rigor, headache, nausea, and vomiting. She also complained of yellowish discoloration of eyes and urine × 10 days, which was gradually progressive and was associated with pruritus. The fever continued to persist after onset of jaundice. There was no history of similar illness in past. No history of hepatobiliary surgery or blood transfusion was noted. Neither was it associated with abnormal behavior, hematemesis or melena, or abdominal distension.

There was no history of diabetes, hypertension, tuberculosis, and chronic and regular drug intake for any disease. Also, there was no history of over-the-counter or alternative medication use.

On examination, the patient was conscious, cooperative, well-oriented to time and place, and for a person lying on the couch with vitals—oxygen saturation (SPO_2) 97% on room air, pulse 90 beats/min regular, blood pressure (BP) 110/70 mm Hg, respiration rate (RR) 16/min, and temperature 100 °F.

On general examination, only icterus was present and systemic examination was within normal limits.

Tropical fever was suspected. Routine investigations were sent, which revealed raised total leukocyte count (TLC) 26,240 (85% N, 13% L), hyperbilirubinemia [total bilirubin (TB)/direct bilirubin (DB) 10/5.5], elevated transaminases [oxaloacetic transaminase (OT)/prothrombin time (PT) 287/239)], raised alkaline phosphatase 1,291, and hyponatremia with hyperkalemia. Ultrasonography (USG) abdomen showed normal sized liver with altered echotexture, portal vein of 10 mm, and mild splenomegaly, common bile duct (CBD) was normal, no intra hepatic biliary radicle dilatation (IHBRD), and no ascites. Evaluation for malaria and dengue was negative, immunoglobulin M (IgM) anti-hepatitis E virus (anti-HEV) antibody turned out to be positive.[1]

But as fever was not subsiding, repeat review of examination revealed a small wound with central eschar **(Fig. 1)**; hence, a

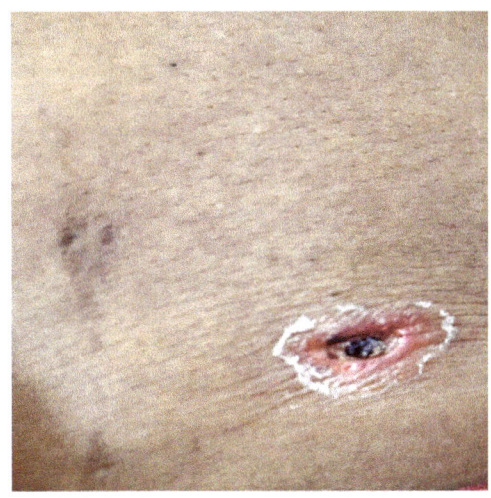

Fig. 1: A small wound with central eschar.

possibility of scrub typhus was entertained.[2] Leptospira IgM and scrub typhus IgM both came positive.

Keeping in view the presence of eschar scrub typhus was kept as first differential and the patient was started on doxycycline along with piperacillin-tazobactam and other supportive medications. She became afebrile after 48 hours and serum test started improving. The patient was discharged after 6 days of hospital stay with stable vitals.[3]

Coinfections of hepatitis A virus (HAV)/HEV with Leptospira, malaria, and dengue are well reported in literature and are not so uncommon, especially in endemic countries. A coinfection of scrub typhus with other viral diseases is very rare. To the best of our knowledge, only one coinfection of HEV with scrub typhus has been reported from PGI Chandigarh in a pregnant lady who succumbed to illness.[4]

Hepatitis E virus coinfection was found in 13 cases of leptospirosis and 1 case of dengue, with one rare case of triple infection with HEV, dengue, and malaria.[5]

This case also highlights the importance of thorough clinical examination. Had the eschar been detected on initial examination, diagnosis would be so evident. Also, this teaches us the importance of going back to review history and examination and existing literature for seeking out missing links if there is no clinical improvement.

■ INVESTIGATION

Date	Hb (gm%)	TLC cells/mm^3	DLC %	Platelet count lakh/mm^3	Bilirubin (T/D) mg/dL	AST/ALT IU/mL	ALP IU/mL	Protein/Albumin g/dL
28/8/22	12.5	26,240	85/13	1.08	10/5.5	287/239	1,291	6.6/3.0
1/9/22	12.24	18,840	53/37	2.37	3/2.5	79/104	849	7.1/2.2
4/9/22	10.3	11,960	22/64	5.17	1.7/1.3	82/72	739	20/0.8

Date	Urea mg/dL	Creatinine mg/dL	Na/K mmol/L	PT/INR seconds
28/8/22	76	1.0	124/6.3	17/1.24
1/9/22	10	1.00	125/5.2	
4/9/22	20	0.8	132/4.8	

(ALP: alkaline phosphatase; AST/ALT: aspartate transaminase/alanine transaminase; DLC: differential leukocyte count; Hb: hemoglobin; PT/INR: prothrombin time/international normalized ratio; TLC: total leukocyte count)

Tests	Result
Anti-HCV/HIV-1 and 2/HBsAg	Non-reactive/NR/NR
IgM anti-HAV/HEV	Negative/positive
Dengue ns1, IgG, IgM, and paracheck	Negative
USG abdomen 30/8/22	Normal sized liver with altered echotexture, mild splenomegaly, PV 10 mm, CBD normal, no IHBRD, and no ascites
HbA1c	5.9
Lepto IgM and scrub typhus IgM antibody	Both positive
Urine routine microscopy	WNL

(CBD: common bile duct; HbA1c: glycated hemoglobin; HBsAg: hepatitis B surface antigen; HCV: hepatitis C virus; HAV: hepatitis A virus; HEV: hepatitis E virus; HIV: human immunodeficiency virus; IgM: immunoglobulin M; IHBRD: intra hepatic biliary radicle dilatation; PV: portal vein; USG: ultrasonography; WNL: within normal limits)

REFERENCES

1. Blanton LS. The Rickettsioses: a practical update. Infect Dis Clin North Am. 2019;33(1):213-29.
2. Devasagayam E, Dayanand D, Kundu D, Kamath MS, Kirubakaran R, Varghese GM. The burden of scrub typhus in India: a systematic review. PLoS Negl Trop Dis. 2021;15(7):e0009619.
3. Anand AC, Garg HK. Approach to clinical syndrome of jaundice and encephalopathy in tropics. J Clin Exp Hepatol. 2015;5(Suppl 1):S116-30.
4. Verma N, Sharma M, Biswal M, Taneja S, Batra N, Kumar A, et al. Hepatitis E Virus-Induced Acute Liver Failure with Scrub Typhus Coinfection in a Pregnant Woman. J Clin Exp Hepatol. 2017;7(2):158-60.
5. Chaudhry R, Das A, Premlatha MM. Serological and molecular approaches for diagnosis of leptospirosis in a tertiary care hospital in north India: a 10-year study. Indian J Med Res. 2013;137:785-90.

Fever, Pain Abdomen, and Altered Liver Tests

Sandeep Nijhawan, Anant Gupta

■ INTRODUCTION

A 66-year-old male presented with fever with chills and continuous, moderate-intensity pain in the right upper quadrant (RUQ) of abdomen and in the right shoulder for 3 days. There was no dyspnea or vomiting. He has had diabetes mellitus since 8 years and is on oral hypoglycemic agents. He consumes about 30 g of alcohol on most days of the week.

On examination, he appeared unwell with a temperature of 101 °F and tenderness in the RUQ. On examination, right hypochondrium was tender, liver and spleen were not palpable, and there was no guarding or rigidity. Blood investigations were done which show: total leukocyte count (TLC) 16,500/mm^3 (neutrophils 86%, lymphocytes 12%), hemoglobin 10.4 g/dL, platelet count 4.5 lakh/mm^3, erythrocyte sedimentation rate (ESR) 64 mm/h, C-reactive protein (CRP) 84 mg/L, total bilirubin 2.4 (direct 1.8, indirect 0.6) mg/dL, alanine aminotransferase (ALT) 92 IU/L, aspartate aminotransferase (AST) 85 IU/L, alkaline phosphatase 256 IU/L, random blood sugar (RBS) 188 mg/dL, and serum creatinine 1.0 mg/dL.

■ WHAT WILL YOU SUSPECT?

In the abovementioned scenario of fever, RUQ pain, tenderness, and deranged liver tests, probable diagnoses will include liver abscess, acute hepatitis, right lobe pneumonia, acute cholangitis, and acute cholecystitis.

Which Investigations Would you Perform to Narrow your Diagnosis?

We would suspect an intra-abdominal infection but will keep possibility of other sources of infections. Thus, ultrasonography (USG) of abdomen, chest X-ray, urine routine, urine, and blood culture were done.

Ultrasound scan **(Fig. 1)** shows a single, poorly demarcated, hypoechoic lesion of 5 cm in maximum diameter in the right lobe of the liver. The gall bladder, common bile duct (CBD), and pancreas appear normal. The chest X-ray and urine routine are within normal limits.

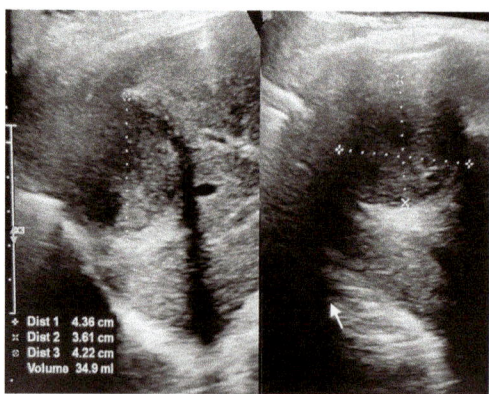

Fig. 1: Ultrasonography image of liver demonstrates a rounded hypoechoic lesion in right lobe of liver with distal acoustic enhancement.

What are the Differential Diagnoses?

- Liver abscesses
- Hepatic tumors (primary or secondary).

The likely primary diagnosis is a liver abscess. Amoebic liver abscess (ALA) is more common than pyogenic liver abscess (PLA). They differ in terms of epidemiology and medical management. However, it may be difficult to distinguish between them based on clinical course (PLA usually has more pronounced systemic features with multiple abscesses) and imaging features (ALA is commonly single and involves the right lobe of liver). Liver abscesses most commonly (nearly 65%) involve the right lobe of the liver, probably because it is larger and has greater blood supply than the left and caudate lobes. Up to 20% of patients may have multiple abscesses.[1-3]

Adequate clinical assessment will guide us towards the right diagnosis. However, abscess must be distinguished from tumors and cysts. Transient perilesional enhancement, which is more frequently associated with a pyogenic abscess, helps exclude hepatic tumors.

WHICH IMAGING MODALITY SHOULD BE USED?

Ultrasonography and computed tomography (CT) [preferred with intravenous (IV) contrast, if feasible] are the imaging modalities usually used for identification of liver abscess. CT (95%) is more sensitive for detection of liver abscesses than USG (85%).[4] Imaging modalities help in achieving a diagnosis and define the size of abscess, location in liver, and its proximity to hepatic surface. It helps to plan the management in such cases.

When is a Cross-sectional Imaging (CT or MRI) Needed?

- High clinical suspicion but USG performed initially does not reveal any lesion. Subdiaphragmatic posterior segment lesions may be difficult to visualize and may be missed, especially in those with fatty liver.
- Atypical appearance on USG (solid appearance) must be distinguished from tumors.
- Need for percutaneous drainage in those with complicated abscesses
- Suspicion of complications—thrombosis of the portal vein and biliary tree obstruction [magnetic resonance imaging (MRI) is preferred to demonstrate communication.]

Typical Appearance on CT (Figs. 2A and B)

The typical finding is a peripherally enhancing, centrally hypoattenuating lesion. The "double-target sign" is a characteristic imaging feature but is present only in a few. Central low attenuation (fluid-filled) lesion is surrounded by a high attenuation (peripheral enhancement of inner rim) and a low attenuation outer ring (surrounding edema).

FINAL CLINICAL DIAGNOSIS

Liver abscess (single, in right lobe)—possibly amoebic

WHAT ARE THE CLINICAL FEATURES OF LIVER ABSCESSES?[5,6]

- Fever (90%)
- Abdominal symptoms (50–75%)—pain, usually localized to the RUQ
- Constitutional symptoms (malaise, anorexia, nausea, and vomiting)
- Diaphragmatic irritation (right shoulder tip pain and respiratory symptoms)
- Jaundice is uncommon and is generally a late finding, unless the abscess is large, causing biliary obstruction to the main duct.

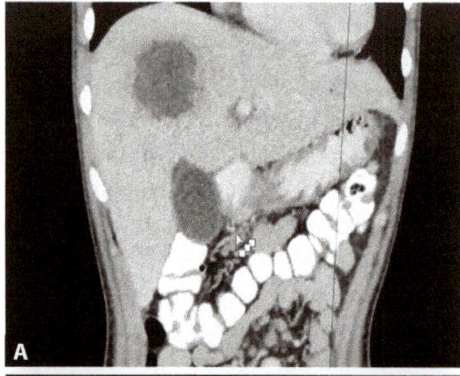

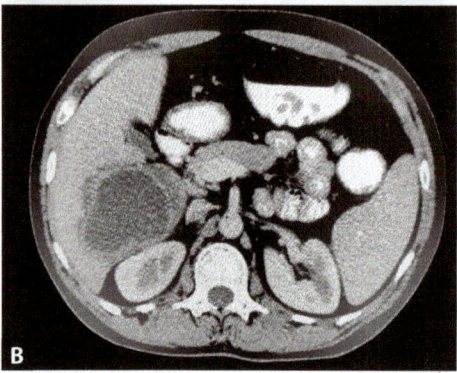

Figs. 2A and B: (A) Coronal computed tomography (CT) image demonstrates hypodense lesion with peripheral enhancement in VII segment of liver with a surrounding rim of 26 mm of liver parenchyma. (B) Axial CT image demonstrates hypodense lesion with peripheral enhancement reaching up to the liver capsule with tenting of liver surface—liver abscess with impending rupture.

WHAT CAN BE THE ETIOLOGY OF HEPATIC ABSCESSES?

Pyogenic: These are frequently polymicrobial. Many of the causative organisms are enteric.
- Enteric Gram-negative bacilli, particularly *Escherichia coli* (*E. coli*) and *Klebsiella pneumoniae* (*K. pneumoniae*) are the most common causes.
- *Staphylococcus aureus* and *Streptococcus pyogenes.*

Amoebic: ALA is commonly seen in the third and fourth decades, with a male preponderance (M:F ratio 4–10:1).[7]

Parasites: Roundworms or flukes can be associated with biliary infection, leading to PLAs.

Fungi: Usually seen in the immunocompromised host and have poor prognosis.

Pathogenesis:[6,8] Majority of PLAs develop after biliary tract infection (cholangitis and acute cholecystitis), abdominal infections (diverticulitis and appendicitis), postprocedural, penetrating wounds, or from hematogenous spread from the systemic circulation.

HOW WILL WE MANAGE THIS PATIENT?

Are Further Investigations Needed?

PLA: Blood cultures are essential in the evaluation of suspected PLAs; they are positive in up to 50% cases.[9]

ALA: Serologic tests are seldom done. They are required when the diagnosis is uncertain. Available serologic tests for EH are antiamoebic immunoglobulin G (IgG) antibody, polymerase chain reaction (PCR), and lectin antigen (not suitable in those where treatment has already been initiated).

Antibodies are detectable at presentation in >90% of patients with ALA.[10] In endemic areas like India, ~30% of presently uninfected individuals will have a positive serology due to prior infection, so a positive serology may not indicate active infection and should be carefully interpreted.[11]

Initial *E. histolytica*-specific IgM rapidly declines to low levels and is replaced with IgG at the time of diagnosis of the disease. IgM is a poor marker and antiamoebic IgG antibodies are thus utilized.[12,13]

Since most ALA patients do not have coexistent amoebic colitis, stool microscopy or antigen detection in stool samples is not helpful for diagnosis.

When to Aspirate the Abscess?

- *Diagnostic aspiration:* During diagnostic uncertainty (i.e., atypical symptoms or imaging) aspiration of purulent material, Gram stain, and culture helps to confirm the diagnosis of abscess. Amoebic abscess, when aspirated, is a thick, brown fluid (called "anchovy paste") and contains acellular debris. Amoebic trophozoites are not seen commonly.
- Therapeutic aspiration/drainage (discussed further under management).

How Will We Treat this Patient?

Mainstay of treatment is antibiotics and drainage of abscess[14] **(Flowchart 1)**.

Antibiotic Therapy

Empiric broad-spectrum antibiotics **(Table 1)** should be started immediately after sending blood cultures and microbiologic culture of abscess contents if aspirated. The empiric regimen should cover enteric Gram-negative bacilli, *anaerobes*, Streptococci, and *E. histolytica,* until the causative pathogens are found on culture or amoebic testing is negative.

To the best of our knowledge, no randomized controlled trials (RCTs) are available that have evaluated antibiotic regimens for treatment of PLA. Treatment should be guided by local bacterial resistance patterns, if available.

The patient was treated with IV antibiotics (ceftriaxone and metronidazole) and other supportive medications. However, he continued to have fever and pain abdomen even after 3 days of antibiotics.

Do We Need to Change Out Plan?

Drainage

Along with antibiotics, drainage of the abscess contents is a standard therapy for treatment of liver abscess. It is attempted under image guidance (mostly USG), or surgical, or endoscopic retrograde cholangiopancreatography (ERCP) guided. Drainage may be with needle aspiration or with catheter placement.

Indication of drainage
- Left lobe abscess
- Abscess with thin hepatic parenchymal rim (<10 mm)
- Impending rupture on imaging
- Nonresponse to medical therapy after 72 hours

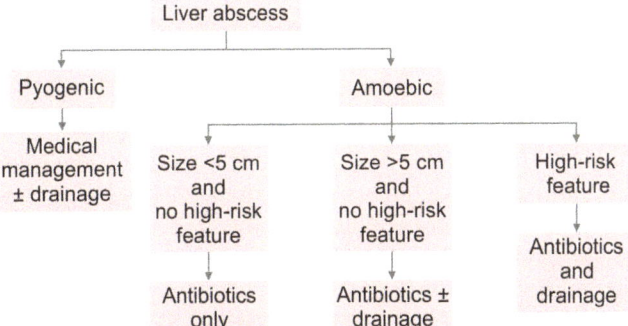

Flowchart 1: Overview of treatment.

TABLE 1: Medications for liver abscess.

Pyogenic liver abscess			Duration 2–6 weeks*
Ceftriaxone with Metronidazole	1 g IV 500 mg IV	Every 12 hourly Every 8 hourly	(Anaerobic coverage)
Special considerations (hemodynamic instability/multi-organ involvement/suspected ESBL			
Piperacillin tazobactam	3.375 or 4.5 g IV	Every 6 hourly	
Ticarcillin–clavulanate	3.1 g IV	Every 4 hourly	
Cefoperazone Sulbactam	2–3 g IV	Every 12 hourly	
Imipenem Cilastatin	500 mg IV	Every 6 hourly	
Meropenem	1–2 g IV	Every 8 hourly	
Ertapenem	1 g IV	Every 24 hourly	
Alternative regimens			
• Ciprofloxacin • Levofloxacin • Metronidazole	• 400 mg IV • 500–750 mg IV • 500 mg IV	• Every 12 hourly • Every 24 hourly • Every 8 hourly	
High suspicion of Gram-positive organism MRSA or resistant Enterococcus (additional antibiotics)			
Vancomycin	1 g IV	Every 12 hourly	
Amoebic liver abscess			
Tissue amoebicidal			
Metronidazole	800 mg oral	Every 8 hourly	7–10 days
Tinidazole	1.2 g oral	Every 24 hours	7–10 days
Luminal amoebicidal (after response to initial tissue amoebicidal)			
Diloxanide furoate	500 mg oral	Every 8 hourly	10 days
Paromomycin	500 mg oral	Every 8 hourly	10 days
Chloroquine DS	• 300 mg oral • 150 mg oral	• Every 12 hourly • Every 12 hourly	• 2 days, then • 14 days

*Usual duration of 2 weeks of IV antibiotics followed by oral antibiotics.
(ESBL: extended-spectrum beta-lactamases; IV: intravenous; MRSA: methicillin-resistant Staphylococcus aureus)

- *Single, unilocular abscess of size 3–5 cm:* Percutaneous needle aspiration (PNA) usually suffices
- *Single, unilocular abscess of size >5 cm:* Percutaneous catheter drainage (PCD) is preferred over needle aspiration. Drainage catheters should remain in place until drainage is minimal (usually up to 7 days). Meta-analysis of five RCTs for large abscesses (>5 cm) suggested that catheter drainage (96%) resulted in a higher success rate and faster recovery as compared with needle aspiration (78%).[15]
- *Multiple or multiloculated abscesses:* Decisions are made on case-to-case basis. Usually, a combination of needle aspiration (for small abscess) and catheter drainage (for larger abscess) are used.

Patient underwent percutaneous catheter placement and drainage for the liver abscess. Symptoms resolved over next 3 days and the drain was removed after 5 days when the daily output was reduced to negligible amount.

When to Suspect Complications?

- Persistence of elevated bilirubin could indicate biliary obstruction.
- Dyspnea, look for lung and cardia complications
- Worsening of pain abdomen and fever. Abscess rupture is a rare complication (<5%).[16] Abscess of diameter >6 cm and coexisting cirrhosis are the main risk factors for rupture, with most ruptures being perihepatic or into the pleural space.

How Should the Follow-up be Planned?

Assessment of symptoms (pain/fever) and general physical examination. Follow-up imaging is needed if persistent clinical symptoms or if drainage catheter gets interrupted. Imaging abnormalities resolve more slowly than clinical and biochemical parameters.

Antibiotics were given IV for 7 days, then orally for next 7 days. After this, a 2-week course of luminal amoebicidal agents was given. Our patient was reviewed every 7 days initially till antibiotics were prescribed.

■ WHAT IS THE PROGNOSIS?

Untreated liver abscesses have a poor prognosis with nearly 100% mortality. Treatment with antibiotics and drainage has reduced the mortality to 2–12%.[5]

Poor prognosis is associated with multiple or large volume liver abscesses, old age, coexisting medical conditions, bilirubin >3.5 mg/dL, albumin <2 g/dL, and encephalopathy.[17]

■ REFERENCES

1. Katzenstein D, Rickerson V, Braude A. New concepts of amebic liver abscess derived from hepatic imaging, serodiagnosis, and hepatic enzymes in 67 consecutive cases in San Diego. Medicine (Baltimore). 1982;61:237-46.
2. Park MS, Kim KW, Ha HK, Lee DH. Intestinal parasitic infection. Abdom Imaging. 2008;33:166-71.
3. Sharma N, Sharma A, Varma S, Lal A, Singh V. Amoebic liver abscess in the medical emergency of a North Indian hospital. BMC Res Notes. 2010;3:21.
4. Halvorsen RA, Korobkin M, Foster WL, Silverman PM, Thompson WM. The variable CT appearance of hepatic abscesses. AJR Am J Roentgenol. 1984;142(5):941.
5. Mohsen AH, Green ST, Read RC, McKendrick MW. Liver abscess in adults: ten years experience in a UK Centre. QJM. 2002;95(12): 797.
6. Huang CJ, Pitt HA, Lipsett PA, Osterman FA Jr, Lillemoe KD, Cameron JL, et al. Pyogenic hepatic abscess. Changing trends over 42 years. Ann Surg. 1996;223(5):600.
7. Lodhi S, Sarwari AR, Muzammil M, Salam A, Smego RA. Features distinguishing amoebic from pyogenic liver abscess: a review of 577 adult cases. Trop Med Int Health. 2004;9(6): 718.
8. Rahimian J, Wilson T, Oram V, Holzman RS. Pyogenic liver abscess: recent trends in etiology and mortality. Clin Infect Dis. 2004;39(11):1654.
9. Chemaly RF, Hall GS, Keys TF, Procop GW. Microbiology of liver abscesses and the predictive value of abscess gram stain and associated blood cultures. Diagn Microbiol Infect Dis. 2003;46(4):245.
10. Stanley SL Jr, Jackson TF, Foster L, Singh S. Longitudinal study of the antibody response to recombinant Entamoeba histolytica antigens in patients with amebic liver abscess. Am J Trop Med Hyg. 1998;58:414-6.
11. Aucott JN, Ravdin JI. Amebiasis and nonpathogenic intestinal protozoa. Infect Dis Clin North Am. 1993;7:467-85.

12. Shetty N, Nagpal S, Rao PV, Schroder H. Detection of IgG, IgA, IgM, and IgE Antibodies in Invasive Amoebiasis in Endemic Areas. Scand J Infect Dis. 1990;22(4):485-91.
13. Jaiswal V, Ghoshal U, Baijal SS, Mittal B, Dhole TN, Ghoshal UC. Evaluation of antigen detection and polymerase chain reaction for diagnosis of amoebic liver abscess in patients on anti-amoebic treatment. BMC Res Notes. 2012;5:416.
14. Sharma S, Ahuja V. Liver Abscess: Complications and Treatment. Clin Liver Dis. 2021; 18:122-6.
15. Cai YL, Xiong XZ, Lu J, Cheng Y, Yang C, Lin YX, et al. Percutaneous needle aspiration versus catheter drainage in the management of liver abscess: a systematic review and meta-analysis. HPB (Oxford). 2015;17(3):195.
16. Jun CH, Yoon JH, Wi JW, Park SY, Lee WS, Jung SI, et al. Risk factors and clinical outcomes for spontaneous rupture of pyogenic liver abscess. J Dig Dis. 2015;16:31.
17. Sharma MP, Dasarathy S, Verma N, Saksena S, Shukla DK. Prognostic markers in amebic liver abscess: a prospective study. Am J Gastroenterol. 1996;91:2584-8.

Fever with Jaundice

Vinod Arora, Anupam Prakash

INTRODUCTION

Fever with jaundice, also called febrile jaundice, can be defined as fever, i.e., temperature >37.5°C in the morning and evening temperature >38°C, accompanied by jaundice recognized clinically as yellow discoloration of skin and mucous membranes.[1] This condition can be of intrahepatic or extrahepatic origin. Jaundice can be secondary to pyrogenic substances, toxin, infections, or obstruction of the biliary system.[2] Fever with jaundice can be a common scenario and understanding the local epidemiology can help in guiding the differential diagnosis. Hepatic involvement can vary from asymptomatic elevation in bilirubin and enzymes to acute liver failure (ALF).[3]

Typically, hepatotropic (Hepatitis A–E) viruses cause ALF; however, a number of nonhepatotropic viruses, bacteria, protozoa, and fungal infections can have hepatic involvement, causing a picture presenting as fever, jaundice, and altered sensorium. In India, malaria, typhoid fever, Leptospira, and dengue are the common infections which present with fever and jaundice and may lead to altered sensorium and hence sometimes can even mimic ALF.[4] Bacteremia or septicemia can sometimes complicate with jaundice and secondary to intrahepatic cholestasis via inhibiting the bile acid or other anionic transporter on the sinusoidal or canalicular membrane.[5]

CAUSES OF FEVER AND JAUNDICE[4]

- Bacterial sepsis
- Malaria
- Typhoid fever (Salmonella typhi or Paratyphi)
- Hepatitis A or E/Epstein–Barr virus (EBV) or herpes simplex virus (HSV)
- Leptospirosis
- Dengue or dengue hemorrhagic fever
- Amoebiasis (biliary communication or complicated abscess)
- Brucella
- Tuberculosis
- Malignancies
- Macrophage activation syndrome
- Cholangitis
- Fungal infection (candida or aspergillus).

CLINICAL APPROACH TO FEVER WITH JAUNDICE

Careful history and physical examination can help in guiding the diagnosis in this group of patients. Features such as pain in right upper abdomen, persistent fever, and presence of hepatomegaly or splenomegaly may help in ruling out ALF.[6] In acute viral hepatitis, fever usually precedes jaundice and by the time patient presents with jaundice, fever is not there.[7] Patient with cholangitis can present with fever, jaundice, pain in abdomen, and have shock or altered sensorium, i.e., Reynold's pentad which can mimic some hepatotropic or nonhepatotropic infection. Infections which can cause hemolysis may present as fever with jaundice, but the bilirubin elevation is usually mild (3–4 mg/dL).[8] Liver function tests which are predominantly cholestatic or hepatocellular can help in guiding the further course of diagnosis and management.

COMMON CAUSES

Malaria Hepatopathy

Malaria leading to liver dysfunction is a common scenario; 8–37% of the patients can have hepatic manifestations.[9] Etiology of jaundice can be multifactorial, from rupture of hepatocytes, hemolysis, sequestration, and cytoadherence in the small vessel, leading to ischemia, occlusion of portal vein branches, intrahepatic cholestasis, and hepatic microvillus dysfunction. Endotoxemia is also intrahepatic cholestasis. Secondary infection with hepatitis A or E can cause jaundice. Disseminated intravascular coagulation (DIC) can also promote hepatic dysfunction and can lead to jaundice.[10]

Increase in jaundice with increase in alanine transaminase (ALT) more than three times upper limit normal (ULN) has been termed malarial hepatopathy.[11]

Clinical presentation that is confused with liver failure has been defined as type B presentation. Patients presenting with fever and jaundice are usually having severe symptoms and they can be associated with kidney failure, sepsis, and DIC.[12] Hepatosplenomegaly can be clinical manifestation. Cerebral malaria, hypoglycemia or hypoxia, and uremia can contribute to altered manifestation. Flapping tremors are usually not noted in complicated malaria, while if there is superimposed viral hepatitis, they can be noted.

Hepatic encephalopathy can be rare in malaria. Delta and triphasic waves may be noted in electroencephalogram. Increase in conjugated bilirubin can be noted up to 50% of the patients. Elevation of aspartate aminotransferase (AST) and ALT up to five times are commonly noted, elevation more than that can be noted too. International normalized ratio (INR) is usually normal but can be elevated in DIC. Persistent fever, anemia, jaundice, and hepatosplenomegaly is the common pointer toward malaria rather than acute viral hepatitis.

Dengue Fever

Dengue virus is usually nonhepatotropic virus and arthropod-borne viral fever. Jaundice in dengue is a poor prognostic factor. Usual manifestation is elevation of AST or ALT without jaundice. Severe dengue can present as fulminant hepatic failure and is associated with high mortality.[13] Incidence of jaundice varies from 2–25% of the patients. Hepatic involvement can be seen in 60–90% of the patients. Majority of the patients have mild elevation in AST/ALT with severe elevation seen in 10% of the patients. AST level is usually more than ALT level in dengue infection.[14]

The injury in dengue can be because of cytopathic effect, destruction of hepatocyte by immune cells, and is exaggerated by sepsis and shock. Liver injury can be precipitated by drugs or herbal medicines.

Zone 2 necrosis and councilman bodies are seen as histological features. Severe injury can be a feature of associated immune response. Jaundice with cytopenia can be a feature of hemophagocytosis (HLH).[15]

The syndrome can mimic ALF; altered sensorium, thrombocytopenia, and hemorrhagic manifestations can be noted.

Typhoid Fever

Typhoid fever usually presents in India as epidemic or sporadic form. Hepatitis or jaundice can be reported with the same. It can be confused with malaria owing to presence of fever and jaundice. Coexistent hepatitis A or E can present as ALF.[16] The damage to the hepatocytes is secondary to endotoxin, damaging the cells. On physical examination, there can be hepatomegaly and raised AST/ALT on biochemical examination.[17] Altered sensorium in enteric fever can sometimes mimic hepatic encephalopathy.[18]

Jaundice in enteric fever is commonly seen during the second week. Hepatomegaly is not commonly seen, and neuropsychiatric manifestations are common during the third week. Raised AST or ALT with no increase in bilirubin can be seen in up to 21–60% of the patients. Hepatocyte balloon, swelling, and degenerative changes can be noted histologically. Increase in conjugated bilirubin can be noted secondary to occlusion of bile canaliculi. Incidence of gastrointestinal (GI) hemorrhage and perforation is more common in icteric patients.

Leptospirosis

Leptospirosis is a spirochetal infection caused by *Leptospira interrogans*. Infection is commonly caused by contaminated water, predominant during the rainy season. Incubation period is usually 10 days, with biphasic presentation with first and second phase, with initial nonspecific febrile illness followed by development of hepatorenal syndrome and pulmonary hemorrhage. These manifestations are common during the second week, with pathology of centrilobular necrosis of liver and acute tubular necrosis.[19] Liver involvement is usually in the form of tender hepatomegaly and jaundice. Bilirubin is very high, with raised bilirubin with normal AST/ALT pointing toward leptospirosis. Conjunctival suffusion with uveitis and muscle tenderness and nonoliguric renal failure are the clinical pointers toward leptospirosis. Confusion, hallucination, and psychosis may complicate the illness. Microscopic agglutination test (MAT) is the gold standard with >1:800 as the diagnostic test.

Sepsis-induced Multiorgan Dysfunction

Sepsis can be complicated by jaundice and encephalopathy as part of multiorgan dysfunction. It can be secondary to pyogenic or amoebic liver abscess or any other infection. It can be secondary to transient hypotension, right-sided heart failure, breakdown of red blood cell (RBC), or drug toxicity.[20] In this, jaundice can be associated with significant mortality and morbidity. Presence of jaundice and encephalopathy is usually associated with poor prognosis.

Brucellosis

Brucellosis is a zoonotic infection caused by *Brucella melitensis* (*B. melitensis*). Exposure to domestic animals is the common mode of transmission, with variable incubation period. Fever and constitutional symptoms are common and hepatomegaly (20–40% of patients) with osteoarticular involvement (23% of cases) is commonly seen. Hepatic involvement is mild and no incidence of ALF is seen. Hepatic abscess is commonly seen. Hepatic granulomas, inflammatory cell infiltrates, and localized parenchymal necrosis are the common histological features. Serological assays are the most common diagnostic test with titer (>1:160).[21]

Hemophagocytic Lymphohistiocytosis

Hemophagocytic lymphohistiocytosis (HLH) is a fatal illness characterized by fever, splenomegaly, and jaundice. It can be primary or secondary to infection, autoimmune diseases, or malignancy. Excessive immune activation or inflammation to upregulation of macrophages and lymphocytes causes multiorgan dysfunction. Immune dysregulation is the underlying pathogenesis behind the etiology. Fever, lymphadenopathy, hepatosplenomegaly with jaundice, and maculopapular rash are the clinical hallmarks of the HLH. Cytopenias, increased triglycerides, hemolysis, marked elevation of ferritin, and lactate dehydrogenase are the biochemical and laboratory features of the disease.[22] Treatment is usually mainly supportive.

■ MANAGEMENT OUTLINE

The aim of the treatment is to treat the underlying cause and provide the supportive care.

Antipyretics are used for fever and paracetamol is the preferred drug; however, they should be used cautiously. Cold sponging may be beneficial. Empirical antimalarials are not routinely recommended even if malaria is the most common etiology for fever and jaundice. Artesunate-based regimens are the drug of choice for complicated malaria. Quinine can be the alternate drug of choice for the management of complicated malaria.

Antibiotics are based on the underlying cause. Third-generation cephalosporins are the most commonly used drug (ceftriaxone) for enteric fever; doxycycline or azithromycin can be used for leptospirosis, enteric, scrub typhus, or brucellosis.

Oral/intravenous (IV) N Acetylcysteine (NAC) at a dose of 140 mg/kg, followed by 70 mg/kg q4h for up to 16 doses can be safely given to patients who present with fever and jaundice complicated by encephalopathy mimicking ALF.[23]

Platelet transfusions are needed if platelet counts are <10,000/mm^3. For DIC or coagulopathy, transfusion of fresh frozen plasma (FFP), or cryoprecipitate may help in correcting coagulopathy. Monitoring for urine output, blood pressure, seizures, encephalopathy, and bleeding should be done.

■ REFERENCES

1. Anand AC, Garg HK. Approach to Clinical Syndrome of Jaundice and Encephalopathy in Tropics. J Clin Exp Hepatol. 2014:1-15.
2. Theodossi A. The value of symptoms and signs in the assessment of jaundiced patients. Clin Gastroenterol. 1985;14(3):545-57.
3. Anand AC, Puri P. Jaundice in malaria. J Gastroenterol Hepatol. 2005;20:1322-32.
4. Kothari VM, Karnad DR, Bichile LS. Tropical infections in the ICU. J Assoc Physicians India. 2006;54:291-8.
5. Aung-Kyaw-Zaw, Khin-Maung-U, Myo-Thwe. Endotoxaemia in complicated falciparum malaria. Trans R Soc Trop Med Hyg. 1988;82:513-4.
6. Anand AC, Garg HK. Approach to clinical syndrome of jaundice and encephalopathy in tropics. J Clin Exp Hepatol. 2015;5(Suppl 1):S116-30.
7. Polson J, Lee WM. ASSLD position paper. Management of acute liver failure. Hepatology. 2005;41(5):1179-97.
8. Patrick Mosler. Management of acute cholangitis. Gastroentrol Hepatol. 2011;7(2):121-3.
9. Devarbhavi H, Alvares JF, Kumar KS. Severe falciparum malaria simulating fulminant hepatic failure. Mayo Clin Proc. 2005;80:355-8.

10. Ghoshal UC, Somani S, Chetri K, Akhtar P, Aggarwal R, Naik SR. Plasmodium falciparum and hepatitis E virus co-infection in fulminant hepatic failure. Indian J Gastroenterol. 2001;20:111.
11. Severe falciparum malaria. World Health Organization, communicable diseases cluster. Trans R Soc Med Hyg. 2000;94:S1-90.
12. Anand AC. Malarial liver failure: myth or reality? Trop Gastroenterol. 2001;22:55-6.
13. Seneviratne SL, Malavige GN, de Silva HJ. Pathogenesis of liver involvement during dengue viral infections. Trans R Soc Trop Med Hyg. 2006;100:608-14.
14. Wong M, Shen E. The utility of liver function tests in dengue. Ann Acad Med Singap. 2008;37:82-3.
15. Nguyen TL, Nguyen TH, Tieu NT. The impact of dengue haemorrhagic fever on liver function. Res Virol. 1997;148:273-7.
16. Anand AC, Kataria VK, Singh W, Chatterjee SK. Epidemic multiresistant enteric fever in eastern India. Lancet. 1990;335:352.
17. Ali G, Kamili MA, Shah MY, Koul RL, Aziz A, Hussain A, et al. Neuropsychiatric manifestations of typhoid fever. J Assoc Physicians India. 1992;40:333-5.
18. Osuntokun BO, Bademosi O, Ogunremi K, Wright SG. Neuropsychiatric manifestations of typhoid fever in 959 patients. Arch Neurol. 1972;27:7-13.
19. Faine S. Clinical leptospirosis in humans. In: Faine S (Ed). Leptospira and Leptospirosis. Boca Raton, Florida, USA: CRC Press: 1994. p. 132.
20. Bansal V, Schuchert VD. Jaundice in the intensive care unit. Surg Clin N Am. 2006;86:1495-502.
21. Akritidis N, Tzivras M, Delladetsima I, Stefanaki S, Moutsopoulos HM, Pappas G. The liver in brucellosis. Clin Gastro Hepatol. 2007;5:1109-12.
22. Larroche C. Hemophagocytic lymphohistiocytosis in adults: diagnosis and treatment. Jt Bone Spine. 2012;79:356-9.
23. Mumtaz K, Azam Z, Hamid S, Abid S, Memon S, Shah HA, et al. Role of N-acetylcysteine in adults with non-acetaminophen-induced acute liver failure in a center without the facility of liver transplantation. Hepatol Int. 2009;3:563-70.

Approach to Dysphagia

Pavan Dhoble, Philip Abraham

■ CLINICAL CASE

A 43-year-old man came with 5-year history of problems with swallowing. He had a sensation of foods, particularly solids but occasionally also liquids, sticking in the upper sternum level. He succeeded in swallowing by taking sips or drinking water. He occasionally regurgitated frothy fluids and undigested food into his mouth, particularly when bending over or lying on his back after a meal. The patient reported being unable to belch but denied heartburn or odynophagia. There was no decrease in weight.

What should be the next step in management?
- Barium swallow
- High-resolution esophageal manometry
- Endoscopy with esophageal biopsies
- Trial of proton-pump inhibitors.

■ INTRODUCTION

The subjective awareness of difficulty moving food from the mouth to the stomach is known as dysphagia. It may be due to mechanical (anatomic) or functional (motor) disorders. It is clinically classified into two types:
1. Oropharyngeal dysphagia (transfer dysphagia) refers to difficulty in passage of a bolus from the mouth to the esophagus.[1]
2. Esophageal dysphagia (transit dysphagia) refers to difficulty in passage of a bolus from the upper esophagus to the stomach.

Odynophagia (painful swallowing) and Globus sensation (constant or sporadic non-painful sensation of a lump, trapped food bolus, or constriction in the throat) may accompany dysphagia.[2]

■ CLINICAL EVALUATION

History

Clinical history helps to distinguish oropharyngeal from esophageal dysphagia and mechanical from functional disorders.

Oropharyngeal Dysphagia Features
- Inability to propel food into the pharynx
- Difficulty initiating the act of swallowing
- Drooling of saliva or food
- Need to swallow repeatedly to clear food from the oropharynx
- Coughing or choking during a meal
- Nasal regurgitation of food or fluid
- Tracheal aspiration and recurrent aspiration pneumonia
- Accompanying dysarthria and dysphonia
- Swallowing with gurgling noise may indicate presence of Zenker's diverticulum.

Esophageal Dysphagia Features
- Symptoms localized to the sternal or epigastric regions
- Dysphagia to both solids and liquids suggests motor disorder; dysphagia to solids only, or dysphagia to solids that is

gradually worsening, suggests mechanical disorder.
- Patients with motor disorders frequently use techniques such as repetitive swallowing, raising the arms over the head, pushing the shoulders back, or applying the Valsalva maneuver to relieve impaction.
- In patients with mechanical disorder, regurgitation is frequently required to relieve food impaction.
- Patients with esophageal spasms may have chest pain and are sensitive to hot or cold beverages.
- Distal esophageal (Schatzki's) ring or esophageal web may be the cause of intermittent, nonprogressive dysphagia to solids without significant weight loss.
- Worsening dysphagia may signal peptic stricture (particularly when accompanied by heartburn or regurgitation) or esophageal cancer. Anorexia, significant weight loss, or quickly deteriorating dysphagia favors esophageal cancer.
- History of ingestion of pill or caustic substance suggests pill-induced esophagitis and corrosive esophageal injury, respectively.
- Medical history taking must include use of nonsteroidal anti-inflammatory drugs (NSAIDs), antibiotics, anticholinergics, sedatives, opiates, and bisphosphonates, as these could impair esophageal motility or increase the risk of reflux or candidiasis.

PHYSICAL EXAMINATION
- Body weight and nutritional status may suggest disease duration and severity.
- Oral cavity inspection for candidiasis, especially in diabetics or those with immune compromise.
- Skin examination for herpetic lesions
- Local examination for neck or supraclavicular lymph nodes, thickening of soft tissue, thyromegaly, neck or oropharyngeal masses, and evidence of previous head and neck surgery or radiation therapy.
- Muscle fasciculation, weakness, or fatigability may suggest motor neuron disease, myopathy, or myasthenia gravis; focal sensory or motor dysfunction suggests cerebrovascular accident.
- Evidence of scleroderma or CREST (calcinosis, Raynaud phenomenon, esophageal dysmotility, sclerodactyly, and telangiectasia) syndrome suggests motor dysfunction.
- AAA syndrome—achalasia, adrenal insufficiency, and alacrimia.
- Acrokeratosis paraneoplastica (Bazex syndrome) and palmoplantar keratosis in case of squamous esophageal cancer.

DIFFERENTIAL DIAGNOSIS
Differential diagnosis of dysphagia is shown in **Table 1**.

INVESTIGATIONS
Videofluoroscopy
Videofluoroscopy offers real-time evaluation of oropharyngeal swallowing using barium-mixed boluses of various consistencies. It is helpful for assessing oropharyngeal function and can direct care to improve oropharyngeal coordination, reduce the risk of pulmonary aspiration, and suggest the best feeding consistencies.[3]

Barium Swallow
In addition to being useful for detecting proximal esophageal lesions including Zenker's diverticulum/pharyngeal pouch, cricopharyngeal bars, and postsurgical and/or radiation-related injuries, it is sensitive for finding esophageal rings and strictures that may be missed on endoscopy.

TABLE 1: Differential diagnosis of dysphagia.

Oropharyngeal	Structural	• Zenker's diverticulum/pharyngeal pouch
		• Extrinsic compression
		  – Cervical osteophytes
		  – Cricopharyngeal bar
		  – Thyromegaly
		  – Lymphadenopathy
		  – Retropharyngeal abscess
		• Oropharyngeal tumor
		• Radiation injury

	Motility	• Central/peripheral nervous system
		  – Cerebrovascular accident
		  – Intracranial mass
		• Neurodegenerative disease
		  – Multiple sclerosis
		  – Parkinsonism
		  – Alzheimer's dementia
		  – Amyotrophic lateral sclerosis
		  – Postpolio syndrome
		• Neuromuscular disease
		  – Botulism
		  – Myasthenia gravis
		  – Lambert–Eaton syndrome
		  – Muscular dystrophies
		  – Myopathies (inflammatory and metabolic)
		• Medications

Esophageal	Structural	• Esophageal webs and rings
		  – Schatzki's ring
		  – Eosinophilic esophagitis
		• Esophageal strictures
		  – Peptic stricture
		  – Caustic ingestion
		  – Pill induced
		  – Radiation induced
		  – Postsurgical/endoscopic submucosal dissection
		• Esophagitis
		  – Eosinophilic
		  – Infectious
		  – Pill or caustic
		  – Gastroesophageal reflux disease
		• Anatomical abnormalities
		  – Hiatus hernia
		  – Esophageal diverticulum
		• Intramural growths
		  – Leiomyoma
		  – Gastrointestinal stromal tumor
		• Extrinsic compression
		  – Mediastinal mass
		  – Aberrant right subclavian artery (dysphagia lusoria)

Contd...

Contd...

	• Malignancy
	  – Primary esophageal tumors (squamous and adenocarcinoma)
	  – Metastatic tumors (e.g., melanoma)

Motility	• Disorders of esophagogastric junction (EGJ) outflow
	  – Achalasia (Types I-III)
	  – EGJ outflow obstruction
	• Disorders of peristalsis
	  – Absent contractility
	  – Distal esophageal spasm
	  – Hypercontractile esophagus
	  – Ineffective esophageal motility
	• Secondary motility disorders
	  – Scleroderma
	  – Other collagen vascular diseases
	  – Amyloidosis

Timed barium swallow has been demonstrated to be superior to endoscopy for evaluating suspected distal esophageal motility disorders such as achalasia cardia. To determine how well a treatment technique for achalasia cardia such as balloon dilatation or myotomy works, the height and area of the barium column are assessed at 1, 2, and 5 minutes following a sip.[4]

Esophagogastroduodenoscopy

Endoscopy offers comprehensive knowledge of the esophagus anatomy as well as allows examination and biopsy sampling of the mucosa. It allows evaluation for eosinophilic esophagitis (EoE) and malignancy or premalignant lesions, such as strictures and dysplasia in Barrett's esophagus. Additionally, it can be used for therapeutic procedures. High-definition endoscopy provides better visualization of the mucosa.[5]

Esophageal Manometry

The gold standard test for the identification of esophageal motility abnormalities is high-resolution manometry (HRM). It entails taking pressure readings of the esophageal musculature and sphincters with solid-state or water-perfused transducers and then utilizing software to create colorimetric pressure graphs[6] (Figs. 1A to D).

Esophageal motility disorders are categorized by the Chicago classification as (i) disorders of esophagogastric junction (EGJ) outflow (achalasia types I, II, and III, and EGJ outflow obstruction) and (ii) disorders of peristalsis (absent contractility, distal esophageal spasm, hypercontractile esophagus, and ineffective esophageal motility). Lower esophageal sphincter (LES) relaxation in response to swallowing is impaired in achalasia. Based on the pattern of esophageal body motility on HRM, achalasia is subclassified[7] (Figs. 1A to D).

Impedance Manometry

The contents of the esophagus reflect in intraluminal impedance, which increases with intraluminal air and lowers with intraluminal liquid. Bolus transit, bolus clearance, intrabolus pressure, and the connections between esophageal pressure

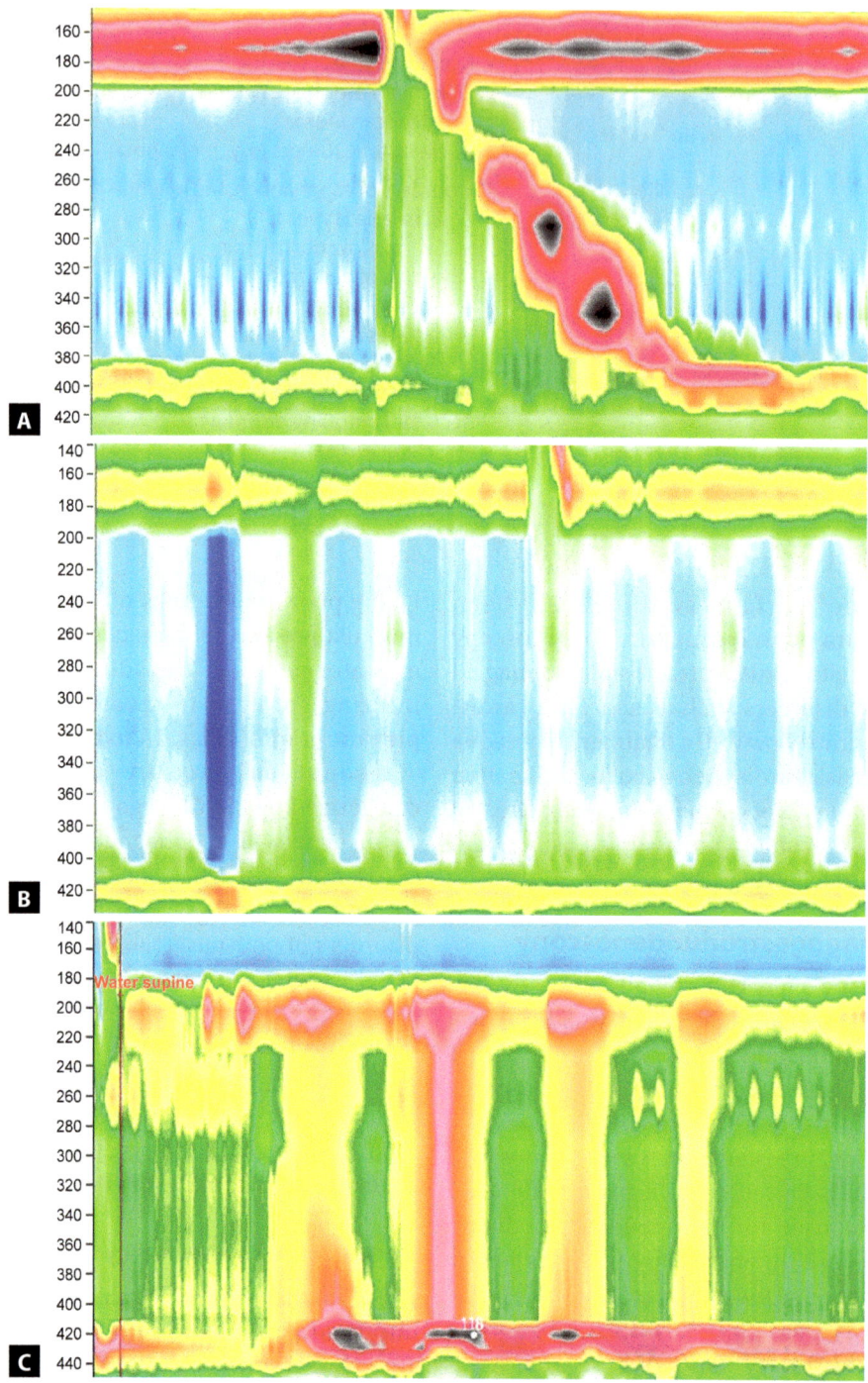

Figs. 1A to C

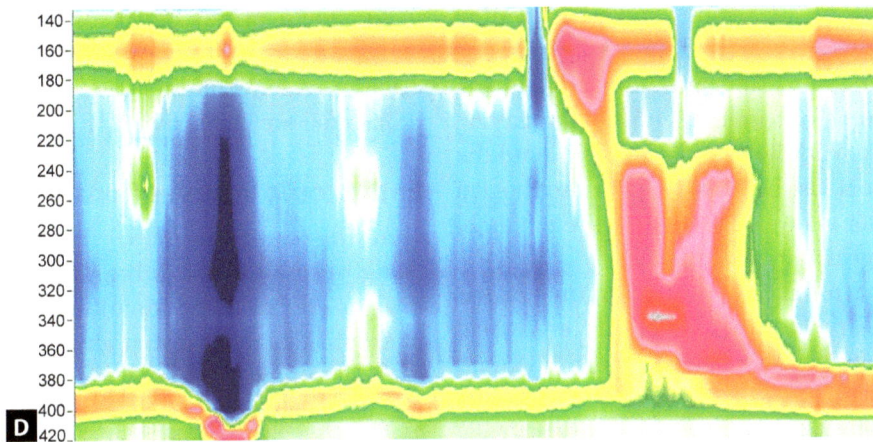

Figs. 1A to D: High-resolution esophageal manometry with color-coded pressure heat maps. Blue color represents low-pressure and red represents high-pressure zones. (A) *Normal swallows:* Landmarks of normal pressure topography with propagation of swallow and relaxation of lower esophageal sphincter. (B) *Type 1 achalasia:* Failed esophageal peristalsis with failure of lower esophageal sphincter relaxation. (C) *Type 2 achalasia:* Uniform, nonpropagating increase in esophageal pressure (panesophageal pressurization) with failure of lower esophageal sphincter relaxation. (D) *Type 3 (spastic) achalasia:* Premature, vigorous contractions of distal esophagus with failure of lower esophageal sphincter relaxation.
Source: Reproduced with permission from Dr Shrikant Mukewar, MIDAS Hospitals, Nagpur.

and bolus flow are all objectively evaluated using high-resolution impedance manometry (HRIM).

Recently, pressure-flow analysis has been applied to HRIM interpretation to objectively measure the components of bolus flow timing, retention, pressurization, and luminal distension. This method is useful in differentiating between healthy controls and patients with post-fundoplication dysphagia and nonobstructive dysphagia. The metrics correlate with symptom scores and clinical outcomes in patients with achalasia and major motor disorders as well as with symptom scores in patients without major motor disorders. Additional novel HRIM metrics of the bolus flow time and esophageal impedance integral quantify trans-EGJ bolus flow and esophageal retention, respectively.

The impedance bolus height measures the height of the residual fluid column 5 minutes after a 200-mL quick liquid consumption in an upright position to quantify esophageal retention. Additionally, HRIM can be used to identify behavioral disorders such as supragastric belching and rumination syndrome.[8]

Functional Luminal Imaging Probe

Functional luminal imaging probe (FLIP) measures the esophagus luminal dimensions and esophageal distensibility in response to controlled volumetric distension using impedance planimetry technology. The 16 cm FLIP offers simultaneous evaluation of the distal esophageal body and EGJ, while the 8 cm FLIP assesses EGJ distensibility. Esophageal body distensibility, contractile response to distension, and EGJ opening mechanics can be evaluated by displaying the changes in esophageal diameter along a space-time continuum with accompanying pressure. Withdrawing the catheter until the balloon is just below the upper esophageal sphincter allows evaluation of the proximal esophageal body's extensibility.

Functional luminal imaging probe panometry is useful to clarify equivocal esophageal motility evaluations on HRM and is useful to confirm a diagnosis of achalasia when achalasia is strongly suspected clinically and on esophagogram but integrated relaxation pressure (IRP) is normal on HRM.[9]

Thoracic Computed Tomography

Computed tomography detects and assesses involvement of adjacent structures or distant spread in esophageal malignancy, esophagus-airway fistula, pseudoachalasia, esophageal injuries, duplication cysts and diverticuli, and esophageal perforation.[10]

■ TREATMENT

Diet

An essential component of treatment, especially for people with oropharyngeal and severe esophageal dysphagia, is swallow rehabilitation with adjustment of food consistency.[11] Although oral feeding is preferred, enteral and parenteral nutrition supplementation may be needed in some circumstances. EoE may need trials with elemental and elimination diets.[12]

Pharmacological Interventions

Patients with gastroesophageal reflux disease and EoE are treated with proton-pump inhibitors. Topical corticosteroids may be tried in patients with chronic eosinophilia.[11] Clinical trials using biologics for EoE have shown promising results.[12] Medical treatments for motility issues include calcium-channel blockers and oral nitrates; prokinetics are ineffective.[11]

Endoscopic Interventions

Esophageal strictures: Push/bougie (longitudinal shear force) and balloon dilators (radial shear force) are two forms of esophageal dilators that give comparable clinical effects.[13] Refractory stricture is defined as inability to maintain luminal diameter of 14 mm after five consecutive dilatation treatments spaced 1-2 weeks apart;[14] recurrent stricture is defined as failure to maintain luminal diameter of 14 mm for 4 weeks after it has been reached. These can be treated with esophageal stents, endoscopic incisional therapy, and intralesional steroid injections.[15]

Palliative care for advanced esophageal malignancies includes the insertion of esophageal stents—covered, partially covered, and uncovered metal, plastic, and biodegradable stents are available.[16]

Achalasia cardia: Per-oral endoscopic myotomy (POEM) is now considered first-line treatment for achalasia, particularly in types II and III achalasia. It involves producing a submucosal tunnel for LES myotomy with outcomes similar to laparoscopic Heller's myotomy (LHM).[17,18] Although it frequently necessitates many sessions and may result in postprocedure reflux, pneumatic (balloon) dilatation (PD) is an acceptable choice for treating achalasia types I and II. However, it carries a risk of up to 8% perforation rate and up to 1% death rate. It is less effective than LHM and POEM.[15,17,18] Those who are not candidates for definitive surgical or endoscopic procedures may have temporary benefit from botulinum-toxin injection into the LES.[17]

In cases where oral feeding is not permitted and the patient needs nutritional support, percutaneous endoscopic gastrostomy is appropriate.

Surgical Interventions

Surgery is recommended for operable malignant esophageal dysphagia. Its function in benign dysphagia is restricted to LHM for achalasia, which has the advantage of being paired with fundoplication to lessen postmyotomy reflux.[18]

■ REFERENCES

1. Sasegbon A, Hamdy S. The anatomy and physiology of normal and abnormal swallowing in oropharyngeal dysphagia. Neurogastroenterol Motil. 2017;29(11):e13100.
2. Aziz Q, Fass R, Gyawali CP, Miwa H, Pandolfino JE, Zerbib F. Esophageal disorders. Gastroenterology. 2016;150(6):1368-79.
3. Ala'A AJ, Katzka DA, Castell DO. Approach to the patient with dysphagia. Am J Med. 2015;128(10):1138-e17-23.
4. Neyaz Z, Gupta M, Ghoshal UC. How to perform and interpret timed barium esophagogram. J Neurogastroenterol Motil. 2013;19(2):251.
5. Pasha SF, Acosta RD, Chandrasekhara V, Chathadi KV, Decker GA, Early DS, et al. The role of endoscopy in the evaluation and management of dysphagia. Gastrointest Endosc. 2014;79(2):191-201.
6. Trudgill NJ, Sifrim D, Sweis R, Fullard M, Basu K, McCord M, et al. British Society of Gastroenterology guidelines for oesophageal manometry and oesophageal reflux monitoring. Gut. 2019;68(10):1731-50.
7. Yadlapati R, Kahrilas PJ, Fox MR, Bredenoord AJ, Prakash Gyawali C, Roman S, et al. Esophageal motility disorders on high-resolution manometry: Chicago classification version 4.0©. Neurogastroenterol Motil. 2021;33(1): e14058.
8. Liu Z, Liao J, Tian D, Liu M, Dan Z, Yu Q. Assessment of esophageal high-resolution impedance manometry in patients with nonobstructive dysphagia. Gastroenterol Res Pract. 2018:6272515.
9. Carlson DA. Functional lumen imaging probe: The FLIP side of esophageal disease. Curr Opin Gastroenterol. 2016;32(4):310-8.
10. Lee KH, Cho SG, Jeon YS, Jeong S, Kim HJ. Spectrum of Esophageal Abnormality Seen on Thoracic CT. J Korean Radiol Soc. 2006;54:273-82.
11. Malagelada J-R, Bazzoli F, Boeckxstaens G, De Looze D, Fried M, Kahrilas P, et al. World gastroenterology organisation global guidelines: dysphagia—global guidelines and cascades update September 2014. J Clin Gastroenterol. 2015;49(5):370-8.
12. Hirano I, Chan ES, Rank MA, Sharaf RN, Stollman NH, Stukus DR, et al. AGA institute and the joint task force on allergy-immunology practice parameters clinical guidelines for the management of eosinophilic esophagitis. Gastroenterology. 2020;158(6):1776-86.
13. Josino IR, Madruga-Neto AC, Ribeiro IB, Guedes HG, Brunaldi VO, de Moura DTH, et al. Endoscopic dilation with bougies versus balloon dilation in esophageal benign strictures: systematic review and meta-analysis. Gastroenterol Res Pract. 2018;2018:5874870.
14. Kochman ML, McClave SA, Boyce HW. The refractory and the recurrent esophageal stricture: a definition. Gastrointest Endosc. 2005;62(3):474-5.
15. Sami SS, Haboubi HN, Ang Y, Boger P, Bhandari P, De Caestecker J, et al. UK guidelines on oesophageal dilatation in clinical practice. Gut. 2018;67(6):1000-23.
16. Rana F, Dhar A. Oesophageal stenting for benign and malignant strictures: a systematic approach. Frontline Gastroenterol. 2015;6(2): 94-100.
17. Esposito D, Maione F, D'Alessandro A, Sarnelli G, De Palma GD. Endoscopic treatment of esophageal achalasia. World J Gastrointest Endosc. 2016;8(2):30.
18. Mundre P, Black CJ, Mohammed N, Ford AC. Efficacy of surgical or endoscopic treatment of idiopathic achalasia: a systematic review and network meta-analysis. Lancet Gastroenterol Hepatol. 2020;6(1):30-8.

5

Approach to Renal Dysfunction in Chronic Liver Disease

Yogesh K Chhabra

■ CLINICAL VIGNETTE

A 56-year-old female with history of hepatitis C virus-(HCV)-related chronic liver disease presented to emergency department with complaints of abdominal distension and decreased urine output for last 2 days. On examination, her blood pressure was 110/70 mm Hg with mild pallor and icterus. On further evaluation, her abdomen was full and had a presence of shifting dullness. She was admitted in the intensive care unit (ICU) and passed urine at 20 mL/h. Her first creatinine after admission was 1.3 mg/dL [baseline serum creatinine (S Cr) done around a week back was 0.8 mg/dL]. She was diagnosed with acute kidney injury (AKI) and nephrology consult was given.

▌DEFINITION OF ACUTE KIDNEY INJURY

As per Kidney Disease Improving Global Outcomes (KDIGO) guidelines 2012, AKI is defined as any of the following:
- Increase in S Cr by >0.3 or more within 48 hours
- Increase in S Cr to >1.5 times of baseline, which is known or presumed to have occurred within 7 days
- Urine volume <0.5 mL/kg/h for 6 hours

Treating team kept following differential diagnosis:
- Prerenal azotemia (PRA)
- Acute tubular necrosis (ATN)
- Hepatorenal syndrome 1 (HRS-1)
- Abdominal compartment syndrome (ACS)
- Acute glomerulonephritis (AGN).

■ EVALUATION OF PATIENT

The patient was further evaluated according to history for the cause of AKI; there was no history of any nephrotoxic agents such as nonsteroidal anti-inflammatory drugs (NSAIDs) and aminoglycosides. There was no history suggestive of excessive blood loss or shock. Patient was hemodynamically stable during her stay in ICU.

Prerenal azotemia was ruled out as the patient did not respond adequately to fluid replacement therapy by 1.5 liter of normal saline. Even after fluid challenge, the urine output of patient remained low in range of 10–15 mL/h. Meanwhile, challenge with albumin 1 g/kg was continued for the next 48 hours.

During further workup, glomerulonephritis was ruled out as there was no evidence of any significant proteinuria (<500 mg/day) and hematuria [RBCs were <50 per high power field (HPF)]. Urinary bladder pressure was 12 mm Hg which ruled out ACS.

To differentiate HRS from ATN, fractional excretion of sodium (FeNa) was calculated and was found to be 0.2% which tilted the diagnosis in favor of HRS. Neutrophil gelatinase-associated lipocalin (NGAL) <220 µg/g Cr supported the diagnosis of HRS in the patient.

After confirming diagnosis of HRS, she was initiated on midodrine 5 mg thrice a day and albumin was continued. Even after above-mentioned therapy, she witnessed further rise in creatinine and urine output remained low. Later midodrine was discontinued and injection Terlipressin was added in dose on 1 mg every 6 hourly along with ongoing albumin management. After 24 hours of treatment, urine output gradually improved and S Cr reversed back to baseline value in next 3–4 days.

INCIDENCE OF ACUTE KIDNEY INJURY

Recent study by Desai et al. with 3.6 million cirrhosis patients, incidence of AKI was 22%. Over time, AKI prevalence doubled from 15% in 2004 to 30% in 2016. Likelihood of death in AKI admissions was 3.75 times more as compared to non-AKI group. As per various studies, HRS–AKI accounts for almost 13–20% of cases of AKI in cirrhotic patients.

PATHOPHYSIOLOGY AND EVALUATION OF VARIOUS DIFFERENTIALS

Prerenal azotemia manifests from some insult before the kidney. Hypoperfusion to kidneys commonly presents as PRA. Common causes of hypoperfusion include physiologic state shock, dehydration, hemorrhage, overdiuresis, burns, and even intravascular depletion from low-oncotic pressure states, such as congestive heart failure and liver failure. There is no or very minimal damage to the tubules.

Acute tubular necrosis, as the name suggests, is because of persistent ischemia or injury to kidney, resulting in tubular damage. Its potential to recover or reaching up to the stage of chronicity will depend upon the type and duration of insult. The typical course of uncomplicated ATN is recovery over 2–3 weeks; however, superimposed renal insults or multiple comorbidities often alter this pattern. Blood urea nitrogen (BUN)/S Cr ratio <20 mg/dL, FeNa >1, and muddy brown casts in urine examination favor ATN as compared to prerenal AKI.

Various histological types of renal diseases are reported in association with HCV infection, including membranoproliferative glomerulonephritis (MPGN), membranous nephropathy, focal segmental glomerulosclerosis, fibrillary glomerulonephritis, immunotactoid glomerulopathy, immunoglobulin A (IgA) nephropathy, renal thrombotic microangiopathy, vasculitic renal involvement, and interstitial nephritis. Glomerulonephritis will usually have significant proteinuria and hematuria. On evaluation, there may be alteration of complement levels or presence of cryoglobulins or presence of autoimmune antibodies. In cases with suspected glomerulonephritis, kidney biopsy might be required to reach up to appropriate diagnosis.

Pathophysiology of Hepatorenal Syndrome

Splanchnic vasodilatation and decline in renal perfusion is the major pathophysiological change, leading to AKI. Splanchnic vessel dilatation is largely mediated by nitric oxide released locally. As the hepatic disease progresses, there is a progressive rise in cardiac output and fall in systemic vascular resistance; the latter change occurs despite local increases in renal and femoral vascular resistance that result in part from hypotension-induced activation from hypotension-induced activation of renin-angiotensin and sympathetic nervous system.

Hepatorenal Syndrome—Acute Kidney Injury: International Club of Ascites Diagnostic Criteria 2019

- Cirrhosis, acute liver failure, and acute-on-chronic liver failure
- Increase in S Cr ≥0.3 mg/dL within 48 hours or ≥50% from baseline value and/or urinary output ≤0.5 mL/kg of body weight for ≥6 hours (requires use of a urinary catheter).
- No full or partial response for ≥2 days of diuretic withdrawal and volume expansion with albumin (dosed at 1 g/kg of body weight/day).
- Absence of shock
- No current or recent treatment with nephrotoxic drugs
- In the absence of chronic kidney disease (CKD), assess for parenchymal disease, as indicated by proteinuria >500 mg/day, microhematuria (>50 RBCs per HPF), urinary injury biomarkers (if available), and/or abnormal renal ultrasonography.
- Suggestion of renal vasoconstriction, with FeNa <0.2% (levels <0.1% are considered highly predictive).

Types of Hepatorenal Syndromes

- *HRS-AKI (previously called type 1 HRS):* This is the classical and more serious form of HRS. Its definition has been modified recently in conundrum with rest of the types of AKI. Previous definition stating rise in S Cr above 2.5 mg/dL is obsolete now. The criteria defining it had been modified in 2019 by the International Club of Ascites (ICA), whereby FeNa <0.2% has been especially emphasized along with the modified definition.
- *Diuretic-resistant ascites (previously called type 2 HRS):* This is a subacute presentation of HRS which happens over weeks and mainly presents as ascites which do not respond easily to diuretics. Overt use of diuretics in this patient can be one of the reasons for AKI in this group of patients.

Management of Hepatorenal Syndrome—Acute Kidney Injury

Diagnosis of HRS-AKI remains a diagnosis of exclusion. Once this diagnosis is being considered, antihypertensive agents especially beta-blockers should be discontinued to minimize further exacerbations.

Especially in ICU settings, initial treatment by norepinephrine and albumin should be taken into consideration. Norepinephrine can be given intravenously in the dose of 0.5–3 mg/h as per requirement with the desired goal of achieving mean arterial pressure (MAP) of 80–85 mm Hg and/or the rise of >10 mm Hg from baseline value. Albumin can be given in dose 1 g/kg/day with maximum dose being 100 g/day. In case of nonavailability, intravenous vasopressin infusion may also be effective; it can be initiated at dose of 0.01 units/min, which can further be titrated.

In relatively more stable patients with HRS-AKI or who have not been admitted to ICU, terlipressin injection along with albumin is the preferred drug combination. Injection Terlipressin can be started at 1–2 mg every 4–6 hours with maximum dose of 12 mg/day. Albumin can be initiated at same dose as with norepinephrine combination but can be tapered to 25–50 mg/day after 2 days and can be continued till terlipressin is going on.

In situations where injection terlipressin is not available, initial treatment with a combination of midodrine and albumin is suggested. Midodrine is started at dose of 7.5 mg thrice a day and can be increased to maximum of 15 mg thrice a day. Octreotide can be added in continuous intravenous infusion (50 µg/h) or subcutaneous (100–200 µg thrice a day) dosage schedule. Head-on trials have shown terlipressin as more effective agent as compared to midodrine or octreotide when given in combination with albumin in patients with more moderate-to-severe category of HRS–AKI. Treatment with terlipressin or midodrine or octreotide is usually recommended for 2 weeks and can be extended further if required in case of partial recovery.

Patients who fail to respond to above-mentioned measures may be suggested to undergo transjugular intrahepatic portosystemic shunt (TIPS) procedure. If successful, this procedure can be considered as a bridging option to liver transplant. Unfortunately, use of contrast during this procedure can further aggravate the AKI.

Hemodialysis or slow low-efficiency dialysis (SLED) can be considered in some patients if the kidney injury is quite strong. Indication for renal replacement therapy can be refractory hyperkalemia, severe metabolic acidosis, or severely reduced urine output, leading to features of fluid overload. S Cr may not rise to a large extent because of hyperbilirubinemia. Dialysis may provide a bridge to the patient where liver transplant is planned in near future. Therapies such as molecular adsorbent recirculating system (MARS) have shown inconclusive results and may require further evaluation. Moreover, heavy cost incurred with MARS therapy remains a serious concern with these therapies.

To conclude, HRS–AKI is a serious and important complication related to cirrhotic liver disease. Diagnosis of HRS–AKI is quite complicated and remains a diagnosis of exclusion. Final treatment would depend upon the cause of AKI in this setting. If diagnosed at early stage, treatment of AKI can be successful in most of the patients.

Section 2

Diseases of the Esophagus

6. **Perplexing Cases of *Candida* Esophagitis**
   Sanjay Banerjee

7. **Refractory Gastroesophageal Reflux Disease**
   VG Mohan Prasad, Vamsi Murthy K, Madhura Prasad, Mithra Prasad

8. **Management of Dysphagia**
   Ashish Chauhan, Soumya Jagannath, Govind Makharia

Chapter 6

Perplexing Cases of *Candida* Esophagitis

Sanjay Banerjee

■ INTRODUCTION

Candida is the most common infectious agent causing esophagitis. Patients generally present with dysphagia, odynophagia, and retrosternal chest pain. Some cases may even be asymptomatic. Diagnosis is usually made during upper endoscopy showing firmly adherent white or yellow plaque-like lesions that leave raw, oozing surface on separation.

Here two unique cases of *Candida* esophagitis are presented that have atypical appearance on endoscopy giving rise to diagnostic dilemma. However, both the cases had uneventful recovery and responded to standard antifungal therapy.

■ CASE PRESENTATION

Case 1: A 23-year-old male presented with hiccup for 7 days and fever for 3 days.

He had a history of coronavirus disease 2019 (COVID-19)-positive severe pneumonia 2 months back for which he was admitted in a hospital for 15 days. The pneumonia was followed by development of postinfectious acute demyelinating radiculoneuropathy for which he was treated with intravenous (IV) methylprednisolone and intravenous immunoglobulin (IVIg). The patient had prompt and successful recovery of neurological disability and was able to walk without any support at the time he came to our hospital.

There was no history of vomiting, pain in abdomen, gastrointestinal bleeding, jaundice, abdominal distension, pedal swelling, shortness of breath, oliguria, or altered mentation. There was no history of diabetes, long-standing pulmonary disease, steroid use, prior abdominal surgery, promiscuous sexual exposure, or any addiction. The rest of the history was unrevealing.

On examination, the patient had a body mass index (BMI) of 22.6 kg/m^2. Vitals were stable. There was no lymphadenopathy, oral ulcer, skin lesions or heart murmurs. Breath sounds were normal, and there was no area of dullness on percussion of chest. Occasional rhonchi were present scattered in both the lung fields. Crepitations were absent. Liver was just palpable with normal hepatic dullness. Hernial sites were normal. Neurological examination revealed normal higher mental functions, no cranial neuropathy, motor power 4/4 in all four limbs, and no sensory or autonomic deficits.

Routine investigations showed low hemoglobin (10.2 g%), normal leukocytes and platelets, an elevated C-reactive protein (CRP) (35 mg/dL), normal serum electrolytes, normal renal parameters, and liver function test. Chest X-ray (CXR) was essentially normal. Abdominal ultrasound showed marginal hepatomegaly (span 14.6 cm).

Esophagogastroduodenoscopy showed extensive esophageal ulceration with

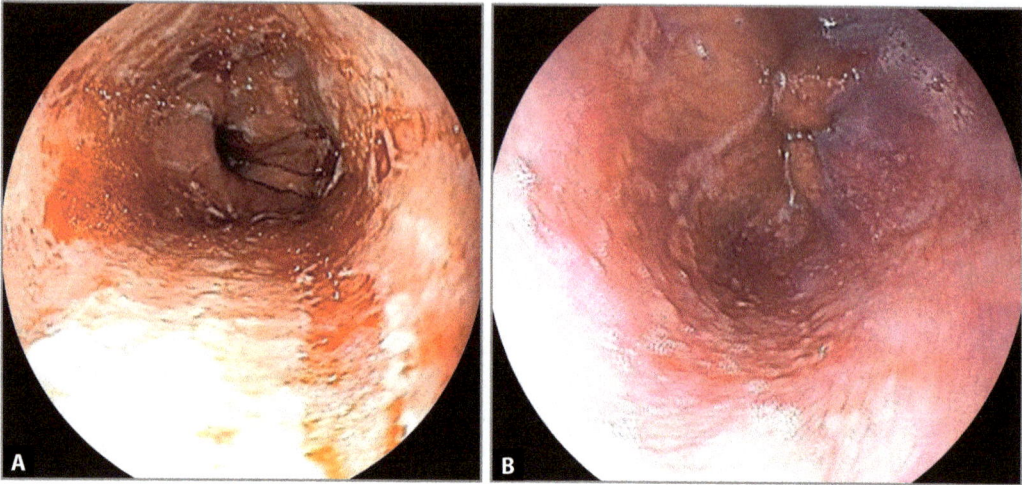

Figs. 1A and B: (A) Endoscopic image of esophageal mucosal ulcers and desquamation; (B) Endoscopic image of significantly healed esophageal ulcers (post-treatment).

sloughing, detachment of mucous membrane, friability, and spontaneous oozing on air insufflation **(Fig. 1A)**. There was no luminal narrowing or mass or resistance felt at gastroesophageal junction. Oral cavity, oropharynx, hypopharynx, stomach, and duodenum (up to second part) all were normal. Brush cytology showed pseudohyphae of *Candida* with background desquamated epithelial cells and few inflammatory cells. Biopsy from the ulcers showed presence of pseudohyphae of *Candida* invading the mucosal cells.

Oral antifungal was started (voriconazole 200 mg daily) along with baclofen for hiccup. Hiccup subsided within next 2 days. Patient was discharged after 7 days, and a follow-up endoscopy after 4 weeks showed complete healing of ulcers with decreased vascularity and increased friability of esophageal mucosa **(Fig. 1B)**.

Case 2: A 55-year-old male, nonsmoker, nonalcoholic, and nondiabetic, presented with repeated episodes of vomiting and regurgitation of food materials for 7 days, with complete cessation of oral intake for last 3 days. Patient has one episode of hematemesis at the emergency during admission. He also complained of indigestion, decreased appetite, nausea, dyspepsia, and dry cough for last 7 days.

Vomiting used to occur immediately after oral intake with occasional streaks of blood. Patient tried to manage the vomiting with oral ondansetron or antisecretory drugs but could not succeed. There was no history of dysphagia, pain abdomen, black stool, hematochezia, or abdominal distension.

On examination, the patient was sick with low blood pressure (80/50 mm Hg), feeble pulse (126 beats/min), tachypnea (30 beats/min), dry mouth, coated tongue, pallor, and cold extremities. Bilateral coarse crepitations were present, more on right infrascapular area. Patent was transferred to intensive care unit (ICU).

On admission, hemoglobin was 8.8 g%, total leukocyte count 32,000/cmm, platelets 1,60,000/cmm, CRP 100 mg/L, sodium 141 mEq/L, potassium 3.3 mEq/L, creatinine 1.5 mg/dL, urea 112 mg/dL. CXR showed perihilar congestion and bilateral reticulonodular lesions. This was further corroborated on computed tomography (CT) that showed active bronchiolitis, perihilar nodules, bronchiolitis obliterans organizing pneumonia **(Fig. 2)**.

The patient had further episodes of hematemesis while in ICU, and an urgent esophagogastroduodenoscopy was planned after blood transfusion and stabilization. It showed extensive necrotic ulcer with adherent mucopus and frank oozing **(Fig. 3A)**. Esophageal lumen was narrowed, and stomach contained blood clots. Brush cytology was taken from the ulcer base, and biopsy was not taken for fear of perforation.

From the third post-admission day, the patient developed intermediate grade fever and blood for infective markers were sent. COVID CBNAAT (cartridge-based nucleic acid amplification test), COVID RT–PCR (real-time reverse transcription–polymerase chain reaction) in nasopharyngeal swab, serology for all hepatitis viruses, IgM anti-hepatitis C virus (HCV), IgM anti-Epstein–Barr virus (EBV) (against capsid antigen), malaria double antigen, dengue NS1 antigen, IgM Typhidot, and HSV DNA-PCR in blood were all negative. The patient was treated with meropenem and doxycycline, given the possibility of bronchopneumonia. Bronchoalveolar lavage (BAL) showed polymorphs only.

Patient subsequently developed hypotension that was managed by pressure support (nor-adrenaline) to which he responded. A possibility of fungal sepsis was considered. Serum 1,3-β-D glucan level (a component of cell wall of *Candida* and related fungi) was elevated (330 pg/mL; normal <60), serum

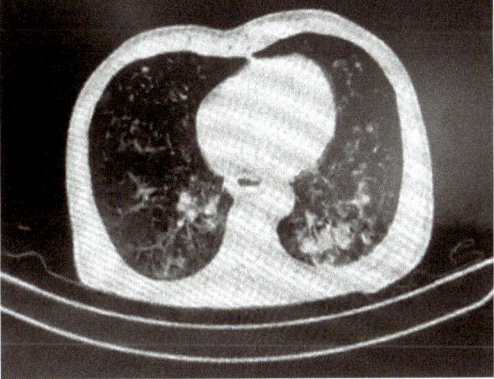

Fig. 2: Computed tomography (CT) thorax showing bilateral reticulonodular opacities.

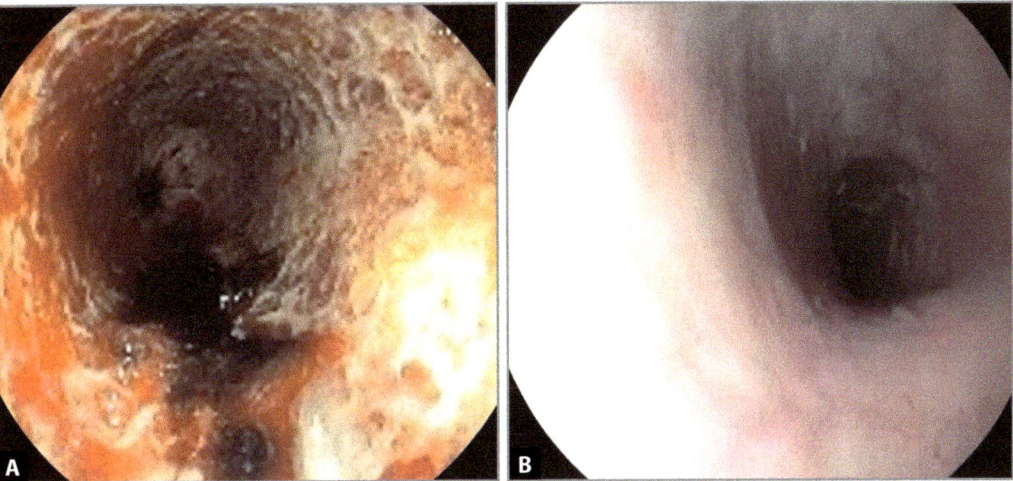

Figs. 3A and B: (A) Endoscopic image showing deep esophageal ulcers and necrotic sloughs; (B) Endoscopic image showing near-complete healing (post-treatment).

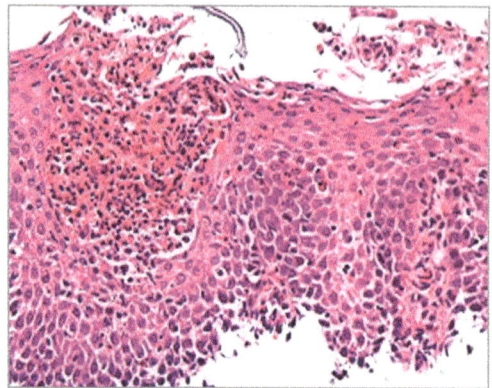

Fig. 4: Photomicrograph showing eosinophilic infiltration in esophageal mucosa.

galactomannan level was normal and anti-SARS CoV2 (severe acute respiratory syndrome coronavirus-2) titer was markedly elevated. By then, the endoscopic brush cytology report was available, and it showed presence of nonpigmented septate hyphae of *Candida* with dichotomous branching at 45°. Patient was treated with micafungin (150 mg/day) and started responding. Gradually pressure support was withdrawn, oral intake resumed, fever subsided, and patient was transferred to the ward. A repeat endoscopy after 7 days showed remarkable improvement in esophageal mucosa with healing longitudinal ulcers **(Fig. 3B)**. This time, multiple biopsies were taken from esophagus and sent for histopathological examination. Both CXR and CT thorax showed improvement.

Klebsiella pneumoniae was grown both on BAL fluid and blood culture. Blood culture also revealed candidemia. Esophageal biopsy revealed extensive eosinophilic infiltration with exudative inflammation **(Fig. 4)**. The patient was discharged after 10 days.

CLINICAL DISCUSSION AND DIFFERENTIALS

Two cases of *Candida* esophagitis are presented here who had atypical presentation.

The diagnosis in the first case was straightforward, though the clinical presentation with fever and hiccup, and the endoscopic findings of extensive esophageal ulceration were unusual. A preceding history of COVID-19 pneumonia, resultant prolonged hospitalization, steroid use, and use of IVIg might have predisposed an otherwise healthy young individual to *Candida* esophagitis. He responded very well to voriconazole for 14 days and had an uncomplicated recovery. No other antimicrobial agent was given and follow-up endoscopy showed complete healing of esophageal lesions.

The second case was more complicated and confusing. First, he presented with features of frank sepsis and required pressure support. Second, the endoscopic finding of necrotic ulcer was unusual for *Candida*. Next, he had an accompanying bronchopneumonia due to *K pneumoniae* which might have contributed to sepsis. Finally, though blood culture and esophageal brushing showed *Candida*, the esophageal biopsy (taken 7 days after the initiation of antifungal) revealed features of eosinophilic esophagitis.

In the general population, incidence rate of esophageal candidiasis is about 4%. *Candida* accounts for the majority of cases (88%) of infectious esophagitis, followed by Herpes simplex virus (10%), and Cytomegalovirus (2%). Patients with *Candida* esophagitis may have entirely asymptomatic or present with dysphagia, odynophagia, and retrosternal pain. *Candida* infections of the esophagus are seen more commonly in immunosuppressed patients, and in them, they are considered to be opportunistic infections. Risk factors for *Candida* esophagitis are increasing age, human immunodeficiency virus (HIV) infection, corticosteroid use (both oral and inhalational), diabetes mellitus, other immunodeficiency states, renal

TABLE 1: Kodsi's grading of esophageal candidiasis.	
Grade	Description
I	Few raised lesions (<2 mm); no surrounding edema or laceration
II	Multiple raised lesions (>2 mm); no surrounding edema or laceration
III	Linear, nodular, and confluent lesions
IV	Same as Grade III plus narrowing of the lumen and/or friability of the mucosa
V	Thick white plaque covering the lumen in circumferential manner with narrowing of the lumen

failure requiring hemodialysis, cancer chemotherapy, prolonged use of proton-pump inhibitors (PPI), gastric outlet obstruction, etc.

Due to impaired cell-mediated immunity, the esophageal epithelial layer is susceptible to infection by *Candida*, which is otherwise present in the normal flora of oral cavity. White–yellow plaques are produced when *Candida* proliferates in the mucosa. These plaques do not wash from the mucosa with water irrigation during endoscopy and may be present throughout the esophagus or be localized. The endoscopic classification proposed by Kodsi et al. is widely used **(Table 1)**.

The differential diagnosis of esophageal ulcer includes cytomegalovirus esophagitis, herpes simplex esophagitis, eosinophilic esophagitis, pill-induced esophagitis, reflux esophagitis, radiation-induced esophagitis, or many other forms of esophageal inflammation. The prevalence of causative agents in infectious esophagitis differs based on the susceptibility of the population and the geographic area studied.

The second case described here presented with acute onset diffuse esophageal ulcer and necrosis. In literature, such endoscopic findings have been described with use of broad-spectrum antibiotics, infections (e.g., *Candida albicans*, cytomegalovirus, herpes virus, and *K. pneumoniae*), Stevens–Johnson syndrome, prolonged vomiting following alcohol binge, diabetic ketoacidosis with vomiting, lactic acidosis, malignancy, cocaine use, and aortic dissection.

Findings of eosinophilia on esophageal mucosa biopsy may be seen in classic eosinophilic esophagitis (a chronic, immune-mediated esophageal disease characterized by symptoms related to esophageal dysfunction and eosinophil-predominant inflammation), reflux disease, allergic vasculitis, Crohn's disease, achalasia, parasitic infections, connective tissue disease, and rarely those on prolonged PPI therapy.

Apart from food and inhalant allergens, microbes have been implicated in the causation of eosinophilic esophagitis. IgE-mediated immune reactions to microbes have been strongly associated with atopic diseases. Eosinophilic esophagitis patients are prone to increased *Candida* colonization, and *Candida* has been shown to induce the production of interleukin-5 further contributing to eosinophil activation in esophagus.

The global pandemic of COVID-19 has predisposed a relatively large number of patients to invasive fungal infections including candidiasis. The estimated mortality attributed to invasive disease may be as high as 40%, even higher (approaching 70%) in critically ill patients. There is an increasing incidence of non-*albicans Candida* species, with de novo resistance to antifungals and/or with a tendency to rapidly acquire antifungal resistance.

■ DIAGNOSTIC STRATEGIES

The gold standard for the diagnosis of *Candida* esophagitis is histologic confirmation of

Candida in the esophagus using hematoxylin and eosin stain of biopsies or brushing of esophageal mucosa. The characteristic finding is pseudohyphae. The mucosa involved may also show desquamated parakeratosis.

Approximately 50% of the invasive candidiasis cases are not identified by blood culture, and the application of nonculture diagnostics like β-D-Glucan (BDG) and galactomannan antigen testing, and molecular tests such as PCR and T2 *Candida* panel are recommended to improve the diagnosis. Combining multiple techniques may improve the yield. BDG is a panfungal marker and, hence, a positive result is not specific for *Candida*. The sensitivity and specificity of BDG for diagnosing invasive candidiasis are nearly 80% and can further be increased when combined with procalcitonin (which helps to differentiate it from bacterial infections).

MANAGEMENT ISSUES

Treatment of *Candida* esophagitis involves the use of antifungal therapy. Unlike oropharyngeal candidiasis (where topical agents are used), esophageal disease should always be treated with systemic agents. Oral fluconazole (200–400 mg per day for 14–21 days) is the most common agent recommended. In patients unable to tolerate orally, IV fluconazole 400 mg daily can be used and then changed to oral fluconazole once the patient can tolerate oral medications. Fluconazole 100–200 mg three times per week can be used to suppress recurrent *Candida* esophagitis. Micafungin 150 mg IV daily has been shown to be noninferior to fluconazole. Itraconazole 200 mg/day orally or voriconazole 200 mg twice daily for 14–21 days are other treatment options.

Amphotericin B deoxycholate 0.3–0.7 mg/kg daily is reserved for patients with refractory *Candida* esophagitis. Liposomal formulation of amphotericin B has better safety profile. Caspofungin may be preferred over amphotericin. Posaconazole 400 mg twice daily has been found to be effective in refractory candidiasis.

Besides effective antifungal therapy, it is also necessary to improve patients' general condition, strengthen the immune function of the body by improving nutrition, and actively treat underlying diseases (including control of blood sugar). Other priorities are to minimize the use of broad-spectrum antibiotics, use of intestinal flora regulator and the application of B vitamins to enhance the resistance of local tissues and inhibit the growth of *Candida*.

SUGGESTED READING

1. Alsomali MI, Arnold MA, Frankel WL, Graham RP, Hart PA, Lam-Himlin DM, et al. Challenges to "classic" esophageal candidiasis: looks are usually deceiving. Am J Clin Pathol. 2017;47(1):33-42.
2. Arastehfar A, Carvalho A, Nguyen MH, Hedayati MT, Netea MG, Perlin DS, et al. COVID-19-associated candidiasis (CAC): an underestimated complication in the absence of immunological predispositions? J Fungi (Basel). 2020;6:211-23.
3. Clancy CJ, Nguyen MH. Diagnosing invasive candidiasis. J Clin Microbiol. 2018:56: e01909-17.
4. Geagea A, Cellier C. Scope of drug-induced, infectious and allergic esophageal injury. Curr Opin Gastroenterol. 2008;24(4):496-501.
5. Gurvits GE. Black esophagus: acute esophageal necrosis syndrome. World J Gastroenterol. 2010;16(26):3219-25.
6. Hoversten P, Kamboj AK, Katzka DA. Infections of the esophagus: an update on risk factors, diagnosis, and management. Dis Esophagus. 2018;31(12).

7. Mohamed AA, Lu XL, Mounmin FA. Diagnosis and treatment of esophageal candidiasis: current updates. Can J Gastroenterol Hepatol. 2019;2019:3585136.
8. Pappas PG, Kauffman CA, Andes DR, Clancy CJ, Marr KA, Ostrosky-Zeichner L, et al. Clinical Practice Guideline for the Management of Candidiasis: 2016 Update by the Infectious Diseases Society of America. Clin Infect Dis. 2016;62(4):e1-50.
9. Pappas PG, Lionakis MS, Arendrup MC, Ostrosky-Zeichner L, Kullberg BJ. Invasive candidiasis. Nat Rev Dis Primers. 2018;4: 18026.
10. Rosołowski M, Kierzkiewicz M. Etiology, diagnosis and treatment of infectious esophagitis. Prz Gastroenterol. 2013;8(6): 333-7.
11. Simon D, Straumann A, Simon HU. Eosinophilic esophagitis and allergy. Dig Dis. 2014;32(1-2):30-3.
12. Takahashi Y, Nagata N, Shimbo T, Nishijima T, Watanabe K, Aoki T, et al. Long-term trends in esophageal candidiasis prevalence and associated risk factors with or without HIV infection: lessons from an endoscopic study of 80,219 patients. PLoS One. 2015;10(7): e0133589.

Refractory Gastroesophageal Reflux Disease

VG Mohan Prasad, Vamsi Murthy K, Madhura Prasad, Mithra Prasad

■ INTRODUCTION

Gastroesophageal reflux disease (GERD) is the most common gastrointestinal disorder affecting a vast number of individuals all around the world. While in most, GERD symptoms can be managed with lifestyle modifications and medications, 20-30% of GERD patients may experience persistent symptoms that are refractory to standard dose of proton-pump inhibitors (PPIs), thus affecting the productivity and quality of life. Patients who exhibit lack of response to PPI twice daily are considered to have failed PPI therapy.[1] Refractory GERD (rGERD) refers to this subset of patients that are difficult to treat. The causes of rGERD are not well understood. Some possible factors that may contribute to the development of rGERD include functional dyspepsia (postprandial distress syndrome with delayed gastric emptying increasing the risk of acid reflux) and functional heart burn. In this chapter, we will explore the clinical considerations, diagnosis, and management of patients with rGERD.

■ CLINICAL CASE

A 35-year-old male presented to the gastroenterology clinic with complaints of persistent and distressing heartburn, despite treatment with PPIs for the past 8 months. He experienced these symptoms everyday regardless of his diet. There was no history of dysphagia or weight loss. The physical examination findings were unremarkable. Further evaluation was done after stopping PPIs for a duration of 7 days. Endoscopy revealed hiatus hernia with Grade B [Los Angeles (LA)] reflux esophagitis **(Figs. 1A and B)**. Esophageal manometry revealed a hiatus hernia **(Fig. 2)**. Impedence pH revealed a DeMeester score of 85.1 (normal <14.7) **(Table 1)**.

■ DISCUSSION

Symptoms of rGERD are similar to those of typical GERD, but they are often more severe and persistent often disrupting the quality of life. These may include severe heartburn, disturbing regurgitation, chest pain, nausea, and vomiting.

■ DIAGNOSIS

To evaluate the potential causes of this patient with rGERD, several diagnostic tests may be considered. Endoscopy can evaluate for peptic ulcer disease, assist in biopsies, and can exclude underlying malignancy or any other structural abnormalities. High-resolution esophageal manometry can evaluate for esophageal motility disorders. pH-monitoring and impedance testing can evaluate the degree of reflux in the esophagus and can differentiate acid and nonacid reflux.

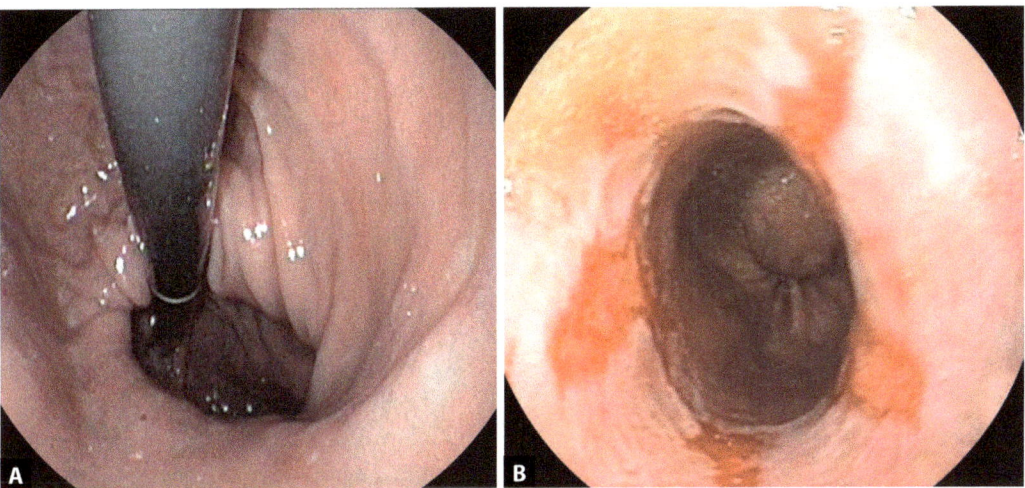

Figs. 1A and B: Endoscopy finding revealing evidence of GERD and a large hiatus hernia.

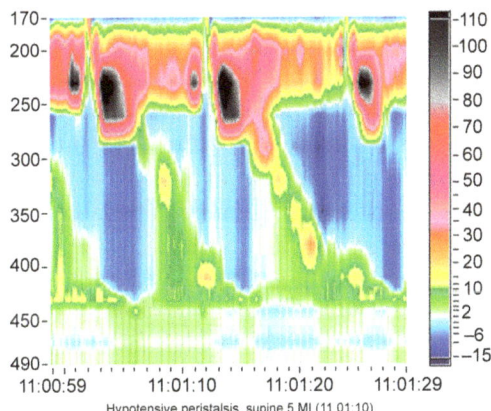

Comments
Basal pressue of LES—hypotensive
Relaxation of LES—present
Esophageal body peristalsis—hypotensive peristalsis in all swallows

Fig. 2: Findings of esophageal manometry in the clinical case. (LES: lower esophageal sphincter)

TABLE 1: Findings of 24-hour impedance pH monitoring in this clinical case.

Acid Reflux Composite Score Analysis (DeMeester) (pH)			
	Patient value	Patient score	Normal threshold
Upright time in reflux	22.6%	9.7	<8.4
Recumbent time in reflux	25.7%	26.1	<3.5
Total time in reflux	24.9%	18.2	<4.5
Episode over 5 minutes	6.3	5.6	<3.5
Longest episode	197.9 minutes	25.3	<19.8
Total episodes	8.4	0.2	<46.9
Composite score		85.1	<14.7

The diagnostic tests for persistent GERD-like symptoms are depicted in **Table 2**.

■ DIFFERENTIAL DIAGNOSIS

The diagnosis of rGERD is considered when there are persistent troublesome symptoms and objective evidence of GERD despite optimized PPI therapy. However, it is also important to note that few individuals who do not have GERD may complain of reflux-like symptoms that are refractory to PPI therapy and this can occur due to diverse etiologies.

TABLE 2: Diagnostic tests for persistent gastroesophageal reflux disease (GERD) like symptoms.

Diagnostic test	Comments
Endoscopy	The Los Angeles (LA) classification is the most widely used and validated scoring system.[2] Endoscopy aids to exclude other conditions that mimic GERD like: • Eosinophilic esophagitis • Infectious esophagitis • Pill-induced esophagitis • Esophageal cancer • Radiation-induced esophagitis • Zollinger–Ellison syndrome • Scleroderma • Caustic agent ingestion
High-resolution esophageal manometry (HREM)	• This can be used to assess motility abnormalities associated with GERD. It should be considered in patients with dysphagia, regurgitation, and prior planning invasive anti-reflux therapies • HREM can exclude underlying esophageal motility disorders,[3,4] e.g., achalasia, hypotensive lower esophageal sphincter, reduced esophageal contractility, supragastric belching, rumination syndrome
24-hour multichannel intraluminal impedance-pH (MII-pH)	• Reflux hypersensitivity • Functional heartburn
Gastric emptying scintigraphy or Electrogastrography	Delayed gastric emptying
Breath tests	Urea breath test, lactose breath test

Alarm features that may be suggestive of a gastrointestinal malignancy include: anemia, gastrointestinal bleeding, unexplained weight loss, dysphagia, odynophagia and gastrointestinal cancer in a first degree relative.

Table 3 enumerates rGERD and its mimickers with clarifying varied response to PPI.

Table 4 guides in differentiating nonerosive reflux disease (NERD) from functional heart burn, if endoscopy is normal. The differential diagnosis for the clinical case is given as follows:

- *Functional heartburn:* Some patients experience symptoms that are consistent with GERD but do not respond to PPIs. This may be caused by esophageal hypersensitivity.
- *Nonacid reflux:* While PPIs are effective in GERD, they may not alleviate symptoms caused by nonacid reflux. This can be evaluated by pH-monitoring or impedence testing.
- *Other causes:* Other potential cases for persistence GERD symptoms include eosinophilic esophagitis, peptic ulcer disease, or malignancy. These can be evaluated with appropriate investigations like endoscopy and biopsy.

TREATMENT OPTIONS FOR REFRACTORY GERD

Refractory GERD warrants further evaluation with repeat endoscopy with mucosal biopsies, esophageal manometry, pH-monitoring, and impedance testing. Endoscopic therapies [anti-reflux mucosectomy (ARMS), anti-reflux mucosal ablation (ARMA), GERDx, etc.] and surgery such as fundoplication may be considered.

Approach to a patient with rGERD are depicted in **Flowchart 1** and the various available options for treating such patients are as follows:

- *Lifestyle changes:* Eating smaller, more frequent meals, avoiding smoking, alcohol, and trigger foods like carbonated

TABLE 3: Refractory gastroesophageal reflux disease (GERD) and mimickers: Clarifying varied response to proton-pump inhibitor (PPI).

Subtypes of GERD	Endoscopy	Esophageal acid exposure	SI%	SAP%	Impedance pH metry Symptom association with acid reflex	Symptom association with nonacid reflex	Response to PPIs
Erosive reflux disease	Mucosal breaks	Abnormal	>50	>95	++	+/–	++
Nonerosive reflux disease	Normal	Abnormal	>50	>95	+	+/–	++
Acid hypersensitive esophagus	Normal	Normal	>50	>95	+	–	+
Nonacid hypersensitive esophagus	Normal	Normal	>50	>95	–	++	–
Functional heart burn	Normal	Normal	<50	<95	Negative	Negative	+/–

Source: Adapted from Rettura et al. (2021).
(GERD: gastroesophageal reflux disease; PPI: proton-pump inhibitor; SAP: symptom association probability; SI: symptom index)

TABLE 4: How to differentiate NERD from functional heart burn (if endoscopy is normal?)

Nonerosive reflux disease (NERD)	• Troublesome heartburn and/or regurgitation • Normal upper gastrointestinal endoscopy and no eosinophilic esophagitis on biopsies • Abnormal impedance pH-monitoring off proton-pump inhibitors (PPIs), with abnormal acid exposure and/or positive symptom association
Functional heartburn	• Retrosternal burning or discomfort (heartburn) • Unsatisfactory or nonresponse to double dose of PPIs after at least 8 weeks of therapy • Normal upper gastrointestinal endoscopy and no eosinophilic esophagitis on biopsies • Normal esophageal manometry • Normal impedance pH-monitoring off PPIs, with normal acid exposure and negative symptom association

Source: Adapted from Rettura et al. (2021).

or citric drinks, and elevating the head of bed by 6–8 inches can help to reduce GERD symptoms.

- *Medications:* Double-dose PPIs in combination with prokinetics may be tried. If the symptoms are due to esophageal hypersensitivity antidepressants, cognitive behavioral therapy, or neuromodulators may help.
- *Endoscopic therapies:* Minimally invasive anti-reflux endoscopic procedures with benefit in treating GERD are as follows:
  - *Stretta procedure:* This involves the application of controlled radiofrequency (RF) energy to the LES and has been shown to have therapeutic benefits.[5]
  - *Transoral incisionless fundoplication (TIF):* TIF 1.0 and TIF 2.0 are now available for management of GERD. TIF 2.0 procedure can reduce PPI use and control symptoms similar to current anti-reflux procedures, with a lower side effect profile and greater safety.[6]

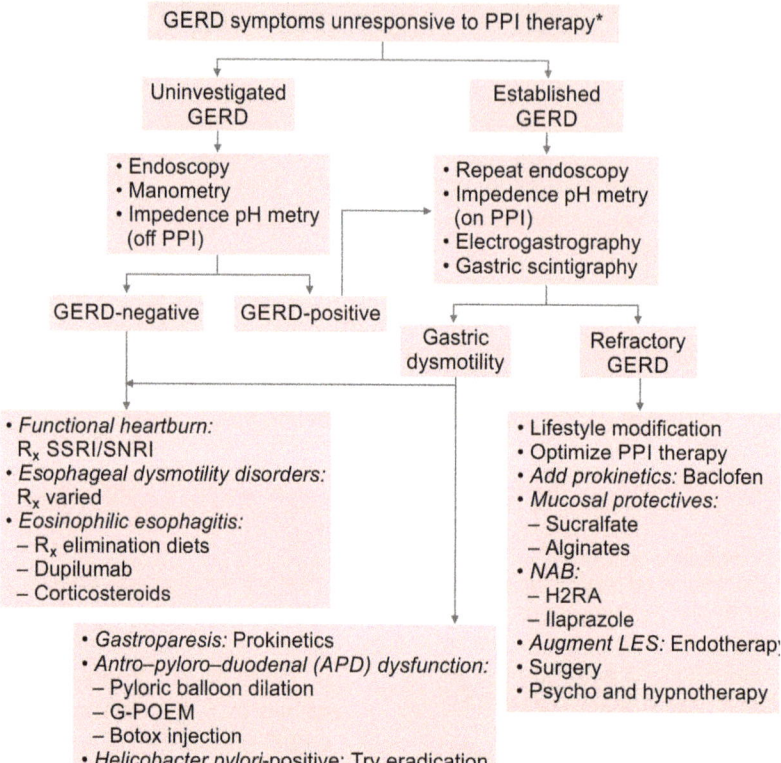

Flowchart 1: Approach to refractory gastroesophageal reflux disease (GERD).

Reasons for PPI failure:
- Noncompliance
- Incorrect dosage time
- Inadequate dosing
- Low drug bioavailability

(G-POEM: gastric peroral endoscopic pyloromyotomy; NAB: nocturnal acid breakthrough; PPI: proton-pump inhibitor; SNRI: serotonin–norepinephrine reuptake inhibitor; SSRI: selective serotonin reuptake inhibitor)

- *Endoscopic plication:* This is a minimally invasive endoscopic procedure used in treating patients with GERD. In a prospective trial, endoscopic plication with the GERDx™ device reduced distal acid exposure of the esophagus, reflux-related symptoms, and improved Gastrointestinal Quality of Life Index (GIQLI) scores.[7]
- *Anti-reflux mucosectomy (ARMS):* This is a novel endoscopic procedure wherein a crescentic endoscopic mucosal resection (EMR) is done over the gastroesophageal junction (GEJ). Anti-reflux mucosectomy seemed effective in improving GERD symptoms at 24 months.[8]
- *Anti-reflux mucosal ablation (ARMA):* This is a simple, safe endoscopic procedure and improves GERD-related symptoms and objective acid reflux parameters. In a pilot study, the median DeMeester score decreased from 33.5 to 2.8 ($p = 0.049$) at 2 months' follow-up after ARMA.[9]

- *Surgery:* Anti-reflux surgery corrects anatomical abnormalities, strengthens the esophageal sphincter, and eliminates the need for long-term PPIs.
- *Novel therapies:* There are numerous ongoing clinical trials investigating new therapies for rGERD, including novel medications and implantable magnetic devices,[10] electric stimulation of LES and neuromodulation of the LES (EndoStim).[11]

CLINICAL CASE (CONTINUATION)

Our patient was prescribed prokinetics along with double dose of PPIs. He improved well but could not stop the drugs even for a day and so, requested for a definitive procedure. We performed laparoscopic Nissen fundoplication. The patient had no further reflux episodes and is off PPIs for 5 years.

CONCLUSION

Refractory GERD is a challenging clinical problem that requires careful evaluation to determine the underlying cause. A detailed history and appropriate diagnostic tests such as endoscopy with biopsy, esophageal manometry, pH-monitoring, and impedance testing may be necessary to determine the cause of symptoms. Testing for the cause of dyspepsia by way of breath tests, electrogastrography, and/or gastric scintigraphy may be required to solve the puzzle. Some of these patients may not benefit with pharmacotherapy alone and may need endoscopic therapies or surgery. The management of rGERD needs a tailored approach to an individual patient, which may be different from the other.

REFERENCES

1. Sifrim D, Zerbib F. Diagnosis and management of patients with reflux symptoms refractory to proton pump inhibitors. Gut. 2012;61:1340.
2. Lundell LR, Dent J, Bennett JR, Blum AL, Armstrong D, Galmiche JP, et al. Endoscopic assessment of oesophagitis: clinical and functional correlates and further validation of the Los Angeles classification. Gut. 1999;45(2):172-80.
3. Gyawali CP, Fass R. Management of Gastroesophageal reflux disease. gastroenterology 2018;154:302-18.
4. Gyawali CP, Roman S, Bredenoord AJ, Fox M, Keller J, Pandolfino JE, et al; International GERD Consensus Working Group. Classification of esophageal motor findings in gastro-esophageal reflux disease: conclusions from an international consensus group. Neurogastroenterol Motil. 2017;29.
5. Triadafilopoulos G. Stretta: a valuable endoscopic treatment modality for gastroesophageal reflux disease. World J Gastroenterol. 2014;20(24):7730-8.
6. Gerson L, Stouch B, Lobonțiu A. Transoral incisionless fundoplication (TIF 2.0): a meta-analysis of three randomized, controlled clinical trials. Chirurgia (Bucur). 2018;113(2):173-84.
7. Weitzendorfer M, Spaun GO, Antoniou SA, Witzel K, Emmanuel K, Koch OO. Clinical feasibility of a new full-thickness endoscopic plication device (GERDx™) for patients with GERD: results of a prospective trial. Surg Endosc. 2018;32(5):2541-9.
8. Laquière A, Trottier-Tellier F, Urena-Campos R, Lienne P, Lecomte L, Katsogiannou M, et al. Evaluation of antireflux mucosectomy for severe gastroesophageal reflux disease: medium-term results of a pilot study. Gastroenterol Res Pract. 2022;2022: 1606944.
9. Inoue H, Tanabe M, de Santiago ER, Abad MRA, Shimamura Y, Fujiyoshi Y, et al. Anti-reflux mucosal ablation (ARMA) as a new treatment for gastroesophageal reflux refractory to proton pump inhibitors: a pilot study. Endosc Int Open. 2020;8(2): E133-8.
10. Bonavina L, DeMeester T, Fockens P, Dunn D, Saino G, Bona D, et al. Laparoscopic sphincter augmentation device eliminates

reflux symptoms and normalizes esophageal acid exposure: one- and 2-year results of a feasibility trial. Ann Surg. 2010;252:857.
11. Stephan D, Attwood S, Labenz J, Willeke F. EndoStim® treatment: a new minimally invasive technology in antireflux surgery. Chirurg. 2018;89(10):785-92.

SUGGESTED READING

1. Hunt R, Armstrong D, Katelaris P, Afihene M, Bane A, Bhatia S, et al; Review Team. World Gastroenterology Organisation Global Guidelines: GERD Global Perspective on Gastroesophageal Reflux Disease. J Clin Gastroenterol. 2017;51(6):467-78.
2. Katz PO, Dunbar KB, Schnoll-Sussman FH, Greer KB, Yadlapati R, Spechler SJ. ACG Clinical Guideline for the Diagnosis and Management of Gastroesophageal Reflux Disease. Am J Gastroenterol. 2022;117(1):27-56.
3. Naik RD, Meyers MH, Vaezi MF. Treatment of refractory gastroesophageal reflux disease. Gastroenterol Hepatol (NY). 2020;16(4):196-205.
4. Rettura F, Bronzini F, Campigotto M, Lambiase C, Pancetti A, Berti G, et al. Refractory Gastroesophageal reflux disease: a management update. Front Med (Lausanne). 2021;8:765061.

Chapter 8

Management of Dysphagia

Ashish Chauhan, Soumya Jagannath, Govind Makharia

■ INTRODUCTION

Swallowing is a complex event requiring neuromuscular coordination along with mechanical factors associated with anatomical organs. Therefore, any alteration in normal anatomy or physiology associated with swallowing can result in dysphagia. Dysphagia is defined as difficulty in swallowing that may be in the form of delayed passage of food or "sticking" of food to the esophagus and is considered as a "red flag" or an alarm symptom. Dysphagia is classified as either oropharyngeal or esophageal dysphagia depending upon the structural or functional origin. Oropharyngeal dysphagia occurs commonly due to neurological disorders such as stroke, Parkinson's disease or amyotrophic lateral sclerosis, or structural lesions such as Zenker's diverticulum, strictures, or webs. Esophageal dysphagia may be due to the structural component or due to motility disorders of esophagus. Moreover, dysphagia needs to be differentiated in terms of motor versus mechanical, oropharyngeal versus esophageal, and malignant versus benign.

■ CLINICAL CASE

A 35-year-old lady presented with a history of intermittent dysphagia to solids and liquids for the past 3 years. She had a weight loss of 8 kg in the past 3 years. Dysphagia was nonprogressive and it was not associated with any odynophagia. She did not have any history of connective tissue disorder. She was subjected to an endoscopy at a private center which showed liquid food residue in esophagus and there was resistance in negotiating lower esophageal sphincter (LES). A timed barium esophagogram was done which showed significant contrast retention at 1 and 5 minutes with grossly dilated esophagus with bird-beak appearance. Esophageal manometry was suggestive of an integrated relaxation period (IRP) of 25 mm Hg with panesophageal pressurization. This patient was diagnosed as achalasia cardia type II.

■ PHYSIOLOGY OF SWALLOWING

The process of swallowing involves a set of sequential events that allows the passage of food from mouth to stomach. The initial step involves crushing of food in the mouth and then the food bolus is pushed into the oropharynx by the tongue. This process involves simultaneous closure of nasopharynx by the soft palate and closure of mouth by the tongue to prevent nasal/oral regurgitation of the food. This pharyngeal phase of swallowing is involuntary and irreversible. Further the food is pushed till the upper esophageal sphincter (UES) which relaxes for the passage of food into the esophagus.

Here, the epiglottis causes the closure of airway to prevent the passage of food into the respiratory tract. There is simultaneous contraction of vocal cords to further prevent the entry of food into the respiratory tract. The pharyngeal phase is modulated by IX, X, XI, and XII nerves. Hence, most common causes of oropharyngeal dysphagia are neurological and the patient commonly presents with nasal/oral regurgitation, choking, or coughing during swallowing. The UES is in contracted state and next step involves relaxation of UES to push the food into esophagus. The peristaltic activity of the esophagus pushes the food forward and LES relaxes to allow food into the stomach.

It is important to note that muscles of oral cavity are supplied by trigeminal and facial nerve, the tongue by XII cranial nerve, and the pharyngeal muscles by IX and X cranial nerves. UES and muscles facilitating its opening are fifth, seventh, tenth, and twelfth. The cervical esophagus has striated musculature and is innervated by lower motor neurons of vagus nerve. In contrast, distal part of esophagus is constituted by smooth muscles and is under the control of excitatory and inhibitory neurons of esophageal myenteric plexus. The function of LES is supplemented by crus of the diaphragm.

APPROACH TO DYSPHAGIA

The approach to dysphagia begins with detailed clinical history with initial distinction directed toward localizing dysphagia to oropharynx or esophagus, differentiating motor from structural dysphagia and malignant from benign causes. Next step involves confirmation of the causes of dysphagia by objective testing. Various causes of dysphagia have been listed in **Table 1**. The objective testing usually starts with endoscopy and we now have radiological contrast studies and manometric evaluation for motility disorders. A structured approach to dysphagia based on clinical history requires us to answer a few questions to ascertain the cause of dysphagia.

IS IT OROPHARYNGEAL OR ESOPHAGEAL DYSPHAGIA? (TABLE 2)

As pointed out earlier, most of the causes of oropharyngeal dysphagia are usually neurological in origin such as stroke, Parkinson's, amyotrophic lateral sclerosis, motor neuron disease, and myasthenia gravis. Anatomical causes such as Zenker's diverticulum, strictures, webs, and malignancies are less common. Oral dysphagia is associated with poor bolus formation and poor bolus control. The patient may present with difficulty in initiating swallow, drooling, or nasal regurgitation. Hence the patient should be inquired about neurological symptoms as drooling of saliva, nasal regurgitation of food, and choking or coughing during swallowing. Apart from dysphagia patient may have other manifestations of underlying neurological disease which may point toward the diagnosis. Dysphagia that is localized to the retrosternal area is usually esophageal, whereas the dysphagia localized by patient to suprasternal notch could be oropharyngeal or esophageal as one-third of esophageal dysphagia may be referred proximally. In a nutshell, patient must be inquired for these accompanying symptoms as follows:

- Difficulty initiating a swallow
- Nasal regurgitation or nasal speech
- Coughing or choking during swallowing
- Drooling of saliva
- Dysarthria and diplopia
- Halitosis in patients (may be seen in a large, residue-containing Zenker's diverticulum with luminal accumulation)
- Recurrent pneumonia.

TABLE 1: Common causes of dysphagia.

Local structural lesions	Neuromuscular disease	Disorders of upper esophageal sphincter (UES)

• *Inflammatory:*
  – Pharyngitis
  – Abscess
  – Tuberculosis
• Neoplastic
• Congenital webs
• Plummer–Vinson syndrome
• *Extrinsic compression:*
  – Thyromegaly
  – Cervical spine hyperostosis
  – Lymphadenopathy
• Surgical resection of the oropharynx
	• *Central nervous system:*
	  – CVA (brain stem or pseudobulbar palsy)
	  – Parkinson's disease
	  – Multiple sclerosis
	  – Amyotrophic lateral sclerosis
	  – Brain stem tumors
	  – Tabes dorsalis
	• *Peripheral nervous system:*
	  – Bulbar poliomyelitis
	  – Peripheral neuropathies (e.g., diphtheria, botulism, rabies, diabetes mellitus)
	• *Motor end plate:*
	  – Myasthenia gravis
	• *Muscle:*
	  – Muscular dystrophies
	  – Primary myositis
	  – Metabolic myopathy (e.g., thyrotoxicosis, myxedema, steroid myopathy)
	  – Amyloidosis
	  – SLE
		• Hypertensive UES (spasm, possibly in globus)
		• *Abnormal UES relaxation or opening:*
		  – Incomplete relaxation (cricopharyngeal achalasia)
		  – Inadequate opening (cricopharyngeal bar, Zenker's diverticulum)
		  – Delayed relaxation (e.g., familial dysautonomia)

(CVA: cerebrovascular accident; SLE: systemic lupus erythematosus)

TABLE 2: Differentiating features of oropharyngeal and esophageal dysphagia.

S. No	Oropharyngeal dysphagia	Esophageal dysphagia
1.	Occurs immediately after swallow (usually within a minute)	Occurs later
2.	May have nasal regurgitation, coughing, choking, and voice change	These symptoms are not seen
3.	Mostly have association with other neurological disorders	No neurological manifestations
4.	Patient may refer to suprasternal notch location of dysphagia	Patient refers to retrosternal location of dysphagia

MECHANICAL OR MOTOR DYSPHAGIA (TABLES 3 AND 4)

Structural dysphagia usually presents with progressive dysphagia more for solids and then gradually progressing to dysphagia for liquids. The normal esophageal diameter is 2 cm in anteroposterior plane and 3 cm in lateral plane. Dysphagia to solids usually starts when luminal diameter decreases to <13 mm. Form therapeutics perspective, patients are able to tolerate a modified diet at a luminal diameter of 15 mm and a normal diet at a diameter of 18 mm. Dysphagia that is progressive over weeks should raise the alarm for structural

TABLE 3: Common causes of mechanical and motor dysphagia.	
Mechanical obstruction	**Motor dysphagia**

• Benign stricture:
  – Peptic
  – Corrosive
  – Drugs
  – Inflammatory
  – Webs and rings
  – Extrinsic compression
• Malignant:
  – Carcinoma
  – Polyp (fibrovascular polyp)
  – GIMT
	• Primary:
	  – Achalasia cardia
	  – Diffuse esophageal spasm
	  – Nutcracker esophagus
	  – Hypertensive LES
	  – Non-specific motility disorder
	  – EGJ outflow obstruction
	• Secondary:
	  – Diabetes
	  – Scleroderma
	  – Hypothyroidism
	  – Chagas disease

(EGJ: esophagogastric junction; GIMT: gastrointestinal mesenchymal tumor; LES: lower esophageal sphincter)

TABLE 4: Differentiating features of mechanical and motor dysphagia.		
Features	**Mechanical**	**Motor**
Course	Progressive	Static or fluctuating (usually)
Duration	Shorter	Longer
Dysphagia	Solids > liquids	Liquids > solids
Temperature of food	No difference	Dysphagia to cold/hot
Relieve with maneuvers	No	Specific maneuvers can relieve dysphagia

TABLE 5: Differentiating features of malignant and benign etiology of dysphagia.		
Features	**Malignant**	**Benign**
Course	Progressive	Static (generally)
Duration	Shorter	Longer
Constitutional symptoms	Present	Generally absent
Etiology	• Esophageal malignancy • Mediastinal tumor	• Peptic stricture • Corrosives • Drugs, inflammatory

MALIGNANT VERSUS BENIGN (TABLE 5)

Malignant dysphagia is progressive and has a shorter duration to development of significant dysphagia, whereas benign dysphagia is usually static and presents with dysphagia of longer duration. Malignant dysphagia usually has constitutional symptoms such as weight loss or loss of appetite.

POINTS TO REMEMBER IN HISTORY FOR VARIOUS ETIOLOGIES

Acute dysphagia is commonly due to food impaction, commonly seen in children. History of dysphagia following a meal might point toward impaction. In adult patients with psychiatric complaints, intentional ingestion (mostly metallic objects) is more common than food impaction. History of heartburn for years preceding dysphagia may suggest peptic stricture. A history of radiotherapy to head and neck, corrosive ingestion, or nasogastric intubation should also be probed. If dysphagia is associated with odynophagia, it usually indicates ulceration or infection. Tubercular lymph nodes can erode in midesophagus causing ulceration presenting as dysphagia and odynophagia with constitutional symptoms.

malignant pathology. Motor dysphagia is characterized by constant dysphagia for both solids and liquids. Episodic dysphagia for solids for years may be due to Schatzki ring or eosinophilic esophagitis (EoE). Patients with motor dysphagia may give the history of passage of food bolus with a particular posture or water.

In a specific clinical setting as human immunodeficiency virus (HIV) infection, candida esophagitis may be considered.

■ DIAGNOSTIC APPROACH

History may provide a pointer toward whether dysphagia is oropharyngeal or esophageal, malignant or benign, and structural or motor. The diagnostic evaluation in the management of dysphagia involves endoscopy, barium studies, esophageal manometry, and cross-sectional esophageal evaluation. We would focus most of the discussion of this approach for esophageal dysphagia.

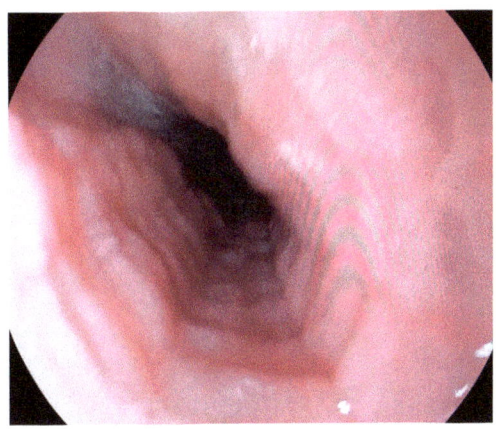

Fig. 1: Endoscopic finding in a patient with eosinophilic esophagitis showing pseudotrachealization of esophageal mucosa.

Endoscopy

Upper gastrointestinal (GI) endoscopy is the first investigation in patients presenting with dysphagia. Endoscopy has a role in diagnosing the etiology of dysphagia whether malignant or benign, assessing the need for any therapy as stenting in malignant obstruction or balloon dilation. Endoscopy will reveal level of obstruction, the severity of obstruction and etiology of obstruction in malignant pathologies. It can also diagnose strictures, rings, retained food as well as mucosal abnormalities. In case of a normal endoscopy, it is recommended to take multiple esophageal biopsies to rule out EoE. The diagnostic yield of endoscopy in patients undergoing endoscopy with an indication of dysphagia reached ~75% in a single-center study with 694 patients and another ~4% with normal endoscopy were diagnosed based on histology[1] **(Figs. 1 and 2)**.

Fluoroscopic Contrast Studies

Fluoroscopic contrast studies as barium esophagogram can delineate the structural anatomy as mucosal abnormalities, strictures, or extrinsic compression of the esophagus as well as can evaluate the esophageal function. Multiple modifications have been done to barium studies as single- or double-contrast timed barium evaluation (TBE). TBE involves ingestion of 200 cc of thinned barium with images taken at 1, 5, and 10 minutes. Esophageal contrast retention at 1 and 5 minutes can be measured from esophagogastric junction (EGJ). Amongst motility disorders, highest accuracy of radiographic studies is seen for achalasia and less for other esophageal motility disorders.[2] Overall the diagnostic accuracy of barium studies is less than endoscopy and it is used as an adjunct tool for assessment of esophageal diameter, stricture length, and location. Fluoroscopic evaluation of upper esophagus can ascertain bolus time and give insight into motility disorders **(Figs. 3A to D)**.

Esophageal Manometry

High-resolution manometry (HRM) is the modality of choice to evaluate esophageal contractility, and to evaluate dysphagia in a setting of normal endoscopy and histology. The standard metrics measured during HRM are IRP, distal contractile interval, distal

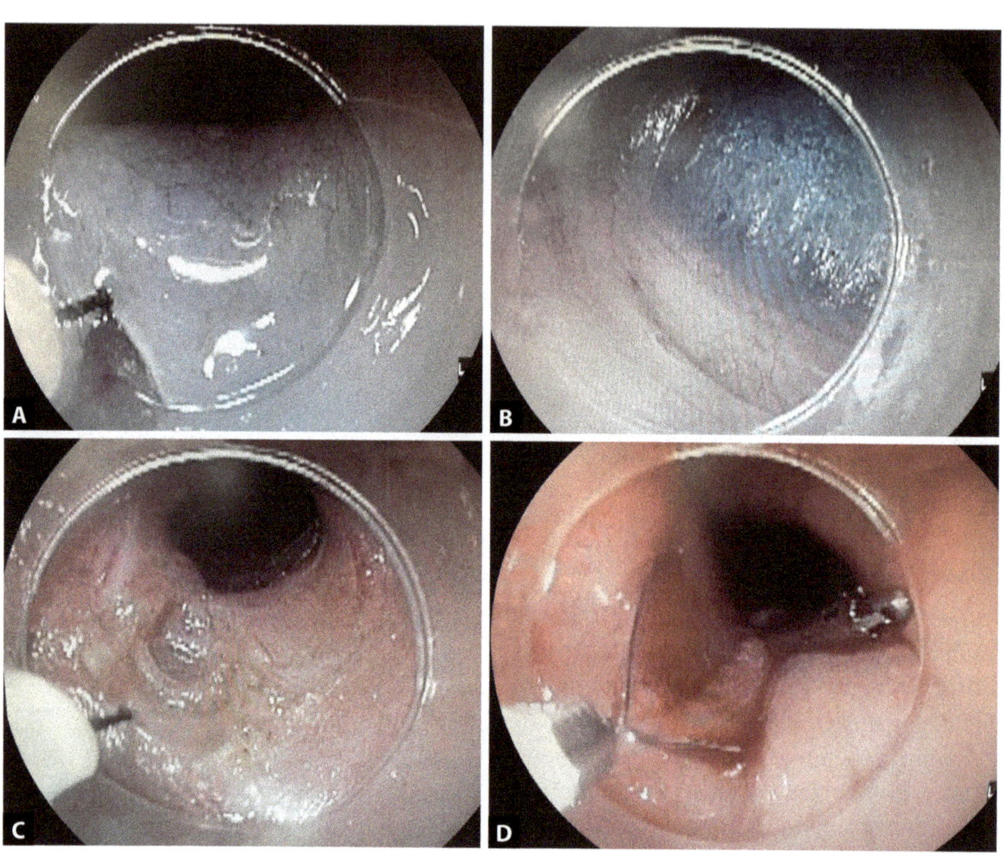

Figs. 2A to D: Peroral endoscopic myotomy being performed for a patient with achalasia cardia. (A) Mucosal incision; (B) submucosal dissection; (C) myotomy; (D) closure of the entry site.

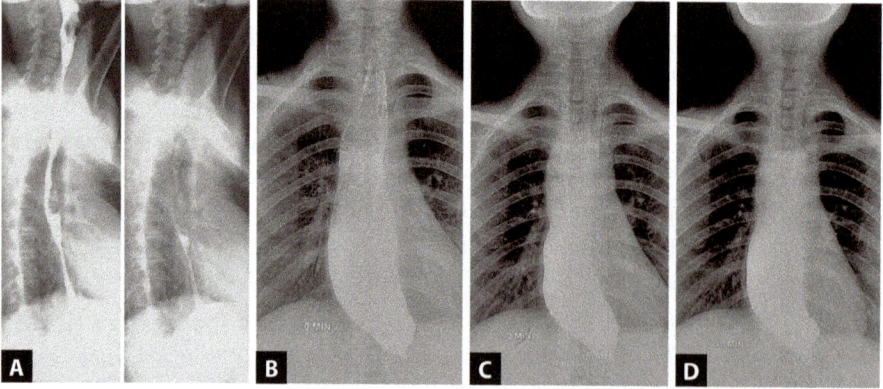

Figs. 3A to D: Fluoroscopic contrast studies for evaluation of dysphagia showing (A) postcorrosive lower esophageal stricture, and (B to D) timed barium evaluation in a case of suspected achalasia cardia. At 2 and 10 minutes there is significant retention of contrast in the dilated esophagus with narrowing at the lower esophageal sphincter.

latency, LES pressure, peristaltic breaks, etc. HRM uses a solid-state catheter assembly with closely places pressure tracers to provide esophageal pressure dynamics and pressure continuum to classify esophageal motility disorders. Chicago classification 4.0 is used to classify motility disorders of esophagus into achalasia of various types, distal esophageal spasm, hypercontractile esophagus, or absent contractility. Achalasia is the most common of all and is characterized by impaired relaxation of LES to swallow with absent or spastic contraction of esophageal body in the absence of any structural abnormality of esophagus or EGJ.

Imaging

Cross-sectional imaging as contrast-enhanced computed tomography of the thorax can provide relevant information in structural obstruction. It can give useful information on nodal metastasis, contiguous organ or vascular involvement, and extent of luminal involvement. CECT can also provide information on strictures whether benign or malignant, length of the stricture, and enhancement with contrast agent.

Newer Technologies—HRIM and FLIP

High-resolution impedance manometry (HRIM) can provide information about bolus transit, intrabolus pressure, bolus clearance, and relationship of bolus movement and pressure. It may provide more insight into motility disorders. FLIP or functional luminal imaging probe measures esophageal dimensions and esophageal distensibility in response to controlled distension. FLIP panometry can provide metrics on EGJ opening, esophageal body distensibility, and the contractile response to distension, that is, secondary peristalsis.[3]

■ CONCLUSION

Dysphagia is a red flag symptom or a danger sign especially in elderly. Approach to dysphagia includes differentiating malignant from benign, mechanical from motor, and localizing dysphagia to oropharynx or esophagus. Endoscopy is the initial investigation of choice for dysphagia. Fluoroscopic contrast study might complement endoscopy. Manometry studies have become quintessential in patients of motor dysphagia.

■ REFERENCES

1. Boeckxstaens GE, Zaninotto G, Richter JE. Achalasia. Lancet. 2014;383:83-93.
2. Patel DA, Yadlapati R, Vaezi MF. Esophageal Motility disorders: current approach to diagnostics and therapeutics. gastroenterology. 2022;162:1617-34.
3. Rengarajan A, Gyawali CP. Functional anatomy and physiology of swallowing and esophageal motility. In: Richter JE, Castell DO, Katzka DA, Katz PO, Smout A, Spechler S, et al. (Eds). The Esophagus, 6th edition. United States: John Wiley & Sons, Ltd.; 2021. pp. 59-96.

Section 3

Gastrointestinal Bleed

9. **Nonvariceal Upper Gastrointestinal Bleed**
   Kunal Das

10. **Obscure Gastrointestinal Bleed**
    Neha Berry, Ajay Kumar

11. **Gastric Variceal Bleed**
    Rajesh Upadhyay, Sagar Tyagi, VS Gaurav Narayan

9. Nonvariceal Upper Gastrointestinal Bleed

Kunal Das

■ CASE

A 63-year-old woman presented in the medical emergency with blood in vomiting for 1 day. She also had weakness, dizziness, and black stools for 2–3 days. There is no history of abdominal pain and fever. She was a known diabetic for the last 10 years and was on oral hypoglycemic medicines. There is no history of alcohol intake or analgesics. On examination she was pale, heart rate (HR)—110 beats/min, thereby low volume, blood pressure (BP)—90/60 mm Hg. No jaundice, peripheral pulses present but low volume, and hands are cold and clammy. *Chest examination:* unremarkable, cardiovascular system (CVS): within normal limits (WNL), per abdomen examination: no organomegaly. *Investigations:* complete blood count (CBC)—hemoglobin (Hb)—7.9 g%, total leukocyte count (TLC)—11,000/cumm, platelets—90,000/cumm, blood urea—101 mg/dL, serum creatinine—1.4 mg/dL, liver function test (LFT)—aspartate aminotransferase (AST) 54 IU/mL, alanine aminotransferase (ALT) 74 IU/mL, serum alkaline phosphatase (SAP) 112 IU/mL, serum bilirubin—2.4 g/mL. Ultrasonography (USG) abdomen—liver shows increased echogenicity, 13-cm span, mild splenomegaly, no ascites, rest—WNL. The patient underwent upper gastrointestinal (UGI) endoscopy which showed grade 2 esophageal varices with mild diffuse portal gastropathy. Duodenum shows a large ulcer with blood clot with active ooze. Endoscopic sclerotherapy was done using injection of adrenaline 2 mL × 5 sites. Further, a hemoclip was applied at the base of the ulcer. Rapid urease testing was done from antral biopsy which was positive for *Helicobacter pylori*. The patient was started on anti-*H. pylori* management.

■ INTRODUCTION

Nonvariceal GI bleeding is a major issue worldwide and causes significant morbidity and mortality and is encountered in both outpatient department (OPD) and emergency situations. It is responsible for large number of admissions in the GI department and has a mortality rate of 2–10%. Bleeding from the GI tract is categorized into UGI bleeding (UGIB) (from esophagus till ligament of Treitz), small bowel bleeding (from ligament of Treitz till distal Ileum) and lower GI (LGI) bleeding (large intestine).

■ DEFINITION

Gastrointestinal hematemesis, melena, or hematochezia are three possible manifestations of bleeding that are clinically evident as visible blood loss.

Hematemesis refers to bleeding close to the Treitz ligament and is defined as the vomiting of either fresh blood or coffee ground emesis.

Melena is characterized as black, tarry stools that may appear hours after a bleeding episode and are brought on by the gut microbes' breakdown of blood into hematin or other hemochromes. It can happen with different amounts of blood loss and becomes obvious with as little as 50 mL of blood.

Hematochezia is the term for red or maroon-colored blood or blood clots in the stool, which indicates a location of ongoing bleeding that is often caused by a right colonic LGI bleed but may also be recognized as heavy bleeding from small intestine.

In this chapter, we will be discussing the initial assessment, causes, diagnostic methods, and management of nonvariceal UGIB.

■ PRELIMINARY ASSESSMENT

The primary evaluation of a patient presenting with GI bleeding, regardless of the cause of bleeding rests on appropriate resuscitation, eliciting a good and relevant history, physical examination, and laboratory tests which will guide decisions regarding triage, empiric medical therapy, and further diagnostic testing and therapeutic interventions **(Table 1)**. It is important to emphasize that the primary assessment involves a detailed review of drugs of a patient presenting with GI bleed, particularly use of painkillers, antiplatelet agents, and anticoagulants.

■ CAUSES

The etiologies of nonvariceal UGIB.

Common Causes

- Peptic ulcer disease (PUD) (20–50%)
- Gastroduodenal erosions (8–15%)
- Esophagitis (5–15%)

TABLE 1: Glasglow-Blatchford Score.

Risk factors at presentation	Threshold	Score
Blood urea nitrogen (mmol/L)	6.5–7.9	2
	8.0–9.9	3
	10.0–24.9	4
	≥25.0	6
Hemoglobin for men (g/L)	120–130	1
	100–119	3
	<100	6
Hemoglobin for women (g/L)	100–120	1
	<100	6
Systolic blood pressure (mm Hg)	100–109	1
	90–99	2
	<90	3
Heart rate (beats/min)	>100	1
Melena	Present	1
Syncope	Present	2
Hepatic disease	Present	2
Cardiac failure	Present	2

Total score (0–23). Patients with scores >0 are considered to be at high risk

Source: With permission from Blatchford O, Murray WR, Blatchford M. A risk score to predict need for treatment for upper-gastrointestinal haemorrhage. Lancet. 2000;356(9238):1318-21.

- Mallory–Weiss syndrome (8–15%)
- Vascular malformations (5%).

Less Common Causes

- Malignancy
- Dieulafoy's lesions
- Gastric antral vascular ectasia (GAVE)
- Hemobilia
- Hemosuccus pancreaticus
- Aortoenteric fistula
- Cameron lesions.

Most important risk factors for gastroduodenal ulcers which are bleeding are *H. pylori* infection, nonsteroidal anti-inflammatory drug (NSAIDs) use, stress, and gastric acid secretion.

DIAGNOSIS

Upper GI endoscopy is most frequently used to diagnose UGIB. Early endoscopy performed within 24 hours after GI bleeding manifestation is linked to shorter hospital stays and reduced transfusion needs. As a result, early endoscopy is strongly advised for individuals who come with nonvariceal bleeding. Endoscopy aids in the diagnosis of conditions including gastric ulcers, duodenal ulcers, Mallory–Weiss Tears, arteriovenous malformations (AVMs), and portal gastropathy that cause UGIB and assists in determining the patient's best course of endoscopic and nonendoscopic treatment. Additionally, endoscopy can locate people with low-risk lesions who can get outpatient care.

Stratification of Risk

In order to identify people at higher risk of bleeding, early risk stratification **(Table 2)** is extremely helpful and strongly advised in patients who complain of acute UGIB.

MANAGEMENT

Common Endoscopic Therapies

Following the GI causes' identification, if bleeding has already started, endoscopic techniques, such as injectable treatment, ablative procedures, or mechanical therapy, can be used to achieve therapeutic hemostasis, depending on the lesion.

Endoscopic Sclerotherapy

This type of hemostasis uses injectable treatment with saline or diluted epinephrine, which works as a local pressure tamponade (1:10,000 to 1:20,000 epinephrine in saline). Local vasospasm is also produced when diluted injection epinephrine is injected into four quadrants within 3 mm of the bleeding region. A clearer field of vision results from this injection technique. Injection absolute alcohol, sodium tetradecyl sulfate, polidocanol, and ethanolamine, among other sclerosants, are really tissue irritants that, when injected into the body, promote endofibrosis and vascular obliteration

TABLE 2: Pre-endoscopic Rockall score.

Item indicators	Categories	Criteria	Score
Age (years)	<60		0
	60–79		1
	≥80		2
Shock	No shock	• SBP >100 mm Hg • Pulse <100/min	0
		• SBP >100 mm Hg • Pulse >100/min	1
		• SBP <100 mm Hg	2
Comorbidity	• No major comorbidity		0
	• Cardiac failure • Ischemic heart disease • Any major comorbidity		2
	• Renal or liver failure • Disseminated malignancy		3

(SBP: systolic blood pressure)

through vascular thrombosis and endothelial damage.

Thermal Coagulation

It often occurs by argon plasma coagulation (APC) or contact heat probes (such as a gold probe). By simultaneously applying pressure and closing the underlying vessel while doing coagulation, contact probes can accomplish hemostasis. APC employs ionized, nonflammable argon gas to give thermal energy that causes the target tissue to coagulate, resulting in hemostasis. APC is a noncontact thermal technique of hemostasis.

Hemoclips

Hemostasis caused by the use of hemoclips is mechanical because the underlying vessel is mechanically sealed between the two hemoclip arms. This method avoids the tissue damage or inflammation brought on by sclerosants or thermal coagulation. The use of hemoclips in the treatment of peptic ulcer bleeding (PUB) may be advantageous.

Hemostatic Powder

The innovative endoscopic hemostatic powder/spray TC-325 is safe and an option for the treatment of UGIB and LGI bleeding. The hemostatic spray, which is applied to actively bleeding lesions using a novel catheter, contains a highly absorbent inorganic mineral nanopowder. This creates a mechanical barrier that can result in immediate hemostasis and has been shown to speed up the coagulation process by encouraging the formation of clots in the bleeding lesions. Hemospray has a success rate of between 75 and 100% for nonvariceal UGIB (including ulcers and other lesions), with rebleeding rates ranging from 10 to 49%. It may also be beneficial for people with malignant GI hemorrhage.

■ MEDICAL MANAGEMENT

Proton-pump Inhibitors

In patients with suspected UGIB, intravenous (IV) proton-pump inhibitors (PPI) are advised as the first line of therapy. Numerous studies demonstrate that an intragastric pH >6 encourages the development and maintenance of clots, while a severely acidic intragastric environment inhibits platelet aggregation, plasma coagulation, and encourages the dissolution of existing clots. Patients on PPI treatment were shown to have less active bleeding, a lower need for endoscopic intervention, but most critically, there were no changes in transfusion needs, hospital stay length, surgical necessity, or death. Pre-endoscopic IV PPI medication lowers the percentage of high-risk lesions (active bleeding, nonbleeding visible vessel, and adherent clot) during index endoscopy in patients with UGIB related to PUD, and occasionally the requirement for endoscopic surgery.

Prokinetics

In situations, where there is a high likelihood of finding new blood or blood clots in the stomach, prokinetic drugs (such as injection metoclopramide/injection erythromycin) are used to increase stomach visualization and improve endoscopic diagnostic yield. Patients with acute UGIB should get injections of erythromycin or metoclopramide at least 20–120 minutes before their endoscopy. This increased mucosal visibility reduced the need for a second look endoscopy to identify the location and origin of the bleeding. However, it has not been demonstrated that this has any advantages in terms of the necessity of blood transfusions, length of hospital stay, or surgical procedure.

Finding individuals with low-risk lesions who may be treated as outpatients via

CHAPTER 9: Nonvariceal Upper Gastrointestinal Bleed

TABLE 3: Forrest classification.

Stage	Characteristics	Rebleeding
Ia	Spurting bleed	60–100%
Ib	Oozing bleed	50%
IIa	Nonbleeding visible vessel	40–50%
IIb	Adherent clot	20–30%
IIc	Flat spot in ulcer crater	7–10%
III	Clean base ulcer	3–5%

Ia	Ib	IIa	IIb	IIc	III
Spurting bleed	Oozing bleed	Nonbleeding visible vessel	Adherent clot	Flat spot in ulcer crater	Clean base ulcer

endoscopy is helpful. The gold standard of care for treating ulcers with stigmata of recent hemorrhage (SRH), which have a greater risk of recurrent bleeding and death, is endoscopic therapy. These stigmata are listed in **Table 3** (Forrest categorization). Endoscopic therapy may not be advised since the majority of individuals with PUB have low-risk Forrest IIc and Forrest III lesions. Both ulcers that are currently bleeding and visible vessels that are not bleeding are advised to undergo endoscopic therapy. If possible, irrigate peptic ulcers with overlaying clots to evaluate and treat the underlying lesion. The use of endoscopy in conjunction with injectable therapy, thermal coagulation, mechanical device, and a PPI is advised by guidelines. endoscopic procedures. Endoscopic sclerotherapy using substances other than epinephrine, such as sclerosants (such as absolute alcohol, polidocanol, and ethanolamine), thermal ablation (bipolar or monopolar electrocoagulation, APC, heater probe, and laser), thrombin/fibrin glue, and hemoclips are all individually effective and noninferior to one another in achieving hemostasis in bleeding ulcers. The use of cautery or hemoclips in conjunction with an epinephrine injection was found to be superior than epinephrine alone (a single operation) in numerous meta-analyses and to minimize the risk of recurrent bleeding, the need for further medical intervention, and death. When endoscopic treatment fails to control active bleeding, Hemospray may be tried.

Mallory–Weiss Tears

Mucosal rips at the gastroesophageal (GE) junction, gastric cardia, or distal esophagus are the hallmarks of Mallory–Weiss tears, which are frequently accompanied by violent retching or vomiting. The majority of the time, bleeding from submucosal arteries that involves the GE junction is self-limited, but in rare occasions, significant bleeding may necessitate endoscopic treatment. Endoscopic procedures such band ligation, heat coagulation, clip implantation, and epinephrine administration. Surgery or angiographic embolization may be needed to stop bleeding that is unresponsive to endoscopic treatment.

Arteriovenous Malformations

These are also known as angiodysplasias, refer to the abnormal blood vessels that are present throughout the GI tract. As a result, 4–7% of people develop UGIB. They are more frequently discovered in conjunction with chronic illnesses, such as aortic stenosis, inherited hemorrhagic telangiectasias, cirrhosis, end-stage renal disease (ESRD), and cirrhosis. Bleeding from AVMs often manifests as long-term blood loss with anemia but may present with overt bleeding. Elective hemostatic therapies include APC, bipolar or heater probe coagulation, ligation, and sclerotherapy.

Dieulafoy Lesion

This refers to a dilated aberrant submucosal artery, often situated in the proximal stomach along the lesser curvature, which erodes the underlying epithelium before rupturing. Normally it is located adjacent to the GE junction, but can be located elsewhere throughout the GI tract. Bruising that comes and goes and extreme pain are the typical clinical manifestations. Effective treatments include endoscopic banding, clipping, electrocautery, laser therapy, heater probe, injection of sclerosants, or epinephrine. While band ligation may be linked to a higher risk of bowel perforation, the use of epinephrine alone is linked to a higher risk of rebleeding.

Gastric Antral Vascular Ectasia (GAVE)

This is also known as "watermelon stomach", is most frequently observed in people with cirrhosis and systemic sclerosis, and generally shows as anemia and ongoing blood loss. The most prevalent form of treatments is APC, and more recently radiofrequency ablation (RFA), other options include endoscopic coagulation with a heater probe, bipolar probe, or laser therapy.

Gastrointestinal Tumors, Benign and Malignant

They account for <3% of cases of UGIB. Neoplasms can cause bleeding from disuse mucosal ulceration or from erosion into an underlying vessel. Standard endoscopic treatment modalities include injection therapy, thermal contact probes, and APC. Hemostatic powder is effective for acute control of active bleeding, however rebleeding in malignant lesions is common.

Endoscopic therapy can effectively control bleeding in the vast majority of patients with UGIB, but persistent or recurrent bleeding may be seen in 7–24% of cases. Repeat endoscopic therapy is recommended and is usually successful. However, if bleeding cannot be controlled endoscopically, angiographic control should be considered.

■ CONCLUSION

Nonvariceal gastrointestinal hemorrhage is a serious medical emergency. Then appropriate, prompt diagnosis and prompt initiation of medical and endoscopic hemostatic treatment enhance results. Additional prognostic improvements are predicted when additional diagnostic and therapeutic endoscopic capabilities develop and find applications.

SUGGESTED READING

1. Mujtaba S, Chawla S, Massaad JF. Diagnosis and management of non-variceal gastrointestinal hemorrhage: a review of current guidelines and future perspectives. J. Clin. Med. 2020;9:402.
2. Sung JJ, Chan FK, Chen M, Ching JY, Ho KY, Kachintorn U, et al.; Asia-Pacific Working Group. Asia-Pacific Working Group consensus on non-variceal upper gastrointestinal bleeding. Gut. 2011;60:1170-7.
3. Ramaekers R, Mukarram M, Smith CA, Thiruganasambandamoorthy V. The predictive value of preendoscopic risk scores to predict adverse outcomes in emergency department patients with upper gastrointestinal bleeding: a systematic review. Acad Emerg Med. 2016;23:1218-27.
4. Odutayo A, Desborough MJ, Trivella M, Stanley AJ, Dorée C, Collins GS, et al. Restrictive versus liberal blood transfusion for gastrointestinal bleeding: a systematic review and meta-analysis of randomised controlled trials. Lancet Gastroenterol Hepatol. 2017;2:354-60.
5. Masci E, Arena M, Morandi E, Viaggi P, Mangiavillano B. Upper gastrointestinal active bleeding ulcers: review of literature on the results of endoscopic techniques and our experience with Hemospray. Scand J Gastroenterol. 2014;49:1290-5.

Chapter 10

Obscure Gastrointestinal Bleed

Neha Berry, Ajay Kumar

■ CLINICAL CASE

A 74-year-old female patient, who is a known case of hypertension, hypothyroidism, and coronary artery disease since 2018 [post-percutaneous transluminal coronary angioplasty (PTCA) status] on aspirin 75 mg, presented at our tertiary care hospital for the first time in 2020 with chief complaints of black, tarry stools on and off for last 3 years for which she had received >5 blood transfusions in the last 2 years. She had a previous history of endoscopy done 3 years back which was normal. General physical examination showed tachycardia and pallor. Baseline investigation revealed anemia [microcytic hypochromic with hemoglobin (Hb) of 4.0 g/dL and mean corpuscular volume (MCV) of 67] with peripheral smear and iron studies suggestive of iron deficiency anemia. Rest of the investigations were unremarkable. Patient received 3 units of packed RBC transfusions and other resuscitative measures. After stabilization, patient underwent upper GI (UGI) endoscopy which was unremarkable, followed by colonoscopy which showed melenic stools till the ileum. In view of active bleed and ongoing tachycardia, computed tomography (CT) angio-whole abdomen was done which revealed no significant bowel wall thickening, active arterial blush, or any polypoidal lesion. Hence, a provisional diagnosis of obscure overt gastrointestinal bleed was made and the patient was subjected to capsule endoscopy (CE). CE **(Figs. 1A to C)** was done which revealed fresh blood in proximal jejunum with active ooze?

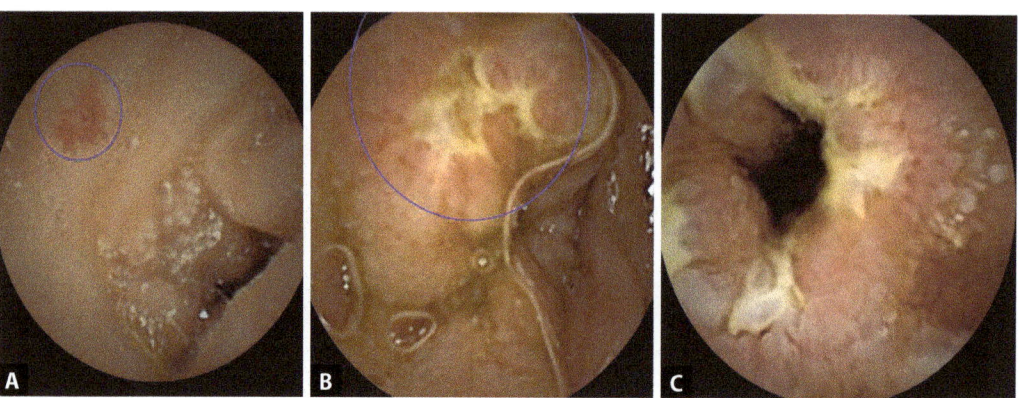

Figs. 1A to C: Capsule endoscopic images. (A) Angioectasia; (B) ulcer; (C) ulcerated stricture.

Angioectasia (AE)? Dieulafoy's lesion (DL). Antegrade enteroscopy was then performed which showed DL in the proximal part of jejunum with intermittent active ooze. Argon plasma coagulation (APC) was done and hemostasis achieved. Subsequently patient passed normal colored stools, maintained Hb levels, and was discharged after 48 hours observation. Hb gradually increased on follow-up with no further melenic episodes in next 6 months of follow-up.

■ POINTS TO DISCUSS

- How do you define obscure gastrointestinal (GI) bleed?
- What are the common etiologies of obscure GI bleed?
- How do you evaluate obscure GI bleed?
- What is endoscopic treatment of small bowel (SB) bleed?
- What options are available for pharmacological management of SB bleed?
- What is algorithm for management of obscure GI bleed?

Question 1: How do you define obscure GI bleed?
Answer: Any bleed where the source is identified distal to ampulla of Vater and/or proximal to the ileocecal valve is defined as a case of SB bleed, and these account for only about 5–10% of all GI bleeds. SB bleed can then be classified as either "overt SB bleed" for patients presenting with overt melena or hematochezia, or "occult SB bleed" for patients presenting with iron deficiency anemia with or without positive stool guaiac test. With the introduction of video capsule endoscopy (VCE) and enteroscopy, majority (>75%) patients previously classified to have obscure GI bleed, are found to have SB as their source, and hence recent American College of Gastroenterology (ACG) guidelines have proposed to reserve the term obscure GI bleed for patients in whom despite comprehensive evaluation of SB, no obvious source of bleed is identified. In the case discussed above, the patient will be defined to have a SB bleed as the CE showed evidence of active bleed in proximal jejunum.

Question 2: What are the common etiologies of obscure GI bleed?
Answer: The most common causes of obscure bleed are vascular lesions, such as angiodysplasia, telangiectasia, phlebectasia, arteriovenous malformation (AVM), DL and varices, while other causes being tumors, inflammatory lesions, drug-induced bleeds [caused by aspirin, nonsteroidal anti-inflammatory drugs (NSAIDs), anticoagulants, other antiplatelet agents] and other rare causes. In a large study of 385 patients with obscure GI bleed by Zhang et al., the common causes in elderly (>65 years of age) were vascular anomalies (54.35%), SB ulcer, predominantly NSAID-induced (13.04%), SB tumors (11.96%), while vascular anomalies (34.82%), tumors (31.25%) and nonspecific enteritis (9.82%) were the major causes in middle age (41–64 years), and Crohn's disease (34.55%), tumors (23.64%), and nonspecific enteritis (10.91%) in young adults (<40 years). **Table 1** shows the common etiologies of SB bleed divided according to age groups. AEs are abnormal dilated tortuous thin-walled vessels, involving small capillaries, veins, or arteries, lined by endothelium with little or no smooth muscle, without any inflammatory component or fibrosis, and are visualized within the mucosa or submucosa. Certain risk factors have shown a positive association with AEs in various studies. These include cardiovascular diseases, liver cirrhosis, respiratory diseases, thromboembolic disease, chronic renal

TABLE 1: Etiology of obscure gastrointestinal bleeding according to age.			
Elderly (>65 years)	**Middle-aged (41–65 years)**	**Young adult (17–40 years)**	**Rare causes**
• Vascular anomalies • Small intestinal ulcer • NSAID enteropathy • Small intestinal tumors • Nonspecific enteritis • Celiac disease	• Vascular anomalies • Small intestinal tumors • Nonspecific enteritis • Small intestinal ulcer	• Crohn's disease • Small intestinal tumors • Meckel's diverticulum • Nonspecific enteritis • Dieulafoy's lesion • Vascular anomalies • Celiac disease • Polyposis syndromes	• Small bowel varices and/or portal hypertensive enteropathy • Amyloidosis • Blue rubber bleb nevus syndrome • Pseudoxanthoma elasticum • Osler–Weber–Rendu syndrome • Kaposi's sarcoma with AIDS • Plummer–Vinson syndrome • Ehlers–Danlos syndrome • Inherited polyposis syndromes (FAP, Peutz–Jeghers) • Malignant atrophic papulosis • Hematobilia • Aortoenteric fistula • Hemosuccus entericus

(AIDS: acquired immunodeficiency syndrome; FAP: familial adenomatous polyposis ; NSAIDs: nonsteroidal anti-inflammatory drugs)

failure, hypertension, hypercholesterolemia, systemic sclerosis, aortic stenosis, and anticoagulant use. DL refers to histologically normal but abnormally large arteries that typically protrude through a small mucosal defect. It is proposed that ischemic injury, probably related to comorbidities (e.g., cardiovascular disease) or drugs (e.g., NSAIDs and antithrombotic drugs) may lead to disruption of the overlying epithelium thus causing massive bleeding from this large submucosal vessel.

Small bowel vascular lesions can be endoscopically classified into four categories based on the Yano-Yamamoto classification. AEs are classified as type 1a: punctuate (<1 mm) erythema or type 1b: patchy (>1 mm) erythema with or without oozing. DLs are classified as type 2a: punctuate lesions with pulsatile bleeding or type 2b: Pulsatile red protrusions without surrounding venous dilatation. Some intestinal AVMs are classified as type 3: pulsatile red protrusions with surrounding venous dilatation. Congenital intestinal AVMs can be large and sometimes appear as a mass or polypoid lesion which can be classified under type 4: lesions not classified into any of the above categories.

Question 3: How do you evaluate obscure GI bleed?

Answer: Small bowel evaluation should be considered when upper endoscopy and colonoscopy and relook procedures when required, are noncontributory. VCE is now considered as the first-line step for SB evaluation, following which push or deep enteroscopy can be performed, depending on the location of probable source of bleed on VCE, as both diagnostic and therapeutic strategy. European Society of Gastrointestinal Endoscopy (ESGE) recommends VCE to be done as soon as possible after the bleeding episode, preferably within 48 hours, to maximize the yield. VCE allows noninvasive visualization of the entire SB with a diagnostic yield of 38–83%. The diagnostic yield is higher for patients with overt bleed (92%) compared to occult bleeders (44%) or those with prior

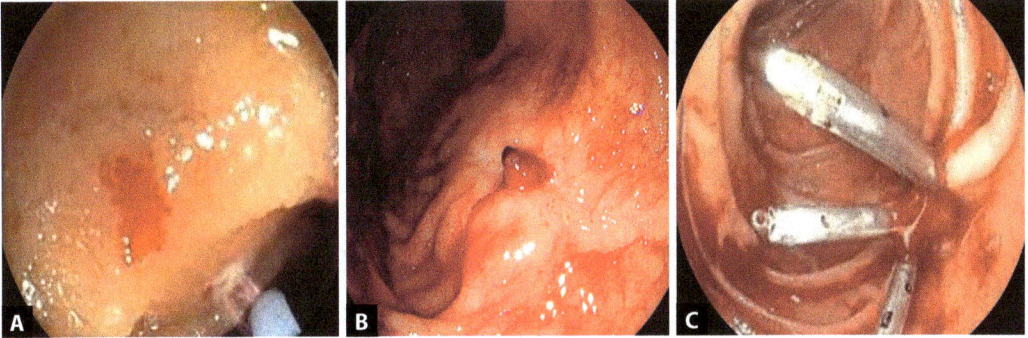

Figs. 2A to C: Argon plasma coagulation (APC) for angioectasia and hemoclips for Dieulafoy.

overt bleeding (67%). VCE can take images at the rate of 2-6 frames per second, over 8-12-hour period, which are transferred to a recording device, downloaded, and viewed on a computer station with VCE software. Although VCE is well tolerated, its main complication is capsule retention, which usually occurs in only about 1.5% patients, but may increase to 13% in patients with SB strictures, such as those with Crohn's disease, thus limiting its use in patients with obstruction or strictures until patency is documented. CT enterography (CTE) or magnetic resonance enterography (MRE) is a safer option in such patients. Hence, patients with a history suggestive of obstructive symptoms should first undergo CTE/MRE, and VCE should be done if CTE is noncontributory with no evidence of obstruction/stricture.

Push enteroscopy allows only limited evaluation of proximal SB, up to 70 cm distal to the ligament of Treitz. Double-balloon enteroscope (DBE) can be advanced to a distance of 240-360 cm distal to pylorus and 100-140 cm proximal to ileocecal valve via retrograde technique, and can be used to obtain biopsies as well as perform therapeutic procedures such as hemostasis, polypectomy, and dilatation. However, its main limitation includes its invasive nature, prolonged procedure time, and difficulty in hemodynamically unstable patients. Spiral enteroscopy can complete the SB evaluation in lesser time compared to DBE, and a diagnostic yield of up to 57% is reported in patients with a positive CE. As a last resort, intraoperative endoscopy can be used with a diagnostic yield reported in the range from 58 to 88%. CT enterography should be performed in patients with suspected SB bleeding and negative CE because of higher sensitivity for detecting mural-based SB masses, and ability to guide subsequent deep enteroscopy. **Figures 2A to C** provides an algorithm on how to approach a patient with suspected SB bleed.

Question 4: What is endoscopic treatment of SB bleed?
Answer: Patients with SB bleeds are treated according to etiology. Patients with NSAID-induced ulcers are advised to avoid NSAIDs, and those with Crohn's disease treated with steroids and immunosuppressants. Patients with SB tumors are advised surgical evaluation. AEs are usually very closely monitored and streamlined into treatment modalities, whether endoscopic, conservative with blood and iron transfusions, or pharmacological, depending on their existing comorbidities. In this chapter, we will discuss

in detail regarding treatment modalities for vascular malformations. Though there is no consensus on the best endoscopic treatment for vascular malformations, APC during enteroscopy is the most common modality for AEs. Even though APC has shown to reduce transfusion requirement and improve mean Hb measurements, studies have shown a significant rebleeding rate as high as 42% despite APC. Hemoclip application, either alone or in combination with epinephrine injection, may be used for DLs and larger AVMs. Injection sclerotherapy with polidocanol has also been tried in patients with type 1b SB AEs, though literature is limited. Superselective transcatheter embolization (SSTCE) after successful delineation of bleeding vessel on mesenteric angiography, has been successfully used to control SB bleed, particularly when endoscopic therapy has failed, however with a risk of bowel infarction and mucosal ischemia. Intraoperative endoscopy for exact localization of AEs with limited segmental resection of the SB is now considered as one of the last therapeutic options for uncontrollable SB bleed, after failure of endoscopic and embolization options.

Question 5: What options are available for pharmacological management of obscure bleed?

Answer: This is particularly useful for patients with recurrent bleeding and those with extensive AEs throughout the SB, where exact origin of bleed cannot be determined.

- *Somatostatin analogs:* Somatostatin is an inhibitory peptide secreted by the D cells in the gastric and intestinal mucosa, and by enteric neurons and islet cells of the pancreas, and causes reduction of acid secretion, pancreatic enzyme release, and bile flow. Somatostatin analogs can reduce bleeding from AEs, via a combination of improved platelet aggregation, decreased splanchnic blood flow, increased vascular resistance, and the inhibition of angiogenesis. Several small studies and one meta-analysis have shown the usefulness of octreotide on bleeding cessation, with doses varying from the short-acting subcutaneous formulation twice a day to the long-acting intramuscular injection every 4 weeks, with improvement in Hb level and reduction in transfusion requirement and rebleeding episodes. Nardone et al. showed that 73.4% patients with recurrent bleeding from AEs achieved a stable Hb level without requiring a blood transfusion after one to three cycles of intramuscular long-acting ocreotide (OCT-LAR). However, the major limitation for prolonged use of somatostatin analogs is cost in addition to the potential for long-term side effects including diarrhea, abdominal pain, constipation, hypothyroidism, gallstone formation, kidney stones, and pancreatic enzyme deficiency which may be seen in up to 30% patients.
- *Thalidomide:* Thalidomide is an immunomodulatory drug with anti-inflammatory and antiangiogenic properties which has been successfully used in the treatment of AEs, including in those who have failed other therapy including endotherapy or in combination. Thalidomide acts by its ability to downregulate the expression of vascular endothelial growth factor (VEGF) both at protein and mRNA level. At low concentrations, it has also been shown to activate mural cells and their proliferation, which form protrusions around blood vessels, thus stabilizing them and decreasing the risk of bleeding.

This antiangiogenic effect can persist even on stopping it, thus having a bleeding-free period even after stopping thalidomide. Doses range from 100–300 mg/day in several studies. In one study, patients received either 100 mg of thalidomide or 400 mg of iron, with response rates in the thalidomide and control groups recorded at 71.4 and 3.7%, respectively. In one retrospective study of 15 patients treated with thalidomide, 38.5% had no recurrent bleed and overall 86.4% had decrease in recurrence of GI bleed, hospitalizations, blood transfusions, and need for endoscopic therapy. Effect of thalidomide becomes prominent usually after 3 months of treatment, likely reflecting the time it takes to change balance between anti and proangiogenic factors. Thalidomide carries the risk of serious adverse events, such as deep vein thrombosis, and common side effects such as fatigue, constipation, dizziness, peripheral neuropathy, and edema.

- *Lenalidomide:* This is a second generation immunomodulatory drug which is more potent than thalidomide and has antimigratory effects on endothelial cells. A case series of five patients with von Willebrand factor (vWF) disease and GI bleed from AEs treated with lenalidomide, has shown that it is effective and relatively well tolerated with significant reduction in number of endoscopic interventions needed and increased bleed-free interval. The starting dose is usually 5 mg/day orally, which can be titrated up to 10–15 mg per day. However, the use of antiangiogenic drugs, thalidomide, and lenalidomide is limited by severe side effects including peripheral neuropathy in up to 50% of patients, teratogenicity, and thromboembolism. Hematological abnormalities such as neutropenia and thrombocytopenia are also common adverse effects. However, these are usually not seen at the doses used for SB bleeds.
- *Bevacizumab:* Bevacizumab (Avastin®) is a humanized monoclonal antibody against VEGF which has been used in refractory AE bleeds at a dose of 5 mg/kg every 2 weeks initially, with maintenance treatment of 5 mg/kg per month. A recent study from Mayo Clinic of 21 patients with at least 6 months of follow-up showed that 52.4% patients remained transfusion-free at 6 months and overall 90 and 86% achieved a positive treatment response (≥50% reduction in RBC transfusion needs) at 6 and 12 months of follow-up, respectively. There was a tenfold reduction in RBC transfusion requirements 1 year post-treatment with over half patients remaining transfusion-free at 6 months. Adverse effects include worsening hypertension, bleeding episodes like epistaxis, and a rate of bowel perforation of up to 5.4% has been reported, mostly in patients with underlying malignancy.
- *Hormonal therapy:* Combination of estrogen and progesterone has been used to treat refractory AEs in several case reports and two randomized trials. Several proposed mechanisms of hormonal therapy in reducing bleeding include an increase in the number of circulating activated platelets, an increase in vascular sensitivity to catecholamines promoting vasoconstriction and promoting the repair of the endothelium. In two randomized double-blind trials, patients with hereditary hemorrhagic telangiectasia (HHT) and AEs who received hormonal therapy or placebo experienced no significant improvement in Hb or bleeding episodes. Meta-analysis

by Swanson et al. also showed no benefit of combination therapy of estrogen and progesterone.

- *Tranexamic acid:* It is an antifibrinolytic agent that can bind reversibly to plasminogen, blocking the binding of plasminogen to fibrin and its activation and transformation to plasmin thus resulting in the stabilization of clots. It is seven to ten times more potent than aminocaproic acid and has a half-life of 80 hours as compared to 4 hours of aminocaproic acid. Doses of up to 4.5 g/day have been used successfully to treat patients with HHT as well as upper GI bleeding and colonic AE bleed. In two case reports, tranexamic acid was used to treat SB bleeding and was proposed as a new potential pharmacological treatment in patients with chronic blood transfusion-dependent AE bleeding who are resistant to currently available therapies. More studies are required before considering routine use of tranexamic acid for this indication.
- *Other drugs:* Drugs such as danazol, desmopressin, and tamoxifen have also been tried in patients with SB AE-related

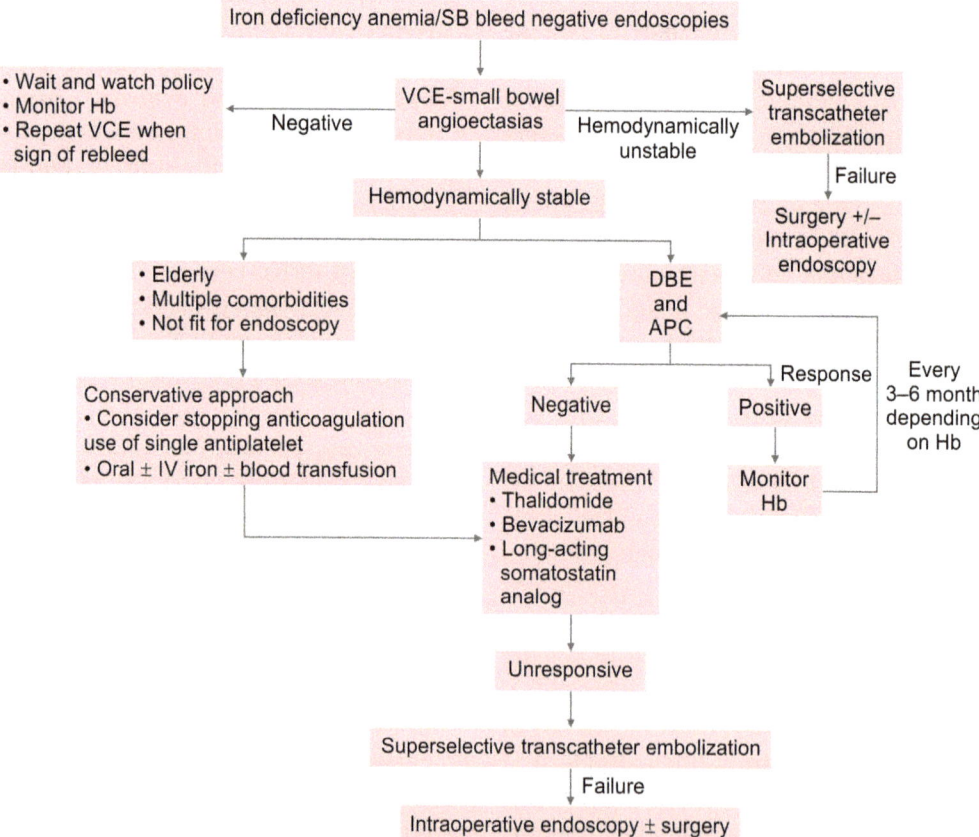

Flowchart 1: Algorithm for evaluation of obscure gastrointestinal (GI) bleed.

(APC: argon plasma coagulation; DBE: double-balloon enteroscope; Hb: hemoglobin; IV: intravenous; SB: small bowel; VCE: video capsule endoscopy)

bleeds. Though there are few case reports, none of these have significant evidence to support their use.

Question 6: What is the algorithm for management of obscure GI bleed?

Answer: Capsule endoscopy is considered the gold standard for diagnosis of SB AEs. Although DBE and APC remain a mainstay in treatment, the presence of multiple AEs, associated comorbidities, and a high rebleeding rate highlights the need to consider other additional modalities of treatment. Patients who respond well to treatment with APC can be monitored regularly with serial Hb measurements, and if clinically indicated, repeat DBE and APC may be performed as guided by repeat CE showing persisting or recurrent SBA. Pharmacological therapy may be considered as salvage therapy for patients who fail to respond to APC as monotherapy or earlier in the management of patients in whom the risks of DBE are high, particularly in elderly and those with multiple comorbidities. **Flowchart 1** shows the approach to management of SB bleed from AEs.

■ CONCLUSION

Obscure GI bleeding, with its origin from SB, is rare cause of gastrointestinal bleeding, with vascular lesions being the most common implicated cause. CE and deep enteroscopy (with spiral enteroscopy) has made it easy to diagnose the causes of SB bleed, with CT is more useful in detecting mural and extraintestinal lesions. Most vascular lesions are now managed endoscopically with APC or clipping, and pharmacological treatment with antiangiogenic drugs and somatostatin analogs reserved for recurrent, refractory, inaccessible angiodysplasias, and in patients at high risk for other interventions. The role of surgery is declining, however, it is last resort in failed endoscopic treatments and recurrent bleeding.

Gastric Variceal Bleed

Rajesh Upadhyay, Sagar Tyagi, VS Gaurav Narayan

CASE PRESENTATION

A 56-year-old male with nonalcoholic steatohepatitis (NASH)-related chronic liver disease (CLD) presented to the outpatient department (OPD) in view of persistently dark, tarry stools. He had undergone two cycles of cyanoacrylate glue injection in the past (1 year and 6 months before presentation) for hematemesis due to gastric fundal variceal bleed. He was compliant with all his medications, including nonselective beta-blockers. On examination, he was tachycardic [heart rate (HR)—120 beats/min] and hypotensive [blood pressure (BP)—100/70 mm Hg] but was conscious and well oriented. The rest of the systemic examination was normal. Initial laboratory analysis revealed anemia—hemoglobin 6.2 g%, total leukocyte count (TLC)—10,200 cells/cumm, platelets—154,000 cells/cumm, creatinine—0.93 mg/dL, urea—43.5 mg/dL, prothrombin time—16.7 seconds [international normalized ratio (INR)—1.45], bilirubin—1.42 mg/dL, and albumin—3.1 g/dL. The patient was transfused with two units of packed red cells, after which his blood pressure improved, and heart rate normalized. On repeating his upper GI endoscopy, he was found to have large, engorged gastroesophageal varices type II (GOV-II) with red color signs, without esophageal varices. Glue casts were seen at the sites of previous injection. However, no active bleeding was noted. In view of the persistent formation of gastric varices despite repeated glue therapy and adequate medical treatment, the option of BRTO (balloon-occluded retrograde transvenous obliteration) of varices was considered.

To get a roadmap of the portosystemic collaterals, a multiphase computed tomography (CT) (MPCT) abdomen was done, which revealed an enlarged and tortuous splenic vein with dilated splenorenal and gastrorenal collaterals, confirming a gastrorenal shunt. The patient subsequently underwent PARTO (plug-assisted retrograde transvenous obliteration) of gastric varices, performed by the interventional radiologist. A postprocedural CT abdominal angiography confirmed stasis in the gastrorenal shunt. The patient did not have any bleeding episodes on follow-up, and his hemoglobin was steady (10 g%) at 2 months post the procedure.

INTRODUCTION

Gastric variceal bleed is an important cause of hospital admission and mortality in patients with liver cirrhosis and other causes of portal hypertension. The prevalence of gastric varices ranges from 17% to 25% in patients with clinically significant

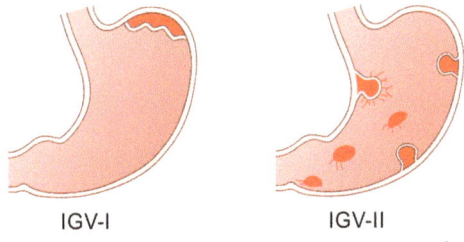

Fig. 1: Sarin's classification of gastric varices.[3]

APPROACH AND MANAGEMENT

There are multiple available modalities for the treatment of gastric varices,[4] which include:
- *Endoscopic:* Direct endoscopic intervention (DEI) and endoscopic ultrasound (EUS)-guided glue injection/coiling
- *Interventional radiology (IR):* BRTO, PARTO, CARTO (coil-assisted retrograde transvenous obliteration), TIPS (transjugular intrahepatic portosystemic shunt), partial splenic embolization
- *Surgical:* Partial/total splenectomy, diversion procedures

There are multiple factors to be considered while choosing the modality of treatment; the presence of liver cirrhosis, the MELD (Model for End-stage Liver Disease) score, the flow within the gastrorenal shunt, economic factors, and the expertise in the chosen modality at the treating center. Most centers advocate DEI as the initial mode of treatment. Injection of sclerosants into the varices was the traditional approach to various types of gastric varices. However, with the advent of n-Butyl cyanoacrylate glue, it has been the preferred agent, due to greater efficacy and lesser adverse events. Glue injection carries the risk of embolism, especially in patients with cardiac shunts. Additionally, multiple injections are required to obliterate the visible gastric varices. A major disadvantage of glue injection is only visible varices can be obliterated, highlighting the importance of the "iceberg effect" in gastric varices. There are multiple collaterals that cannot be visualized and obliterated on routine endoscopy.[5]

Endoscopic ultrasound-guided glue injection is advantageous in this context, as visualization and injection into feeder vessels is possible. Additionally, this procedure can be coupled with placement of vascular coils,

portal hypertension (as compared to 85% prevalence of esophageal varices). Bleeding form gastric varices are dependent upon their size, wall thickness, and the presence of red color sign. Additionally, gastric varices can bleed even at low portal pressures.[1] Treatment of gastric varices is indicated when the patient has an active bleed, has a history of bleed or has incidentally found high-risk gastric varices on endoscopy. There are multiple classification systems for gastric varices. The most widely used, Sarin's classification **(Fig. 1)** is based on the anatomic location of the varices, and classifies them into GOV-I and II, and isolated gastric varices (IGV) I and II.[2] However, a major drawback of this classification is that it fails to address the underlying nature of the portosystemic shunt. Kiyosue and Saad–Caldwell classification systems **(Fig. 2)** classify gastric varices based on the presence of inflow and outflow channels, which provide a better anatomical landmark for interventional therapy.

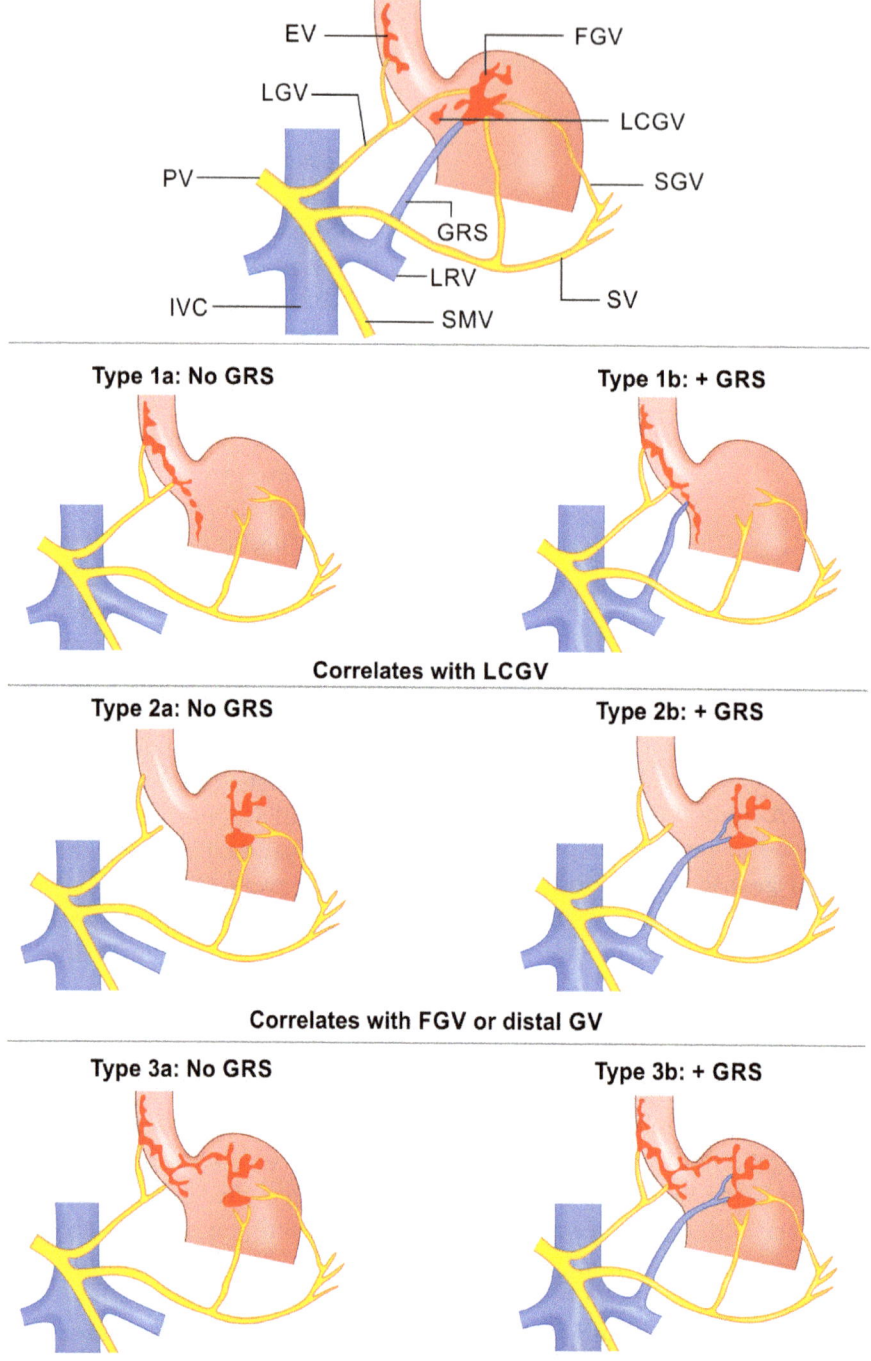

Fig. 2: Saad–Caldwell classification of gastric varices.[1] (EV: esophageal varices; FGV: fundal gastric varices; GRS: gastrorenal shunt; LCGV: lesser curve gastric varices; LGV: left gastric vein; LRV: left renal vein; IVC: inferior vena cava; PV: portal vein; SGV: short gastric vein; SMV: superior mesenteric vein; SV: splenic vein)

which also act as a scaffold for glue, thus reducing the risk of embolization, and enhancing the efficacy of the same. EUS is also a one-stop solution for measuring portosystemic pressure gradient (PPG), performing a liver elastography, and a liver biopsy if required.[6] Both DEI and EUS-guided procedures do not alter the underlying portal pressure, or have an impact on hepatic function. There is also a significant risk of rebleed in high-risk patients.

TIPS placement is often used as a salvage therapy in refractory esophageal and gastric variceal bleed. It carries the advantage of effectively reducing the portal pressure, and greatly reducing rebleeding rates. It has the additional advantage of resolving refractory ascites. The largest drawback is the increased incidence of hepatic encephalopathy post TIPS. Additionally, due to shunting of portal flow to the systemic circulation, there is often a deterioration of hepatocellular function. Thus, placement of TIPS should be limited to patients with a MELD score of <10, as TIPS in patients with MELD 18 and 25 carry a 35% and 66% 3 months' risk of mortality, respectively.[7] Needless to say, TIPS is not appropriate as a stand-alone procedure in patient with prehepatic type of portal hypertension (splenic or portal vein thrombosis), unless it is coupled with vascular recanalization. Contraindications, and adverse hepatic events with TIPS have led to the advent of other minimally invasive interventional radiological procedures, like BRTO.

BRTO is a minimally invasive technique devised by Kanagawa for the treatment of gastric varices. Olson et al. published the first study on attempted balloon-occluded sclerotherapy of the gastrorenal shunt, in 1984. BRTO has demonstrated considerable efficacy in controlling gastric variceal bleeding with surprisingly low rebleed rates.

It can be performed on patients with poor hepatic reserve and encephalopathy, which may even improve post BRTO.[8] However, it requires exhaustive postprocedural monitoring and can have complications related to balloon rupture and adverse effects of sclerosing agents.

Hence, modified BRTO techniques have been developed like vascular PARTO, CARTO, or antegrade techniques like balloon occluded antegrade transvenous obliteration.

A vascular plug has few important benefits as compared to balloon occlusion. The Amplatzer vascular plug on its own provides some embolic effect. Balloon rupture during BRTO can also result in symptomatic pulmonary embolism, recurrent variceal bleeding, and treatment failure which are avoided by the same. CARTO and PARTO are similar procedures. The major difference between the two is that PARTO uses a plug to occlude the shunt outflow vessel, instead of a coil pack which is used in CARTO. Studies have revealed BRTO and allied procedures to be an effective method to treat gastric varices, with a technical success ranging from 84% to 100%.[9]

A study by Lee et al. on CARTO for the Treatment of Portal Hypertensive Variceal Bleeding revealed that CARTO is a technically feasible and safe alternative to traditional BRTO.[10] However, BRTO and related procedures should be reserved for patients with a high flow gastrorenal shunt. Its technical feasibility is limited in patients who do not have a significant gastrorenal shunt. Hence, a preprocedural MPCT is mandatory to assess the nature and size of shunts and collaterals.

Partial splenic embolization aims to reduce the splenic size, thus reducing portal venous inflow, and reducing portal pressure. It is efficacious even in patients with sinistral portal hypertension. However, there is limited literature on its use in patients with cirrhosis and decompensated chronic liver disease. Splenic embolization can be coupled with vascular embolization and/or DEI and may have a synergistic effect on reducing portal pressure. However, further studies are required to assess the same.[11]

Partial or total splenectomy acts similarly by reducing splenic size and reducing portal inflow. However, surgery is invasive, and carries a risk of adverse events and longer hospital stay. IR-guided splenic embolization has greatly reduced the need of splenectomy. Surgical diversion procedures are efficient in reducing portal pressure and reducing the risk of variceal rebleed. However, similar to TIPS, it can cause an increased risk in mortality, encephalopathy, and hepatic function deterioration on patients with advanced liver disease.[12]

CONCLUSION

Direct endoscopic intervention has been the traditional approach to managing gastric varices. However, it neither mitigates the underlying portal hypertension, nor obliterates the feeder vessels. EUS-guided and vascular coil placement has several advantages in this regard. TIPS is a frequently used salvage therapy, but is limited by the high mortality in patients with advanced chronic liver disease. BRTO and related procedures are relatively newer interventional procedures that have demonstrated high efficacy and safety, and can often be advocated as a standalone initial therapy in patients with GOV-II and IGV-I, with a high-flow gastrorenal shunt. They carry the additional advantage of potentially improving hepatic function and lowering the risk of hepatic encephalopathy. Splenic embolization is another efficient adjuvant procedure and can be used as a standalone procedure in sinistral and prehepatic portal hypertension. Surgical procedures, although effective in reducing portal pressure and mitigating bleeds, are limited by their high incidence of adverse events and increased hospital stay. The choice of therapy should be decided based on the location of the gastric varices, the underlying etiology of portal hypertension, the nature of the portosystemic shunt, and the experience of the treating physician.

REFERENCES

1. Maydeo A, Patil G. How to approach a patient with gastric varices. Gastroenterology. 2022;162(3):689-95.
2. Bhat R, Wani Z, Bhadoria A, Maiwall R, Choudhury A. Gastric varices: classification, endoscopic and ultrasonographic management. J Res Med Sci. 2015;20(12):1200.
3. Luo X, Hernández-Gea V. Update on the management of gastric varices. Liver Int. 2022;42:1250-8.
4. Goral V, Yılmaz N. Current approaches to the treatment of gastric varices: glue, coil application, TIPS, and BRTO. Medicina (Kaunas). 2019;55(7):335.
5. Guo YW, Miao HB, Wen ZF, Xuan JY, Zhou HX. Procedure-related complications in gastric variceal obturation with tissue glue. World J Gastroenterol. 2017;23(43):7746-55.
6. Thiruvengadam SS, Alireza Sedarat. The role of endoscopic ultrasound (EUS) in the management of gastric varices. Curr Gastroenterol Rep. 2021;23(1):1.
7. Parvinian A, Gaba RC. Outcomes of TIPS for Treatment of Gastroesophageal Variceal Hemorrhage. Semin Intervent Radiol. 2014;31(03):252-7.
8. Saad W. Balloon-occluded retrograde transvenous obliteration of gastric varices: concept, basic techniques, and outcomes. Semin Intervent Radiol. 2012;29(02):118-28.
9. Kim DJ, Darcy MD, Mani NB, Park AW, Akinwande O, Ramaswamy RS, et al. Modified

Balloon-Occluded Retrograde Transvenous Obliteration (BRTO) Techniques for the Treatment of Gastric Varices: Vascular Plug-Assisted Retrograde Transvenous Obliteration (PARTO)/Coil-Assisted Retrograde Transvenous Obliteration (CARTO)/Balloon-Occluded Antegrade Transvenous Obliteration (BATO). Cardiovasc Intervent Radiol. 2018;41(6):835-47.
10. Lee EW, Saab S, Gomes AS, Busuttil R, McWilliams J, Durazo F, et al. Coil-Assisted Retrograde Transvenous Obliteration (CARTO) for the Treatment of Portal Hypertensive Variceal Bleeding: Preliminary Results. Clin Transl Gastroenterol. 2014;5(10):e61.
11. Henry Z, Patel K, Patton H, Saad W. AGA Clinical Practice Update on Management of Bleeding Gastric Varices: Expert Review. Clin Gastroenterol Hepatol. 2021;19(6):1098-107.e1.
12. Henderson JM, Anderson CD. The surgical treatment of portal hypertension. Clin Liv Dis (Hoboken). 2020;15(Suppl 1):S52-S63.

Section 4

Diseases of the Liver

12. **Nonalcoholic Fatty Liver Disease**
    Ashish Kumar

13. **Alcoholic Hepatitis**
    Rajesh Upadhyay, VS Gaurav Narayan, Priyanka Ojha

14. **IgM Anti-HEV Positivity in a Patient with Suspected Severe Alcoholic Hepatitis: Cause or a Red Herring?**
    Harshil Trivedi, Kaushal Madan

15. **Acute on Chronic Liver Failure**
    Akash Roy, Mahesh Kumar Goenka

16. **Intrahepatic Cholestasis**
    Rajesh Upadhyay, VS Gaurav Narayan

17. **Herb-induced Liver Injury**
    Bhabadev Goswami, Preeti Sarma

18. **Autoimmune Hepatitis**
    Reethesh SR, Manav Wadhawan

19. **Recompensation and Reversal of Cirrhosis: Myth or Reality?**
    Naveen Bhagat, Arka De, Ajay Duseja

20. **Sickle Hepatopathy**
    AC Anand, Shivam Kalia, Dibyalochan Praharaj, Preetam Nath, Sarat Chandra Panigrahi, Bipadabhanjan Mallick, Saroj Kant Sahu

Nonalcoholic Fatty Liver Disease

Ashish Kumar

CASE PRESENTATION

Mr S, a 55-year-old obese male presents to the outpatient department (OPD) with complaints of fatigue, right upper abdominal discomfort, and unintentional weight loss over the past few months. His medical history is significant for type 2 diabetes mellitus (10 years), hypertension (6 years), and dyslipidemia (3 years). He has a sedentary lifestyle, nonsmoker, and denies alcohol consumption. At the time of presentation, he was on the following medications: metformin 1,000 mg twice daily, sitagliptin 100 mg once daily, insulin glargine 20 units once daily (subcutaneous injection), telmisartan 40 mg once daily, and amlodipine 5 mg once daily. The physical examination revealed hepatomegaly and tenderness in the right upper quadrant of the abdomen. He weighed 105 kg and had a body mass index (BMI) of 39 kg/m².

Laboratory tests **(Table 1)** reveal elevated liver enzymes, including alanine aminotransferase (ALT) and aspartate aminotransferase (AST), suggesting liver inflammation and injury. Additional blood tests show abnormal lipid profiles, including elevated triglycerides and low-density lipoprotein cholesterol (LDL-C). Tests for viral hepatitis (such as hepatitis B and C) were negative, ruling out viral causes of liver disease. The ultrasound **(Fig. 1)** revealed the presence of grade III fatty liver. However, to confirm the diagnosis of nonalcoholic steatohepatitis (NASH) and assess the severity of liver damage, a liver biopsy was recommended, which he refused.

TABLE 1: Laboratory investigations of the patients.

Investigation	Result
Alanine aminotransferase (ALT)	75 U/L
Aspartate aminotransferase (AST)	60 U/L
Alkaline phosphatase	90 U/L
Total bilirubin	1.2 mg/dL
Gamma-glutamyl transferase (GGT)	40 U/L
Total cholesterol	250 mg/dL
LDL cholesterol	160 mg/dL
HDL cholesterol	35 mg/dL
Triglycerides	200 mg/dL
Fasting blood glucose	130 mg/dL
Hemoglobin A1c (HbA1c)	7.5%
Viral hepatitis serology (hepatitis B and C)	Negative
Abdominal ultrasound	Grade III fatty liver
FibroScan®	
• Liver stiffness measurement (LSM)	10.3 kPa
• Controlled attenuation parameter (CAP)	333 dB/m

(LDL: low-density lipoprotein; HDL: high-density lipoprotein)

The FibroScan® revealed a liver stiffness measurement (LSM) value of 10.3 kPa and a controlled attenuation parameter (CAP) value of 333 dB/m **(Fig. 2)**. Based on the diagnostic findings, the patient was diagnosed with NASH (although in the absence of a biopsy).

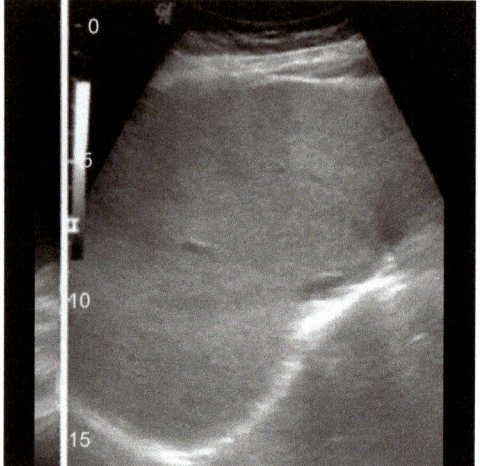

Fig. 1: Ultrasound of abdomen showing brighter (more "echogenic") liver suggesting fatty liver.

The primary goals of treatment are to manage his metabolic risk factors, reduce liver inflammation, and prevent disease progression. The treatment plan involves a multidisciplinary approach, including lifestyle modifications and pharmacotherapy. The patient was advised weight loss, and a gradual weight loss approach is recommended to achieve a healthy body weight and reduce hepatic fat accumulation. A combination of caloric restriction and regular physical activity tailored to his capabilities was advised. He was also encouraged to follow a balanced, low-fat, and low-sugar diet. Increased consumption of fruits, vegetables, whole grains, and lean protein sources was emphasized. He was advised to limit processed foods, sugary beverages, and saturated fats. He was also advised increased physical activity. Regular aerobic exercise, such as brisk walking or swimming, is recommended for at least 150 min/week to improve insulin sensitivity and promote weight loss.

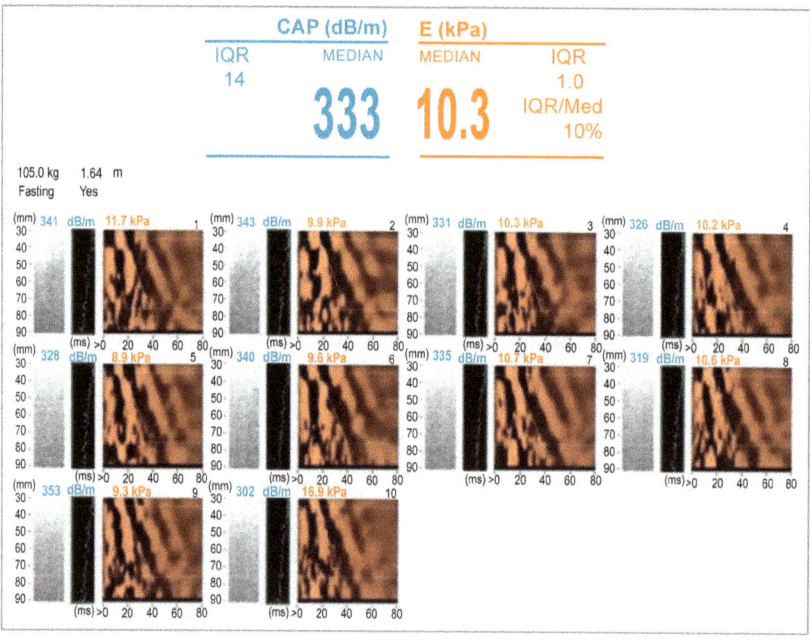

Fig. 2: FibroScan® report of the patient. (IQR: interquartile range)

Given the patient's underlying conditions and the presence of NASH with fibrosis, pharmacotherapy was considered to target specific aspects of the disease. He was prescribed saroglitazar 4 mg to address NASH and a statin to manage dyslipidemia and reduce the risk of cardiovascular events. Semaglutide was added to his current antidiabetic medications to improve his diabetic control and aid in weight management. The initial dose of Semaglutide was 3 mg/day, with the intention to increase it to 7 mg after 4 weeks, and then to 14 mg after an additional 4 weeks. His existing antihypertensive medication was continued.

The patient was closely monitored with regular follow-up visits to assess his response to treatment and disease progression. Periodic laboratory tests, including liver function tests and imaging studies, were conducted to evaluate his liver health. Lifestyle modifications were reinforced, and adjustments to medications were made as needed.

The prognosis for NASH varies depending on the severity of liver fibrosis and the patient's ability to make sustainable lifestyle changes. With early intervention, adherence to treatment plans, and diligent management of metabolic risk factors, Mr S has the potential to slow or even reverse the progression of liver disease, improving his overall health and quality of life. Regular monitoring and ongoing support from a multidisciplinary healthcare team will be crucial in his long-term management.

DISCUSSION

Nonalcoholic fatty liver (NAFL) disease (NAFLD) is a condition characterized by the accumulation of excess fat in the liver of individuals who consume little to no alcohol. Obesity, type 2 diabetes, and metabolic disorders contribute significantly to its development. NAFLD affects not only the liver but also other body systems, with cardiovascular disease (CVD) being the leading cause of death in NAFLD patients. The prevalence of NAFLD is increasing globally and is now the leading cause of chronic liver disease in many countries. In India, NAFLD is a significant cause of unexplained liver enzyme elevation, cryptogenic cirrhosis, and non-hepatitis B virus (HBV), non-hepatitis C virus (HCV) hepatocellular carcinoma (HCC). NAFLD is also becoming an important indication for liver transplantation. NAFLD is associated with an increased risk of HCC, even in the absence of cirrhosis or advanced fibrosis. Most patients with NAFLD are asymptomatic or have nonspecific symptoms. Lifestyle interventions are currently the main approach for NAFLD treatment, but their effectiveness is limited. This article provides an overview of diagnostic methods and investigational therapeutic drugs for NAFLD, focusing on targeted pathways. It also discusses the current status of drug development and combination therapy for NAFLD.

NONALCHOHOLIC FATTY LIVER DISEASE SPECTRUM

The spectrum of NAFLD includes various conditions **(Figs. 3A to F)** given as follows:
- *NAFL:* This is the initial stage of NAFLD, characterized by the accumulation of fat in the liver without inflammation or significant liver damage.
- *NASH:* NASH is a more advanced form of NAFLD, where along with fat accumulation, there is inflammation and liver cell damage. It can progress to more severe liver diseases such as fibrosis, cirrhosis, and HCC.
- *NASH–fibrosis:* In this stage, fibrosis, which is the scarring of liver tissue, starts to develop. The degree of fibrosis can

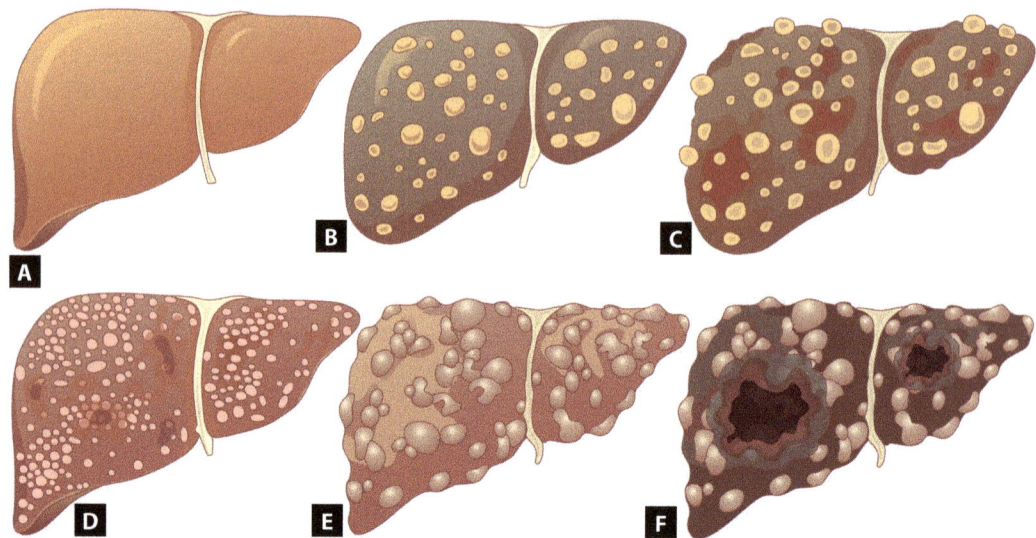

Figs. 3A to F: Spectrum of nonalcoholic fatty liver disease (NAFLD). (A) Normal liver; (B) NAFL; (C) Nonalcoholic steatohepatitis (NASH); (D) Nonalcoholic steatohepatitis with liver fibrosis (NASH–fibrosis); (E) Nonalcoholic steatohepatitis with liver cirrhosis (NASH–cirrhosis); (F) Nonalcoholic steatohepatitis with hepatocellular carcinoma (NASH–HCC).
Courtesy: BioRender.com.

range from mild to severe, indicating the progression of liver damage.
- *NASH-cirrhosis:* Cirrhosis is the advanced stage of liver disease characterized by extensive scarring and irreversible damage to liver tissue. NASH-cirrhosis occurs when NASH progresses to this severe stage.
- *NASH–HCC:* HCC is a type of liver cancer. NASH–HCC refers to the development of liver cancer in individuals with NASH, either with or without cirrhosis.

The progression from NAFL to NASH is not linear, and fibrosis progression can be faster in patients with NASH. Fibrosis is a key determinant of outcomes, and while most patients have slow fibrosis progression, some may experience rapid progression.

Pathogenesis

The development of NAFLD is a complex process influenced by multiple factors and genetic predisposition. It is characterized by a series of metabolic stress and inflammatory events, accompanied by reparative responses aimed at reducing inflammation. Recent advancements in our understanding of NAFLD have shed light on the genetic determinants, such as *PNPLA3*, *TM6SF2*, *HSD17b*, and *MOAT7*, that contribute to its development. Additionally, the identification and validation of biomarkers have provided valuable tools for assessing disease severity and prognosis. Despite these advancements, there are still significant gaps in our knowledge regarding individual susceptibility and the variability in disease progression.

Diagnosis

The diagnostic criteria for NAFLD involve the presence of fat in >5% of liver cells, without excessive alcohol consumption or other chronic liver diseases. Ultrasound of abdomen is the most basic test for demonstrating liver fat. However, ultrasound has limited sensitivity for mild cases and cannot detect steatohepatitis or fibrosis. Various other diagnostic methods include computed tomography (CT), magnetic resonance imaging (MRI), liver biopsy, and laboratory testing. CT has similar sensitivity but is limited by cost and radiation exposure. MRI is the most sensitive method for detecting fat in liver cells, but its accuracy may be affected by fibrosis.

In cases where noninvasive imaging is inconclusive, liver biopsy can provide an accurate diagnosis of NAFLD and its subtype. The specific diagnosis of NASH and NASH-fibrosis requires histological documentation of inflammation and fibrosis, respectively, by liver biopsy. However, liver biopsy acceptance in clinical practice is low, and various noninvasive tests have been developed to replace liver biopsy (see below). Noninvasive methods can also diagnose the advanced stages of NAFLD, viz., NASH–cirrhosis and NASH–HCC but require the exclusion of other etiologies.

Nonalcoholic fatty liver disease is frequently associated with extrahepatic diseases, including chronic kidney disease (CKD) and CVD. Screening for CKD and CVD in NAFLD patients is suggested, but there is no consensus on the screening modalities. NAFLD is also associated with other conditions, such as osteopenia, osteoporosis, sleep apnea, hypothyroidism, polycystic ovarian syndrome, and an increased risk of various malignancies. NAFLD can coexist with other liver diseases, such as chronic hepatitis B (CHB), chronic hepatitis C (CHC), and alcohol-associated liver disease (ALD), and worsen their outcomes. Dual etiology fatty liver disease or steatohepatitis (DAFLD/DASH) comprising alcohol and metabolic risk factors is not uncommon and aggravates liver disease severity. In addition to treating the underlying liver disease, attention should be given to controlling metabolic risk factors in these patients.

NONINVASIVE EVALUATION OF NAFLD

Noninvasive Detection of Hepatic Steatosis

Ultrasound is a simple method for detecting hepatic steatosis by evaluating the brightness or echogenicity of the liver caused by fat deposits. CAP using FibroScan® is another noninvasive technique that measures the absorption of ultrasound waves by the liver to quantify fat content. CAP provides a reliable and quantitative assessment of liver steatosis, however, CAP alone cannot determine liver inflammation or fibrosis, and additional tests may be necessary. CT can also be used, with the liver attenuation index (LAI) being a common method. LAI compares the density of the liver to the spleen on CT scans, providing a quantitative measurement of liver steatosis. However, routine use of CT scans for steatosis assessment is limited due to radiation risk and cost considerations in clinical practice. Magnetic resonance–proton density fat fraction (MR-PDFF) is accurate in detecting steatosis but less commonly recommended due to cost and availability.

Noninvasive Detection of Hepatic Fibrosis

Evaluating liver fibrosis in advanced NAFLD is crucial. Noninvasive methods such as the NAFLD Fibrosis Score (NFS), Fibrosis-4 (FIB-4) score, and Enhanced Liver Fibrosis (ELF) test have been developed to assess fibrosis without the need for a liver biopsy. These methods consider various factors such as age, BMI, hyperglycemia, platelet count, albumin, and AST/ALT ratio to predict advanced fibrosis. Among these, NFS, FIB-4, and ELF have shown better performance compared to other indices. Blood-based tests like platelet count and AST/ALT ratio as well as elastography techniques like FibroScan® and magnetic resonance elastography (MRE) are accurate tools for assessing fibrosis, although they may have limitations in terms of availability and cost.

Noninvasive Detection of Hepatic Inflammation

Noninvasive tests have very limited effectiveness in evaluating hepatic inflammation. Inflammation is a complex aspect to assess, and there is a recognized need for improved noninvasive markers for this purpose. Although serum liver enzymes such as AST and ALT are commonly used, they are not entirely reliable in diagnosing NASH due to their limited correlation with hepatic inflammation. Promising alternative markers like CK-18 and FibroScan-AST (FAST) score have shown potential, but further validation studies are necessary to establish their effectiveness in accurately detecting and evaluating hepatic inflammation in NASH patients.

OVERVIEW OF THE MANAGEMENT OF NAFLD

Management of NAFLD involves a comprehensive approach that includes lifestyle modifications, addressing underlying metabolic risk factors, regular monitoring, and, in some cases, medication or interventions. The primary focus is on promoting weight loss through a combination of healthy diet, increased physical activity, and behavioral changes. Managing obesity, diabetes, and dyslipidemia is essential. Regular follow-up visits, noninvasive assessments of liver fibrosis, and screening for complications like NASH–cirrhosis and NASH–HCC are crucial for monitoring disease progression. Medications such as vitamin E, saroglitazar, pioglitazone, and bariatric surgery may be considered in specific cases. Patient education and support play a vital role in ensuring adherence to treatment and sustaining lifestyle changes. Individualized management plans, collaboration with a multidisciplinary team, and patient-centered care are essential for optimal management outcomes in NAFLD.

LIFESTYLE MODIFICATIONS

Lifestyle modifications form the cornerstone of treatment for NAFLD. These modifications aim to address the underlying risk factors associated with the disease and promote overall liver health. The main components of lifestyle modifications for NAFLD include weight reduction, dietary changes, increased physical activity, and behavior modification. It is important to note that lifestyle modifications for NAFLD should be individualized based on the patient's specific needs, preferences, and medical conditions. Regular monitoring and follow-up with healthcare professionals are crucial to track progress, provide support, and make necessary adjustments to the treatment plan.

Weight Reduction

Achieving and maintaining a healthy weight is a key goal in NAFLD treatment. Weight loss of about 7–10% of total body weight has shown significant improvements in liver health. This can be achieved through a combination of dietary modifications and increased physical activity. However, weight loss should be gradual and sustainable to avoid potential adverse effects.

Dietary Modifications

A healthy diet is crucial in managing NAFLD. The emphasis is on consuming a well-balanced diet that is low in saturated fats, refined carbohydrates, and added sugars. Instead, the focus is on incorporating whole grains, fruits, vegetables, lean proteins, and healthy fats, such as those found in nuts and avocados. Portion control and avoiding excessive calorie intake are important. It is also recommended to limit the consumption of sugary beverages and alcohol **(Box 1)**.

Increased Physical Activity

Regular physical activity is beneficial for NAFLD management. Engaging in aerobic exercises, such as brisk walking, jogging, cycling, or swimming, for at least 150 min/week is recommended. Strength training exercises that target major muscle groups should also be included. Physical activity helps in weight management, improves insulin sensitivity, and reduces liver fat accumulation.

Behavior Modification

Changing unhealthy behaviors and adopting healthy habits is essential in the long-term management of NAFLD. This includes addressing factors such as emotional eating, stress management, improving sleep patterns, and reducing sedentary behavior. Working with a registered dietitian, behavioral therapist, or counselor can provide valuable support and guidance in making sustainable behavior changes.

■ PHARMACOTHERAPY OF NAFLD

There is currently no Food and Drug Administration (FDA)-approved treatment for NASH, but with advancements in understanding its pathogenesis, novel targets and strategies have emerged and are being investigated in clinical trials **(Table 2)**. The drugs which are currently available in India are being discussed below.

Vitamin E

Vitamin E has been investigated for its potential role in the treatment of NAFLD. Administered at a dose of 800 IU/day, divided into two doses in the PIVENS trial, vitamin E has shown clinical benefits including a decrease in ALT levels, reduction in hepatic steatosis, lobular inflammation, ballooning, and NAFLD activity score (NAS). However, its effect on fibrosis remains debatable. As an antioxidant, vitamin E helps reduce oxidative stress and inflammation in the liver, key contributors to NAFLD progression. Clinical trials have demonstrated improvements in liver enzyme levels and decreased

> **BOX 1:** Dietary advice for patients with non-alcoholic steatohepatitis (NASH).
>
> - Calorie intake should be reduced by 500–1,000 kcal for overweight or obese patients with nonalcoholic fatty liver disease (NAFLD)
> - Energy intake should be balanced with energy expenditure for lean individuals
> - Calorie restriction is more important than the specific type of diet
> - Total fat intake should not exceed 30% of total energy intake
> - Saturated fats intake should be <10% of total energy intake
> - Transfats intake should be <1% of total energy intake
> - Shift from saturated fats and transfats to unsaturated fats
> - Limit-free sugars intake to <10% of total energy intake
> - Consider reducing free sugars intake to <5% of total energy intake for additional health benefits
> - Curtail fructose and sweetened beverage consumption
> - Moderate consumption of caffeinated coffee (>2 cups per day) may be beneficial for NAFLD

TABLE 2: Currently available and future drugs for nonalcoholic steatohepatitis (NASH).

Class of drugs	Name of drugs	Current status
Antioxidants	Vitamin E	Available in India
Peroxisome proliferator-activated receptor agonists	• Saroglitazar (α/γ) • Fenofibrate (α) • Pioglitazone (γ) • Pemafibrate (α) • Lanifibranor (α/δ/γ) • Elafibranor (α/δ) • Rosiglitazone (γ)	• Available in India; approved by Drug Controller General of India (DCGI) for use in NASH • Available in India for dyslipidemia • Available in India for type 2 diabetes mellitus • Undergoing trials • Undergoing trials • Failed phase 3 trial • Discontinued in India
Farnesoid X receptor (FXR) agonists	Obeticholic acid (OCA)	Available in India for primary biliary cholangitis
Sodium–glucose cotransporter 2 inhibitors	• Empagliflozin • Dapagliflozin	• Available in India for type 2 diabetes mellitus • Available in India for type 2 diabetes mellitus
Glucagon-like peptide 1 (GLP-1) agonists	• Semaglutide • Tirzepatide	• Available in India for type 2 diabetes mellitus • Completed phase 2 trial • Undergoing trials
Thyroid hormone receptor beta (THR-β)	Resmetirom	Completed phase 3 trial
Fibroblast growth factor analogs	• Aldafermin • Efruxifermin • Pegbelfermin	• Completed phase 2 trial • Completed phase 2 trial • Undergoing trials
Acetyl-CoA carboxylase inhibitors	Firsocostat	Undergoing trials
Chemokine receptor (CCR) antagonist	Cenicriviroc	Failed phase 2 trial

hepatic fat accumulation with vitamin E supplementation. It holds potential in improving liver histology by reducing hepatocellular ballooning and inflammation. However, long-term safety and optimal dosing regimens require further investigation. Vitamin E is widely available, of low cost, and recommended by various international societies for biopsy-proven NASH in patients without diabetes. It is important to note that vitamin E may not be suitable for everyone and should be used under medical supervision. Potential adverse effects of long-term use include an increased risk of prostate cancer and hemorrhagic stroke, with no significant increase in all-cause mortality.

Saroglitazar

Saroglitazar, a dual peroxisome proliferator-activated receptor (PPAR) agonist, has shown promise in the treatment of NAFLD. By activating PPAR-α and PPAR-γ receptors, saroglitazar improves lipid metabolism, reduces hepatic fat accumulation, and enhances insulin sensitivity. It was being primarily used in patients with diabetic dyslipidemia. However, recent clinical trials have demonstrated its efficacy in improving liver function, decreasing liver enzymes, and reducing liver fat content in NAFLD patients. It also exhibits benefits in improving dyslipidemia and reducing liver inflammation. However, further research is needed to establish its role, long-term safety, and optimal use in NAFLD management. Saroglitazar is approved by the Drug Controller General of India (DCGI) for use in NASH with F1–F3 fibrosis and NAFLD with comorbidities such as obesity, diabetes mellitus, dyslipidemia, or metabolic syndrome. Although its effect on fibrosis is debatable, the availability and cost of the drug should be considered as factors. Saroglitazar is currently available only in India, and further studies are required to assess its broader efficacy and safety profile.

Pioglitazone

Pioglitazone, a PPAR-γ agonist, has been investigated for its potential role in the treatment of NAFLD. Clinical trials, including the PIVENS study, have shown that pioglitazone at a dose of 30 mg/day can improve liver function by decreasing ALT levels and improving insulin resistance. It has also demonstrated benefits in reducing hepatic steatosis and lobular inflammation, increasing the resolution of NASH, and improving histological features of NAFLD. However, pioglitazone has no significant effect on fibrosis and may be associated with weight gain as a side effect. Careful consideration of its use is necessary due to potential adverse effects. The suggested minimum duration of treatment with pioglitazone is 2 years. Pioglitazone is recommended by various international societies for biopsy-proven NASH in patients without diabetes, but its effect on fibrosis remains debatable. Long-term use of pioglitazone may increase the risk of weight gain and certain conditions, such as bladder cancer and heart failure.

Sodium–glucose Cotransporter 2 Inhibitors

Sodium–glucose cotransporter 2 (SGLT2) inhibitors, such as canagliflozin, dapagliflozin, and empagliflozin, are a class of medications commonly used for the treatment of type 2 diabetes. Recent studies have shown their potential as therapeutic options for NAFLD. SGLT2 inhibitors work by inhibiting glucose reabsorption in the kidneys, leading to increased glucose excretion in the urine. This mechanism not only helps control blood sugar levels but also has beneficial effects on liver health. Clinical trials have demonstrated that SGLT2 inhibitors can decrease hepatic fat content, improve liver function parameters, and reduce markers of liver inflammation in patients with NAFLD and type 2 diabetes. Furthermore, these medications may offer additional benefits, including weight loss and improvements in cardiovascular outcomes. However, further research is still needed to fully understand the impact of SGLT2 inhibitors on insulin resistance and hepatic function in NAFLD. Trials are underway to assess the efficacy and safety of SGLT2 inhibitors, such as dapagliflozin, in NAFLD treatment, with promising initial results showing improvements in liver function parameters and metabolic outcomes. Empagliflozin has also shown positive effects on body composition, insulin resistance, liver fibrosis, and hepatic enzymes in NAFLD patients. Although these findings are encouraging, more research is required to validate the long-term efficacy and safety of empagliflozin as a therapeutic option for NAFLD.

Glucagon-like Peptide 1 Agonists

Glucagon-like peptide 1 (GLP-1) receptor agonists, also known as incretin mimetics, have shown promise in the treatment of NAFLD. These medications, including exenatide, liraglutide, and semaglutide, stimulate insulin secretion, decrease insulin resistance, inhibit glucagon release, and promote weight loss. In clinical trials, exenatide has been found to reduce hepatic triglyceride content, liraglutide has shown histological resolution of NASH and a decrease in fibrosis progression, and semaglutide has demonstrated significant improvement in NASH resolution and weight loss. These GLP-1 receptor agonists have beneficial effects on liver health, improving insulin sensitivity, reducing liver fat accumulation, and exhibiting anti-inflammatory properties. Gastrointestinal side effects have been reported, but discontinuation rates have been low. However, further research is needed to determine the long-term efficacy, safety profile, and optimal dosing regimens of GLP-1 receptor agonists for NAFLD treatment. Semaglutide, a more potent GLP-1 receptor agonist, has shown significant improvement in NASH resolution and weight loss. Gastrointestinal side effects were reported with these medications, but discontinuation rates were low. Further studies are needed to assess the long-term efficacy and safety of GLP-1 receptor agonists in NAFLD treatment, including their effects on liver fibrosis. Ongoing trials, such as the ESSENCE trial evaluating semaglutide, will provide more insights into the effectiveness of these medications in resolving steatohepatitis and improving fibrosis in NAFLD patients.

Obeticholic Acid

Farnesoid X receptor (FXR) agonists, particularly obeticholic acid (OCA), have shown promise in the treatment of NAFLD. OCA is a potent and selective FXR agonist that has demonstrated an insulin-sensitizing effect in patients with type 2 diabetes. Clinical studies have consistently shown that OCA at 25 mg daily can induce histological regression of fibrosis, resolution of NASH, and reduce hepatocyte ballooning and inflammation. However, OCA is associated with side effects such as pruritus and increases in LDL-C. To address these issues, second-generation FXR agonists with nonbile acid structures are being developed. These newer agonists show potential in minimizing side effects while maintaining histological efficacy. Further research is needed to evaluate the long-term efficacy, safety, and optimal dosing of FXR agonists for NAFLD treatment. Ongoing trials, including the REVERSE trial evaluating OCA in patients with compensated cirrhosis due to NASH, will provide valuable insights into the effectiveness of FXR agonists in NAFLD management. While OCA represents a promising therapeutic option, its safety and long-term effectiveness are still being evaluated, and careful monitoring is required due to potential side effects. Additional research is necessary to fully establish the role of OCA and optimize its use in the management of NAFLD.

■ CONCLUSION

Nonalcoholic fatty liver disease is a significant health concern characterized by the accumulation of fat in the liver. It is strongly associated with obesity, type 2 diabetes, and metabolic disorders, and its prevalence is increasing globally. NAFLD not only affects the liver but also poses a risk for CVD, making it a leading cause of chronic liver disease and a significant indication for liver transplantation. The pathogenesis of NAFLD is complex, involving multiple factors and genetic predisposition. Advances in understanding the genetic determinants and biomarkers have improved our knowledge of the disease and provided tools for disease stratification. However, there are still gaps in understanding individual susceptibility and disease progression.

Accurate diagnosis of NAFLD involves various methods, including noninvasive imaging techniques such as ultrasound, CT, and MRI. Liver biopsy remains the gold standard for definitive diagnosis but may not always be feasible due to patient refusal or other factors. Noninvasive tests, such as the NFS, FIB-4 score, and ELF test, can assess liver fibrosis without the need for biopsy. CAP using FibroScan is a valuable tool for quantifying liver steatosis. However, there is a need for improved noninvasive markers to assess hepatic inflammation accurately.

The management of NAFLD primarily focuses on lifestyle modifications, including weight reduction, dietary changes, increased physical activity, and behavior modification. These interventions aim to address underlying risk factors and promote overall liver health. Pharmacotherapy options are being explored, including vitamin E, saroglitazar, pioglitazone, SGLT2 inhibitors, GLP-1 agonists, and FXR agonists such as OCA. These medications have shown potential in improving liver function and reducing liver fat content in NAFLD patients, although further research is needed to establish their long-term efficacy and safety profiles.

Nonalcoholic fatty liver disease is a complex and multifaceted disease that requires a comprehensive approach to management. Continued research and advancements in diagnostic methods and therapeutic options are necessary to improve patient outcomes and address the growing burden of NAFLD worldwide.

■ SUGGESTED READING

1. Brennan PN, Dillon JF, McCrimmon R. Advances and emerging therapies in the treatment of non-alcoholic steatohepatitis. touchREV Endocrinol. 2022;18(2):148-55.
2. Cusi K, Isaacs S, Barb D, Basu R, Caprio S, Garvey WT, et al. American Association of Clinical Endocrinology Clinical Practice Guideline for the Diagnosis and Management of Nonalcoholic Fatty Liver Disease in Primary Care and Endocrinology Clinical Settings: Co-Sponsored by the American Association for the Study of Liver Diseases (AASLD). Endocr Pract. 2022;28(5):528-62.
3. Duseja A, Singh SP, De A, Madan K, Rao PN, Shukla A, et al. Indian National Association for Study of the Liver (INASL) Guidance Paper on Nomenclature, Diagnosis and Treatment of Nonalcoholic Fatty Liver Disease (NAFLD). J Clin Exp Hepatol. 2023;13(2):273-302.
4. Isaacs S. Nonalcoholic fatty liver disease. Endocrinol Metab Clin North Am. 2023;52(1): 149-64.
5. Yang Z, Wang L. Current, emerging, and potential therapies for non-alcoholic steatohepatitis. Front Pharmacol. 2023;14: 1152042.

Alcoholic Hepatitis

Rajesh Upadhyay, VS Gaurav Narayan, Priyanka Ojha

■ INTRODUCTION

A 38-year-old male presented to the emergency department with jaundice, abdominal distension, and swelling of both legs. The symptoms were sudden in onset, and progressed over a period of 2 weeks. There was no history of fever or any localizing symptoms suggestive of an infection. His urine output was fairly normal, and there was no history suggestive of altered mentation or a gastrointestinal (GI) bleed. He had no other previous comorbidities. He reported a history of chronic alcohol intake, amounting to >5 standard drinks a day for >12 years. However, his last drink was 35 days prior to admission.

On examination, he was well oriented, and his vital parameters were stable. There was scleral icterus and bilateral pitting pedal edema. His abdomen was distended but the flanks were not full, and there was no shifting dullness on percussion. Review of other systems were normal. His initial laboratory evaluation revealed a hemoglobin level of 11 g%, total leukocyte count (TLC)—12,700 cells/cumm, platelets—199 × 10^9/L, creatinine of 0.7 mg/dL, total bilirubin of 9.6 mg/dL (direct—4.11 mg/dL), aspartate aminotransferase (AST)—72 IU/L, alanine aminotransferase (ALT)—21 IU/L, alkaline phosphatase (ALP)—134 IU/L, gamma-glutamyl transpeptidase (GGT)—75 IU/L, total protein—5.4 g/dL, albumin—2.79 g/L and prothrombin time of 21.8 seconds. Within 2 days, the patient's bilirubin rose to 35.68 mg/dL, with a concurrent rise in transaminases (AST—200, ALT—43 IU/L). There was a concomitant rise in the TLC to 30,000 cells/cumm. Suspecting an infection, blood, and urine cultures, a serum procalcitonin level and a chest X-ray were done. An ultrasonographic study of the abdomen revealed hepatosplenomegaly (liver—22 cm, spleen—18 cm), a prominent portal vein (12.8 mm) and absent free fluid in the abdomen. The cultures subsequently came out to be sterile, and the procalcitonin level was normal. Considering the sudden rise in bilirubin, serum lactate dehydrogenase (LDH), a peripheral smear, and haptoglobin levels were done. However, these reports did not reveal any evidence of hemolysis.

■ DIAGNOSTIC CONSIDERATIONS

It was imperative to ascertain whether the patient had severe alcoholic hepatitis (SAH), acute on chronic liver failure (ACLF) or a decompensated chronic liver disease (DCLD). It was important to note that the patient had no prior history of hepatic decompensation. There was also an absence of coagulopathy and encephalopathy. Abdominal ultrasound revealed an enlarged liver with altered echotexture. These factors suggested a diagnosis of SAH, rather than

ACLF or DCLD. The presence of an acute hepatic insult, in the absence of a prior history of decompensation, which may include infections or a binge alcohol intake, may favor a diagnosis of ACLF. A patient with a prior history of decompensation, with features of decompensation including clinical ascites, an upper GI bleed, encephalopathy or jaundice favors a diagnosis of DCLD. There is heterogeneity in the definition of ACLF. The APASL (Asian Pacific Association for the Study of the Liver) defines ACLF as an "acute hepatic insult manifesting as jaundice (total bilirubin levels of 5 mg/dL or more) and coagulopathy [international normalized ratio (INR) of 1.5 or more, or prothrombin activity of <40%] complicated within 4 weeks by clinical ascites, encephalopathy, or both". This definition excludes patients with a prior history of hepatic decompensation. However, the EASL (European Association for the Study of the Liver) definition also includes patients who have had a prior decompensating event.[1]

A CT scan of the abdomen is a useful tool in differentiating SAH from DCLD. A shrunken liver, with florid features of portal hypertension, including ascites and portal collaterals suggests DCLD. However, an enlarged liver, with/without mild ascites may favor a diagnosis of SAH in the appropriate clinical setting.[2] It is essential to exclude infections, as they are one of the most common causes of ACLF, and the presence of an infection may also impose exclusion of certain therapies like steroids.[3]

SCORING SYSTEMS

The Maddrey's discriminant function (MDF) **(Table 1)** is one of the most commonly used bedside scoring systems to prognosticate SAH. The MDF score in this patient was 83, which confirmed the severity of alcoholic hepatitis (MDF score >32 is suggestive of SAH[5]). Another commonly used scoring system is MELD (Model for End-stage Liver Disease), which utilizes the INR, creatinine, and bilirubin levels. Certain other scoring systems are the Glasgow Alcoholic Hepatitis Score [age, bilirubin, prothrombin time (PT), blood urea nitrogen (BUN), TLC]

TABLE 1: Prognostic scoring systems for alcoholic hepatitis.[4]

Score	Formula				Interpretation
MDF	4.6 × (PT−control PT) + bilirubin (mg/dL)				Severe: ≥32
MELD	3.8 × [ln (bilirubin (mg/dL)] + 11.2 × [ln (INR)] + 9.6 × [ln (creatinine (mg/dL)] + 6.4				Severe: ≥21
ABIC	(Age × 0.1) + (Bilirubin × 0.8)				• Low risk: ≤6.71 • Severe: >9.0
GAHS		1	2	3	Severe: ≥9
	Age	<50	≥50	–	
	WBC count	<15	≥15	–	
	Urea, mmol/L	<5	≥5	–	
	INR	<1.5	1.5–2.0	>2.0	
	Bilirubin, mg/dL	<7.3	7.4–14.6	>14.6	

(ABIC: Age/Bilirubin/INR (international normalized ratio)/Creatinine; GAHS: Glasgow Alcoholic Hepatitis Score; MDF: Maddrey's discriminant function; MELD: Model for End-stage Liver Disease; PT: prothrombin time; WBC: white blood cell)

and the ABIC score (Age, Bilirubin, INR, Creatinine).

MANAGEMENT ISSUES

In the absence of any evidence of infection, the rising TLC was attributed to SAH in this patient. In view of the high MDF score, multiple treatment options were discussed with the patient. The patient was initiated on 40 mg/day of prednisolone under strict supervision. However, despite starting steroids, the patient's bilirubin continued to rise after 3 days of therapy. It was accompanied by a rise in TLC and creatinine, to a level of 1.6 mg/dL. In view of the worsening renal parameters and rising TLC, steroids were stopped and the patient was initiated on broad-spectrum antibiotics to cover possible infections. The Lille score could not be calculated at this point as the patient did not complete 1 week of steroid therapy. Other treatment options were considered at this point. The large splenic size and rising TLC obliviated the use of granulocyte colony-stimulating factor (G-CSF). The option of liver transplant was discussed with the patient, but was met with denial from the patient and his relatives. Hence, we considered the use of plasma exchange (PLEX).

In conjunction with the nephrology team, the patient underwent three cycles of PLEX (1.5 L/day) on alternate days, with strict monitoring of renal and liver function tests. After three cycles of PLEX, the patient's creatinine had improved from 1.9 to 1.1 mg/dL. This was associated with a rapid fall in bilirubin from 35 to 12 mg/dL. The patient's TLC had also improved significantly from 30,000 to 14,000 cells/cumm.

Nutritional therapy is of paramount importance in the management of SAH, as it is an inflammatory condition that can result in catabolism. A high calorie (25–30 kcal/kg/day) and high protein (1.2–1.5 g/kg/day) diet is recommended. Enteral nutrition is favorable as compared to total parenteral nutrition (TPN), so as to reduce the risk of bacterial translocation and systemic inflammation.[6]

Steroids have been the conventional therapy for SAH, despite being met with common hurdles like infections and renal dysfunction. However, nearly 30% of patients with SAH have some contraindication to steroid therapy. Secondly, the failure rate with steroid therapy is also significant (40%).[7] A Lille score > 0.54 at 1 week necessitates cessation of steroid therapy, due to the risk of sepsis. A Lille score > 0.45 at day 4 has been associated with >7.2 times elevation in the risk of mortality.[8] Also, inadvertent usage of steroids in ACLF can worsen the risk of mortality, and make liver transplantation impossible or highly risky.

Pentoxifylline is a phosphodiesterase inhibitor therapy that was commonly used in SAH due to its inhibitory effect on tumor necrosis factor alpha (TNF-α). Over the last few years, multiple studies have demonstrated a lack of improvement in short- and long-term mortality with the use of pentoxifylline. However, it continues to be used by multiple practitioners as it can be administered in the presence of sepsis and renal dysfunction. The STOPAH trial is one of the major trials comparing mortality in patients with SAH in four groups: placebo/placebo, placebo/prednisolone, placebo/pentoxifylline, pentoxifylline/prednisolone. This study did not demonstrate significant short-term (28 days) mortality benefit in the prednisolone or pentoxifylline group. However, the mortality was lower in the prednisolone group (14%) as compared to the placebo group (17%). Interestingly, steroids have only demonstrated improvement in short-term but not long-term mortality (6 months).[9]

Granulocyte colony-stimulating factor is a relatively new option available in the treatment of patients with SAH. There have been multiple studies involving the use of G-CSF in patients with ACLF and SAH. The results have been varying, and most of the studies demonstrating benefit have been of small scale. G-CSF works on the principle of homing of hematopoietic stem cells in the liver, and potentiating regeneration of hepatocytes. There have been reports of an increased incidence of infections and sepsis with the use of G-CSF. Also, the use of G-CSF in patients with an enlarged splenic size has been associated with spontaneous splenic rupture, thus making splenic size an important limiting factor in choosing this therapy.[10,11] More large-scale studies are required to recommend the use of G-CSF in SAH.

N-acetyl cysteine (NAC) is an antioxidant and free radical scavenger that has shown benefit in some studies in patients with SAH. Nyugen-Khac et al. have demonstrated better short-term (28 days) mortality and lower incidence of hepatorenal syndrome (HRS) in patients receiving a combination of prednisolone and NAC as compared to placebo. However, NAC administration had no significant effect on long-term mortality.[12] Large-scale studies are required to further understand the efficacy of NAC in treating SAH.

Plasma exchange has recently emerged as a newer treatment modality for SAH. It has also been studies in patient with ACLF, as a bridge to transplant, and has demonstrated increased transplant-free survival.[13] PLEX has been studied at varying volumes and frequencies in different studies. In contrast to the previously discussed medical modalities, PLEX has demonstrated improvement in long-term mortality (90 days). Kumar et al. have demonstrated better transplant-free survival [54.6%—PLEX group vs. 18.1%—standard medical treatment (SMT) group] at 1 year in a study performed on 109 patients with SAH.[14] Additionally, renal dysfunction and sepsis are not absolute contraindications to PLEX.

In clinical practice, nearly 40% of patients with SAH do not respond to medical therapy, hence necessitating liver transplant. Transplanted patients with SAH who do not respond to steroids showed a favorable 6-month survival (77%) as compared to those who did not get transplant (23%).[15]

Patients with ACLF should be directly referred to transplant centers for further management as their response to medical therapy is often dismal. However, liver transplant is limited by economic factors, availability of a donor liver, and general aversion to major surgery by patients and their relatives, thus making other options like PLEX attractive.

Postliver transplant, patients with SAH and ACLF III have demonstrated a survival rate of nearly 80% at 1 year.[16] However, the post-transplant period is challenging in many aspects. Risk of recidivism by relapsing into alcohol addiction is a major concern in our country, considering the scarcity of de-addiction centers and lack of compliance by patients. Compliance to immunomodulatory agents, and their adverse effects on long-term usage are other limiting factors.

There are multiple newer modalities of treatment for SAH that are now emerging. There has been a substantial amount of data on fecal microbiota transplant (FMT) in alcoholic hepatitis. Alcohol induces gut dysbiosis and a leaky gut syndrome, which promotes a pro-inflammatory state in the liver by introducing "pathogen-associated molecular patterns" (PAMPs) into the system. The gut of an alcoholic patient contains lesser amount of short-chain fatty acid producing bacteria. Also, there is a loss of gut mucosal integrity, which propagates this pro-inflammatory state. The principle of using FMT in SAH is that it potentially improves in gut dysbiosis and subsequently modulates hepatic and systemic inflammation. FMT has demonstrated an increase in survival in small-scale studies, with an improvement in 1 year mortality up to 87% in patients with SAH.[17-19] Similarly, Han et al. demonstrated reduction in serum lipopolysaccharide and improvement in short-term outcomes (7 days) in patients who received *Lactobacillus/Streptococcus*-based probiotics as compared to placebo.[20]

The use of hepatoprotective agents in SAH has been a matter of debate, although practitioners use it commonly in their daily practice. Ursodeoxycholic acid (UDCA) has been one of the most extensively used agents in this regard, although there has been no proven benefit on survival. There has been limited data on the use of metadoxine as an antioxidant in the treatment of SAH. Higuera-de la Tijera et al. demonstrated an improved survival at 90 days (68% vs. 20%) when metadoxine was used in combination with steroids, as compared to steroids alone in patients with SAH.[21] Certain other newer agents like interleukin 22 (IL-22) infusion have been used in small-scale studies. A Mayo Clinic study on 18 subjects with SAH demonstrated a reduction in the MELD score by 6 and 5 points at 28 and 42 days, respectively, when patients were infused with F-652 (IL-22 human recombinant protein). The drug was well tolerated, and 83% of subjects attained a Lille score of <0.45 at 7 days.[22] Similarly, anakinra (IL-1 receptor antagonist) when used in conjunction with zinc and pentoxifylline demonstrated similar survival to patients on methylprednisolone in multicenter double-blinded randomized controlled trials (RCTs).[23]

Alcohol de-addiction plays a major role in the management of SAH, and may need to be continued in the post-transplant period. Multiple drugs such as acamprosate [N-methyl-d-aspartate (NMDA) receptor agonist], naltrexone (opioid antagonist), baclofen [gamma-aminobutyric acid B (GABA-B) agonist] have been used with variable results for the same.[24] The involvement of a counselor and psychiatrist with experience in rehabilitation is essential for the maintenance of effective abstinence.

CONCLUSION

Our patient was followed up after month of discharge, and he showed significant clinical improvement. His physical status had improved and he was back to his usual work routine. His renal function normalized and the creatinine level reduced to 0.8 mg/dL. The total bilirubin level had come down to 6 mg/dL, and the transaminases were normal. However, after a period of 2 months, he was readmitted to the hospital with tense ascites, increasing bilirubin levels, and hepatic encephalopathy. The patient was put on the transplant list, and is currently awaiting liver transplant.

Severe alcoholic hepatitis is a condition with very high mortality rates that requires immediate attention and management. Multiple modalities have demonstrated variable efficacy in the treatment of SAH. Corticosteroids continue to be the mainstay in its treatment, despite its limitations. PLEX has emerged as a new promising therapy, especially as a bridge to transplant. FMT is showing promise as a noninvasive modality for treating SAH, although larger trials are required to determine the same. Anti-inflammatory drugs like Anakinra and IL-22 analogs need to be studied extensively to incorporate them in general practice. Hence, the management of SAH should be tailored on an individual basis based on the patient characteristics, associated comorbidities, the presence of complications like sepsis, renal dysfunction and GI bleed, and economic factors.

■ REFERENCES

1. Hernaez R, Solà E, Moreau R, Ginès P. Acute-on-chronic liver failure: an update. Gut. 2017;66(3):541-53.
2. Kudo M, Zheng RQ, Kim SR, Okabe Y, Osaki Y, Iijima H, et al. Diagnostic accuracy of imaging for liver cirrhosis compared to histologically proven liver cirrhosis. Intervirology. 2008;51(1):17-26.
3. Kumar R, Mehta G, Jalan R. Acute-on-chronic liver failure. Clin Med (Lond). 2020;20(5):501-4.
4. Rachakonda V, Bataller R, Duarte-Rojo A. Recent advances in alcoholic hepatitis. F1000Res. 2020;9:97.
5. Owens RE, Snyder HS, Twilla JD, Satapathy SK. Pharmacologic Treatment of alcoholic hepatitis: examining outcomes based on disease severity stratification. J Clin Exp Hepatol. 2016;6(4):275-81.
6. Dasarathy S. Nutrition and Alcoholic Liver Disease: Effects of alcoholism on nutrition, effects of nutrition on alcoholic liver disease, and nutritional therapies for alcoholic liver disease. Clin Liver Dis. 2016;20(3):535-50.
7. Sarin SK, Sharma S. Predictors of steroid non-response and new approaches in severe alcoholic hepatitis. Clin Mol Hepatol. 2020;26(4):639-51.
8. Foncea CG, Sporea I, Lupușoru R, Moga TV, Bende F, Șirli R, et al. Day-4 Lille score is a good prognostic factor and early predictor in assessing therapy response in patients with liver cirrhosis and severe alcoholic hepatitis. J Clin Med. 2021;10(11):2338.
9. Thursz MR, Richardson P, Allison M, Austin A, Bowers M, Day CP, et al; STOPAH Trial. Prednisolone or pentoxifylline for alcoholic hepatitis. N Engl J Med. 2015;372(17):1619-28.
10. Shasthry SM, Sharma MK, Shasthry V, Pande A, Sarin SK. Efficacy of granulocyte colony-stimulating factor in the management of steroid-nonresponsive severe alcoholic hepatitis: a double-blind randomized controlled trial. Hepatology. 2019;70(3):802-11.
11. Marot A, Singal AK, Moreno C, Deltenre P. Granulocyte colony-stimulating factor for alcoholic hepatitis: A systematic review and meta-analysis of randomised controlled trials. JHEP Rep. 2020;2(5):100139.
12. Nguyen-Khac E, Thevenot T, Piquet MA, Benferhat S, Goria O, Chatelain D, et al; AAH-NAC Study Group. Glucocorticoids plus N-Acetylcysteine in severe alcoholic hepatitis. N Engl J Med. 2011;365(19):1781-9.
13. Ramakrishnan S, Hans R, Duseja A, Sharma RR. Therapeutic plasma exchange is a safe and effective bridge therapy in patients with alcohol-associated ACLF not having immediate prospects for liver transplantation-A case-control, pilot study. J Clin Apher. 2022;37(6):553-62.
14. Kumar SE, Goel A, Zachariah U, Nair SC, David VG, Varughese S, et al. Low volume plasma exchange and low dose steroid improve survival in patients with alcohol-related acute on chronic liver failure and severe alcoholic hepatitis—preliminary experience. J Clin Exp Hepatol. 2022;12(2):372-8.
15. Herrick-Reynolds KM, Punchhi G, Greenberg RS, Strauss AT, Boyarsky BJ, Weeks-Groh SR, et al. Evaluation of early vs standard liver transplant for alcohol-associated liver disease. JAMA Surg. 2021;156(11):1026-34.
16. Sundaram V, Mahmud N, Perricone G, Dev Katarey, Wong RJ, Karvellas CJ, et al; Multi-Organ Dysfunction, Evaluation for Liver Transplantation (MODEL) Consortium. Long-term outcomes of patients undergoing liver transplantation for acute-on-chronic liver failure. Liver Transpl. 2020;26(12):1594-602.

17. Shasthry SM. Fecal microbiota transplantation in alcohol related liver diseases. Clin Mol Hepatol. 2020;26(3):294-301.
18. Sharma A, Roy A, Premkumar M, Verma N, Duseja A, Taneja S, et al. Fecal microbiota transplantation in alcohol-associated acute-on-chronic liver failure: an open-label clinical trial. Hepatol Int. 2022;16(2):433-46.
19. Philips CA, Ahamed R, Rajesh S, Abduljaleel JKP, Augustine P. Long-term Outcomes of stool transplant in alcohol-associated hepatitis—analysis of clinical outcomes, relapse, gut microbiota and comparisons with standard care. J Clin Exp Hepatol. 2022; 12(4):1124-32.
20. Han SH, Suk KT, Kim DJ, Kim MY, Baik SK, Kim YD, et al. Effects of probiotics (cultured *Lactobacillus subtilis/Streptococcus faecium*) in the treatment of alcoholic hepatitis: randomized-controlled multicenter study. Eur J Gastroenterol Hepatol. 2015;27(11):1300-6.
21. Higuera-de la Tijera F, Servín-Caamaño AI, Cruz-Herrera J, Serralde-Zúñiga AE, Abdo-Francis JM, Gutiérrez-Reyes G, et al. Treatment with metadoxine and its impact on early mortality in patients with severe alcoholic hepatitis. Ann Hepatol. 2014;13(3):343-52.
22. Arab, JP, Sehrawat TS, Simonetto DA, Verma VK, Feng D, Tang T, et al. An open-label, dose-escalation study to assess the safety and efficacy of IL-22 agonist F-652 in patients with alcohol-associated hepatitis. Hepatology. 2020;72(2):441-53.
23. Szabo G, Mitchell M, McClain CJ, Dasarathy S, Barton B, McCullough AJ, et al. IL-1 receptor antagonist plus pentoxifylline and zinc for severe alcohol-associated hepatitis. Hepatology. 2022;76(4):1058-68.
24. Williams SH. Medications for treating alcohol dependence. Am Fam Physician. 2005;72(9):1775-80.

IgM Anti-HEV Positivity in a Patient with Suspected Severe Alcoholic Hepatitis: Cause or a Red Herring?

Harshil Trivedi, Kaushal Madan

■ INTRODUCTION

We discuss here a case of 39-year-old male with history of significant alcohol use, who presented with painless progressive jaundice preceded by prodrome of fever and loss of appetite of 1 month duration. Patient was a shopkeeper by profession and had been consuming 80–100 g of alcohol daily for last 15 years. Initial blood investigations revealed direct hyperbilirubinemia with parenchymal pattern of liver injury on liver function test (LFT) profile and mild leukocytosis **(Table 1)**. Immunoglobulin M (IgM) antibodies to hepatitis E virus (IgM anti-HEV) were positive. Hepatitis B surface antigen (HBsAg), antibodies to hepatitis C virus (anti-HCV), and IgM antibodies to hepatitis A virus (IgM anti-HAV) were negative. Standard management with nutritional rehabilitation, thiamine, s-adenosyl methionine, and ursodeoxycholic acid was started. However, after initial improvement in LFT profile, the bilirubin continued to remain high. Multiphase computed tomography (CT) scan abdomen revealed multiple hypo-enhancing lesions suggestive of regenerating nodules with hepatosplenomegaly and signs of portal hypertension (PHT). Upper gastrointestinal endoscopy (UGIE) revealed small low-risk esophageal varices. He had mild ascites on admission which increased in volume during hospitalization requiring large-volume paracentesis. Diagnostic analysis of ascitic fluid showed serum ascitic albumin gradient (SAAG) of >1.1 with no evidence of spontaneous bacterial peritonitis (SBP). Since the history and initial laboratory investigations were suggestive of alcoholic hepatitis, but IgM HEV was positive, a transjugular biopsy was done to confirm the final diagnosis. In addition, we also did HEV RNA to rule out active viremia, as we were planning to start the patient on steroids for severe acute alcoholic hepatitis (SAAH). Liver biopsy was suggestive of alcoholic hepatitis without evidence of cirrhosis (METAVIR stage 2) **(Figs. 1A to D)**. Blood culture and urine culture were sterile and serum procalcitonin was <0.5 ng/mL. He was started on tablet prednisolone 40 mg once a day and he started showing progressive improvement in his clinical and LFT profile. The Lille score was 0.148 and 0.051 on day 4 and 7, respectively which was suggestive of response to steroids which were then continued for 4 weeks. He was discharged on oral steroids prednisolone 40 mg/day and followed up regularly with clinical and laboratory monitoring which showed progressive improvement **(Tables 1 and 2)**.

■ DISCUSSION

Ours is a case of painless progressive jaundice with signs and LFT profile reports suggestive

TABLE 1: Serial monitoring of laboratory parameters (before oral prednisolone therapy).

Investigations	Day 0	Day 1	Day 3	Day 5	Day 7
Hb%	10.8	10.9	10.3	10.4	10.5
TLC/mm^3	9,000	10,400	10,800	9,000	12,000
PLT × 10^3/mm^3	337	294	271	296	352
Bilirubin (mg/dL)	33.5	29.6	26.2	27.5	27.9
AST (IU/L)	92	91	94	106	95
ALT (IU/L)	82	78	82	89	81
ALP (IU/L)	82	78	82	89	81
GGTP (IU/L)	70	72	73	80	82
INR	2.47	2.97	3.15	3.05	3.22
Albumin (g/dL)	3.6	3.7	3.3	3.5	3.6
Creatinine (mg/dL)	0.5	0.5	0.6	0.7	0.5

(ALP: alkaline phosphatase; ALT: alanine transaminase; AST: aspartate transaminase; Hb: hemoglobin; GGTP: gamma-glutamyl transpeptidase; INR: international normalized ratio; PLT: platelet count; TLC: total leukocyte count)

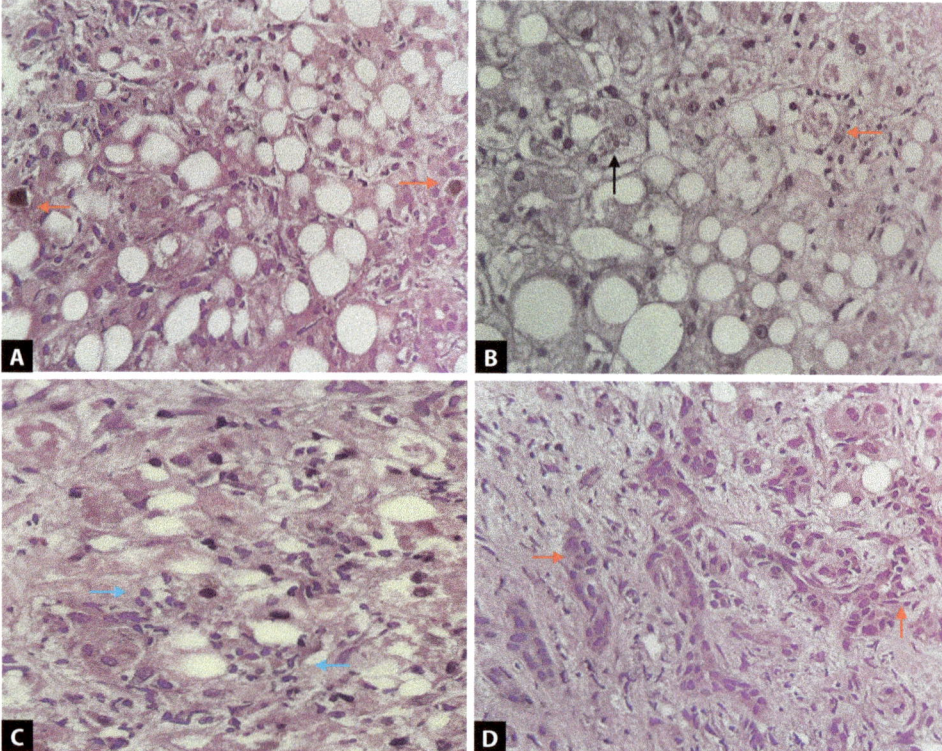

Figs. 1A to D: Liver biopsy 40x view showing (A) Macrovesicular steatosis and cholestasis: Bile pigments (red arrows); (B) Ballooning degeneration (black arrow) and Mallory–Denk bodies (red arrow); (C) Satellitosis: neutrophilic infiltrate surrounding ballooned hepatocytes (blue arrows); (D) Ductular reaction (red arrows).

CHAPTER 14: IgM Anti-HEV Positivity in a Patient with Suspected Severe Alcoholic Hepatitis...

TABLE 2: Serial laboratory parameters monitoring (after steroid therapy: day 11 is day 4 of steroid therapy).

Investigations	Day 11	Day 14	Day 21	Day 28	Day 67	Day 90	Day 115	Day 150
Hb%	11.8	–	11.6	11.2	11.0	11.1	11.1	11.1
TLC/mm^3	13,400	–	15,830	9,900	3,990	5,160	4,630	4,180
PLT × 10^3/mm^3	366	–	140	165	135	120	115	118
Bilirubin (mg/dL)	25.2	21.6	16.1	9.9	3.4	2.5	2.3	1.7
AST (IU/L)	277	231	215	185	78	68	66	41
ALT (IU/L)	134	145	212	176	39	54	46	34
ALP (IU/L)	111	94	175	116	135	149	–	–
GGTP (IU/L)	134	150	138	133	–	–	40	43
INR	2.18	2.13	1.71	1.85	1.68	1.85	1.84	1.6
Albumin (g/dL)	3.9	3.5	3.7	3.3	3.2	3.3	–	–
Creatinine (mg/dL)	0.6	–	0.6	0.5	0.6	0.7	–	–

(ALP: alkaline phosphatase; ALT: alanine transaminase; AST: aspartate transaminase; Hb: hemoglobin; GGTP: gamma-glutamyl transpeptidase; INR: international normalized ratio; PLT: platelet count; TLC: total leukocyte count)

of liver dysfunction. Physical examination did not reveal any stigmata of cirrhosis. The dilemma in the current case was the strong history and LFT profile suggestive of alcohol consumption but the positive IgM HEV serology was not letting us make a definitive diagnosis of SAAH.

Steroids have been recommended as the most effective modality for reducing short-term mortality in patients with SAAH.[1] However, only a small proportion one-fourth to one-third are actually eligible for steroid therapy. Most of them have contraindications to the use of steroids in such a setting, such as active GI bleeding, evidence of sepsis or renal failure. Fortunately, our patient did not have any of these, though he did have self-limited hemorrhoidal bleed in the initial days of hospitalization. However, the positive IgM HEV serology was not letting us go ahead with steroid treatment.

A possibility of a false-positive serology of HEV cannot be ruled out. According to a large hospital-based study, 9% of healthy, asymptomatic controls may have positive markers of HEV infection including positive HEV RNA at any given time in India.[2] In another blood donor healthy population IgM anti-HEV positivity was demonstrated in 0.2–2.6% subjects.[3] It would also have been possible that acute HEV infection was responsible for the recent worsening in a case of underlying alcoholic cirrhosis, leading to acute on chronic liver failure (ACLF). Acute HEV infection over underlying cirrhosis has been described earlier as an important cause of ACLF in the Indian subcontinent.[2,4,5] Since we were contemplating treatment with steroids, it was important to rule out the concomitant presence of HEV. In presence of immunosuppressed state, HEV may be associated with accelerated viral replication and chronicity of liver injury.[6]

We were able to resolve this issue by two laboratory investigations. One was testing for HEV RNA in patient's serum. Even though IgM HEV was positive in our patient, it is not considered a marker of active viremia and may only reflect recent HEV infection or even a false-positive result. Anti-HEV IgM can be positive for up to 12 months after acute infection making anti-HEV IgM as an unreliable marker for diagnosis of acute hepatitis E.[7] Anti-HEV IgM has sensitivity of 27% and specificity of 92%. Anti-HEV IgM has considerable cross reactivity especially with Epstein–Barr virus (EBV) and cytomegalovirus (CMV).[8] In study of acute liver failure in United States of America, only 13.8% of patients who had anti-HEV IgM positivity were also positive for HEV RNA making it an unreliable marker of HEV infection especially in presence of liver failure.[9] HEV RNA positivity usually denotes active viremia. HEV viremia has been described to last for a short duration only in acute HEV infection, but it has been shown to persist for many weeks to months in some patients, where it may be associated with chronic liver injury or chronic hepatitis.[10] Although, as mentioned above, 4.5% of asymptomatic controls may also be positive for HEV RNA in an endemic area like ours. In our patient HEV RNA was undetectable, suggesting absence of active HEV RNA viremia.

The second was a transjugular liver biopsy (TJLB). Liver biopsy showed evidence of fatty infiltration with ballooning degeneration with satellitosis, pericellular fibrosis which were suggestive of acute alcoholic hepatitis. Studies have earlier described macrovesicular fat, neutrophilic infiltration, well-formed Mallory–Denk bodies, ductular reaction, and pericellular fibrosis to be typical features of alcoholic steatohepatitis on a liver biopsy.[11-13] The features which define viral hepatitis, such as rosette formation and lobular disarray were absent.

The combination of history, negative HEV RNA and liver biopsy findings suggestive of acute alcoholic hepatitis allowed us to start the patient on steroids. Alcoholic hepatitis can range from mild to severe disease, with severe disease being defined as: Maddrey's discriminant function (MDF) ≥32 or Model for End-stage Liver Disease (MELD) ≥21. The MDF and MELD scores of our patient were 97.9 and 30, respectively. Of all the treatment options, only steroids have been able to demonstrate survival benefit over short-term. Before starting steroids, sepsis was excluded by sterile blood and urine cultures, normal chest X-ray, and normal procalcitonin levels. However, the data on the use of steroids for severe acute alcoholic hepatitis is conflicting. There have been a number of trials and their meta-analyses which have provided opposing results regarding survival benefit of steroids in this group of patients.[14-16] The largest randomized controlled trial (RCT) done till date, called the STOPAH trial, also demonstrated no survival advantage of the use of steroids, either alone or in combination with pentoxifylline.[17] Subsequently another meta-analysis did demonstrate short-term survival benefit (28 days), but had no impact on survival over a 6 months' duration.[18]

The key to steroid treatment for severe alcoholic hepatitis (SAH), is the patient selection. The presence of acute GI bleed, acute kidney injury and sepsis are considered contraindications for the use of steroids. Recently a window based on the MELD score has been proposed for the use of steroids in SAH. Arab et al. have suggested that survival benefit was seen among patients with SAH, who have a MELD score between 21 and 51 and the best survival could be achieved by patients with MELD score between 25 and 39.[19] After starting steroids, patients can be selected out early during the first week by calculating the Lille score, which guides whether the treatment should be continued or discontinued. The survival was demonstrated to be the best in patients whose Lille score at day 7 of steroid treatment was <0.45.[20] It was also demonstrated that patients who are considered nonresponders as per the Lille score are more likely to develop infection-related complications if the steroid treatment is continued. Among 246 SAH patients treated with steroids, infectious complications developed in 11.1% and 42.5% of responders and nonresponders, respectively.[21] Recently, Lille score calculated at day 4 has also been demonstrated to provide similar information.[22] The patient improved rapidly after starting steroids, with Lille score at day 4 (0.148) and day 7 (0.051) suggesting effective response. At the last follow-up the patient's LFTs have completely normalized.

■ CONCLUSION

This case highlights the importance of utilizing all available tools that help in resolving diagnostic dilemmas and therefore help in making a crucial management decision. The decision to start steroids (despite its controversial role) proved to be life-saving for this patient. In the absence of this decision, and ongoing liver injury, the patient might have continued to have a simmering ongoing liver inflammation and might have ended up requiring a liver transplantation. This case also highlights the importance of proper selection of cases before starting steroids.

■ REFERENCES

1. Louvet A, Thursz MR, Kim DJ, Labreuche J, Atkinson SR, Sidhu SS, et al. Corticosteroids Reduce Risk of Death Within 28 Days for Patients With Severe Alcoholic Hepatitis, Compared With Pentoxifylline or Placebo-a Meta-analysis of Individual Data From Controlled Trials. Gastroenterology. 2018; 155:458-68.
2. Kumar Acharya S, Kumar Sharma P, Singh R, Kumar Mohanty S, Madan K, Kumar Jha J, et al. Hepatitis E virus (HEV) infection in patients with cirrhosis is associated with rapid decompensation and death. J Hepatol. 2007;46:387-94.
3. Al-Absi ES, Al-Sadeq DW, Younis MH, Yassine HM, Abdalla OM, Mesleh AG, et al. Performance evaluation of five commercial assays in assessing seroprevalence of HEV antibodies among blood donor. J Med Microbiol. 2018;67(9):1302-9.
4. Radha Krishna Y, Saraswat VA, Das K, Himanshu G, Yachha SK, Aggarwal R, et al. Clinical features and predictors of outcome in acute hepatitis A and hepatitis E virus hepatitis on cirrhosis. Liver Int. 2009;29(3):392-8.
5. Hamid SS, Atiq M, Shehzad F, Yasmeen A, Nissa T, Salam A, et al. Hepatitis E virus superinfection in patients with chronic liver disease. Hepatology. 2002;36:474-8.
6. Ma Z, de Man RA, Kamar N, Pan Q. Chronic hepatitis E: advancing research and patient care. J Hepatol. 2022;77:1109-23.
7. European Association for the Study of the Liver. EASL Clinical Practice Guidelines on hepatitis E virus infection. J Hepatol. 2018;68:1256-71.
8. Hyams C, Mabayoje DA, Copping R, Maranao D, Patel M, Labbett W, et al. Serological cross reactivity to CMV and EBV causes problems in the diagnosis of acute hepatitis E virus infection. J Med Virol. 2014;86:478-83.
9. Anastasiou OE, Thodou V, Berger A, Wedemeyer H, Ciesek S. Comprehensive Evaluation of Hepatitis E Serology and Molecular Testing in a Large Cohort. Pathogens. 2020;9(2):137.
10. Kamar N, Izopet J, Tripon S, Bismuth M, Hillaire S, Dumortier J, et al. Ribavirin for chronic hepatitis E virus infection in transplant recipients. N Engl J Med. 2014;370:1111-20.
11. Sakhuja P. Pathology of alcoholic liver disease, can it be differentiated from nonalcoholic steatohepatitis? World J Gastroenterol. 2014;20:16474-9.
12. Singh DK, Rastogi A, Sakhuja P, Gondal R, Sarin SK. Comparison of clinical, biochemical and histological features of

alcoholic steatohepatitis and non-alcoholic steatohepatitis in Asian Indian patients. Indian J Pathol Microbiol. 2010;53:408-13.
13. Pinto HC, Baptista A, Camilo ME, Valente A, Saragoça A, de Moura MC. Nonalcoholic steatohepatitis. Clinicopathological comparison with alcoholic hepatitis in ambulatory and hospitalized patients. Dig Dis Sci. 1996;41:172-9.
14. Christensen E, Gluud C. Glucocorticoids are ineffective in alcoholic hepatitis: a meta-analysis adjusting for confounding variables. Gut. 1995;37:113-8.
15. Rambaldi A, Saconato HH, Christensen E, Thorlund K, Wetterslev J, Gluud C. Systematic review: glucocorticosteroids for alcoholic hepatitis—a Cochrane Hepato-Biliary Group systematic review with meta-analyses and trial sequential analyses of randomized clinical trials. Aliment Pharmacol Ther. 2008; 27:1167-78.
16. Mathurin P, O'Grady J, Carithers RL, Phillips M, Louvet A, Mendenhall CL, et al. Corticosteroids improve short-term survival in patients with severe alcoholic hepatitis: meta-analysis of individual patient data. Gut. 2011;6:255-60.
17. Thursz MR, Richardson P, Allison M, Austin A, Bowers M, Day CP, et al. STOPAH Trial. Prednisolone or pentoxifylline for alcoholic hepatitis. N Engl J Med. 2015;372:1619-28.
18. Louvet A, Thursz MR, Kim DJ, Labreuche J, Atkinson SR, Sidhu SS, et al. Corticosteroids Reduce Risk of Death Within 28 Days for Patients With Severe Alcoholic Hepatitis, Compared With Pentoxifylline or Placebo-a Meta-analysis of Individual Data From Controlled Trials. Gastroenterology. 2018; 155:458-468.
19. Arab JP, Díaz LA, Baeza N, Idalsoaga F, Fuentes-López E, Arnold J, et al. Identification of optimal therapeutic window for steroid use in severe alcohol-associated hepatitis: a worldwide study. J Hepatol. 2021;75:1026-33.
20. Louvet A, Naveau S, Abdelnour M, Ramond MJ, Diaz E, Fartoux L, et al. The Lille model: a new tool for therapeutic strategy in patients with severe alcoholic hepatitis treated with steroids. Hepatology. 2007;45:1348-54.
21. Louvet A, Wartel F, Castel H, Dharancy S, Hollebecque A, Canva-Delcambre V, et al. Infection in patients with severe alcoholic hepatitis treated with steroids: early response to therapy is the key factor. Gastroenterology. 2009;137:541-8.
22. Foncea CG, Sporea I, Lupușoru R, Moga TV, Bende F, Șirli R, et al. Day-4 Lille score is a good prognostic factor and early predictor in assessing therapy response in patients with liver cirrhosis and severe alcoholic hepatitis. J Clin Med. 2021;10:2338.

Acute on Chronic Liver Failure

Akash Roy, Mahesh Kumar Goenka

INTRODUCTION

Traditionally, cirrhosis has been classified as a binary of compensated and decompensated cirrhosis with ascites, variceal hemorrhage, and hepatic encephalopathy (HE) being the classical decompensation.[1] However, with improvement in understanding of the pathophysiology of cirrhosis, the concept of various acute insults which dramatically alter the natural history of cirrhosis emerged. The concept culminated in a seminal paper by Sen et al. in 2002, who suggested a new syndrome of acute on chronic liver failure (ACLF), which they attempted to define as: "An acute deterioration of liver function over a period of 2–4 weeks usually associated with a precipitating event leading to severe deterioration in clinical status with jaundice and HE and/or hepatorenal syndrome with high Sequential Organ Failure Assessment (SOFA) and Acute Physiology and Chronic Health Evaluation II (APACHE) II scores".[2] Following, this there has been an exponential rise in knowledge about ACLF leading to multiple definitions, prognostic scores, and therapeutic options. In the subsequent sections, we explore the concept of ACLF in a case-based approach taking a stepwise approach to management with the available evidence.

CASE VIGNETTE

A 38-year-old male with a history of alcohol use disorder (consuming whiskey, 100–150 g/day about 4 days a week for last 6 years with a history of a binge on weekends) presented with progressive jaundice for 1 month followed by abdominal distension for 10 days. He was diagnosed with type II diabetes mellitus 3 years back. He has no history of major surgeries and denies any chronic medicine use or any intake of complementary and alternative medications. Although he had malaise concurrent with jaundice onset, there is no history of fever, abdominal pain, vomiting, change in stool color, pruritis, gastrointestinal bleeding, or alteration in sensorium. There was no history of decreased urine output, shortness of breath on activity or lying down. He was normotensive [blood pressure (BP) 110/70 mm Hg], and had tachycardia (pulse rate 112 beats/min), and tachypnea (respiratory rate 26). On examination, he is deeply icteric and has parotid enlargement with bilateral pedal edema. His body mass index (corrected for ascites and edema) was 28 kg/m^2. His mini-mental status examination yields a score of 27, and has no clinical focal neurological deficit or asterixis. The per abdominal examination is remarkable for an enlarged, firm, irregular liver (liver span 18 cm), presence of significant ascites elicited with a positive shifting dullness test, and splenomegaly (spleen palpable 3 cm below left costal margin). His respiratory and cardiovascular examination was unremarkable. The laboratory findings and their dynamic changes are shown in **Table 1**.

TABLE 1: Dynamic changes in laboratory findings.

Laboratory parameter (units)	On admission	Day 4	Reports Post five sessions PLEX	Discharge	Reference values
Hemogram					
Hemoglobin (g/dL)	10.5	10.9	9.8	9.1	12–18
Total leukocytic count ($\times 10^3/mm^3$)	18	26	13	11	4.0–11.0
Platelet count ($\times 10^3/mm^3$)	132	100	75	90	150–400
Liver function tests					
Bilirubin (mg/dL):					
• Total	23.4	31.4	8.1	4.1	0.3–1.3
• Direct	14.2	18.6	4.2	2	0.1–0.4
• Indirect	9.2	12.8	3.9	2.1	0.2–0.9
ALT (U/L)	90	92	72	70	7–41
AST (U/L)	300	295	112	100	12–38
Alkaline phosphatase (IU/L)	112	120	100	90	30–120
Protein, total (g/dL)	5.1	5.7	6	6.2	6.3–8.2
Albumin (g/dL)	2.6	3.0	3	3.2	3.5–5.0
Globulin (g/dL)	2.5	2.7	3	3	1.5–3.0
Coagulation profile					
Prothrombin time (s)	30.1	38.7	21	21	12.7–15.4
INR	3.2	3.5	2.5	2.1	1.34
Renal profile					
Serum creatinine (mg/dL)	1.1	1.5	1	1	0.5–0.9
Blood urea (mg/dL)	90	108	44	40	10–50
Sodium (mEq/L)	128	128	130	132	135–145
Potassium (mEq/L)	3.6	3.8	4.2	4	3.5–5.5
Blood glucose, random (mg/dL)	88	108			70–140
Blood/urine culture	Sterile				
HIV/HBsAg/anti-HCV	Nonreactive				
Lactate (mmol/L)	1.7	3.2			
Procalcitonin	1.1	1			
CLIF-C ACLF score	46	48	No ACLF	No ACLF	
AARC score	10	13	7	7	

Etiological workup: IgM HAV, IgM HEV, ANA, SMA, IgM CMV, IgM HSV all negative
Ceruloplasmin 24 mg/dL, ferritin 346 µg/L, transferrin saturation 33%

(AARC: APASL (Asian Pacific Association for the Study of the Liver)-ACLF Research Consortium; ACLF: acute on chronic liver failure; ALT: alanine aminotransferase; ANA: antinuclear antibodies; AST: aspartate aminotransferase; CLIF-C: chronic liver failure consortium; CMV: cytomegalovirus; IgM: immunoglobulin M; INR: international normalized ratio; HAV: hepatitis A virus; HBsAg: hepatitis B surface antigen; HCV: hepatitis C virus; HEV: hepatitis E virus; HIV: human immunodeficiency virus; HSV: herpes simplex virus; PLEX: plasma exchange; PT: prothrombin time; SMA: smooth muscle antibodies)

STEP 1: WHAT SYNDROMIC DIAGNOSIS DOES THIS PATIENT FIT INTO?

As evident from history, the patient did not have any liver-related complications in the past. However, there appears to be an acute deterioration that has led to the development of jaundice and ascites, which are manifestations of liver failure and a decompensated state. Hence, this fits into the clinical picture of the scenario described by Sen et al.[2] Hence, the syndromic diagnosis of ACLF is suitable to describe this entity. There are differences in the definition of the syndrome based upon European and Asian guidelines **(Table 2)**, although the central theme remains the same of an acute deterioration of underlying chronic liver disease (CLD) with extremely high short-term mortality.

STEP 2: IDENTIFYING THE ACUTE INSULT AND UNDERLYING CHRONIC LIVER DISEASE ETIOLOGY?

Since ACLF centers around an acute deterioration, it is imperative to identify an acute insult since intervention and cessation of the acute insult can lead to interruption of the downhill course. In our given case, the patient has significant alcohol intake with a history of binge intake, possibly indicating severe alcoholic hepatitis as the acute insult. However, prior to labeling an acute insult detailed history (especially of complementary and alternative medicines) and a search for other common etiologies should be instituted with appropriate sequential tests which are as follows:

- *Hepatotropic viruses:*
  - *Typical:* Immunoglobulin hepatitis A virus (Ig HAV), hepatitis E virus (HEV),

TABLE 2: Understanding the differences in the definition of ACLF according to Asian and European consensus.

Parameter	APASL-ACLF[3]	EASL-CLIF consortium[1]
Definition	Acute hepatic insult manifesting as jaundice and coagulopathy, complicated within 4 weeks by ascites and/or encephalopathy in a patient with previously diagnosed or undiagnosed CLD associated with a high 4 week mortality	An acute deterioration of preexisting CLD usually related to a precipitating event and associated with increased mortality at 4 weeks due to multi-system organ failure
Duration between acute insult and development of liver failure	4 weeks	Not defined
Acute insult	Only hepatic insults (hepatotropic viruses, alcohol, DILI)	Both hepatic and extrahepatic insults including infections and sepsis
Definition of CLD	Any CLD with or without cirrhosis (excludes previously decompensated cirrhosis)	Only cirrhosis including those with past decompensated disease

(ACLF: acute on chronic liver failure; APASL: Asian Pacific Association for the Study of the Liver; EASL-CLIF: European Association for the Study of the Liver–Chronic Liver Failure consortium; CLD: chronic liver disease; DILI: drug-induced liver injury)

hepatitis B virus [HBsAg (hepatitis B surface antigen), IgM anti-HBc (hepatitis B core antigen), and HBV (hepatitis B virus) DNA if positive]
- *Atypical:* Herpes simplex virus, cytomegalovirus, Epstein–Barr virus
- *Autoimmune hepatitis:* Antinuclear antibodies, anti-smooth muscle antibodies, soluble liver antigen
- *Wilson's disease:* Ceruloplasmin levels, Kayser–Fleischer ring assessment, 24 hours urine copper
- *Hemochromatosis:* Ferritin, transferrin saturation
- *Drug-induced liver injury:* Detailed drug history and liver biopsy in confounding cases
- *Sepsis:* Site-specific cultures, C-reactive protein, procalcitonin.

Besides these, in countries with prevalent tropical infections, in the appropriate clinical setting, common tropical febrile syndrome work-up, including malaria, dengue, scrub typhus, and leptospirosis, should also be carried out.

Identifying the Underlying Chronic Disease

In the given case, the patient appears to have underlying CLD, possibly cirrhosis, as exemplified by a nodular liver, splenomegaly, and presence of ascites. One should carefully look for other stigmata of CLD. The sequential tests that aid in corroborating a diagnosis of underlying cirrhosis would be an ultrasound (US) (liver nodularity, portal vein diameter, splenomegaly, and presence of collaterals) and an upper gastrointestinal endoscopy to screen for varices and other signs of portal hypertension. A US when combined with a Doppler study also provides evidence of any presence of portal vein thrombosis or hepatic venous outflow tract obstruction. A contrast-enhanced computed tomography (CT) scan is usually additive in outlining the liver status, presence of collaterals, and portosystemic shunts as well as excluding any presence of hepatocellular carcinoma. The etiology of CLD again appears to be alcohol-related but the patient also has additional risk factors of diabetes and obesity, and it has been shown that the presence of metabolic syndrome has additive detrimental effects and accelerates liver disease progression in those with alcohol-related liver disease.[5]

STEP 3: DETERMINATION OF ORGAN FAILURES AND DISEASE SEVERITY

Since ACLF is an acutely deteriorating state and centers around progressive organ failures (OFs), it is cardinal to assess the OF and assess disease severity scores. Hence, prognostic scoring systems are of paramount importance in management and predicting outcomes. Furthermore, these systems have a day-to-day variation, and the dynamicity of changes in score also needs close attention. Two commonly used scoring systems again with a "west and east" perspective are the Chronic Liver Failure Consortium (CLIF-C) Organ Failure Score[6] and the APASL (Asian Pacific Association for the Study of the Liver)-ACLF Research Consortium (AARC) Scoring and Grading system[7] which are readily available as web-based applications. To simplify, the EASL-CLIF Consortium system, which is based upon the traditional SOFA scoring system divides ACLF into three grades, i.e., grade 1, 2, and 3. ACLF-1 is associated with a 28-day mortality rate of 22%, ACLF-2 of 32%, and ACLF-3 of 73%. In contrast mortality rate in patients without ACLF-1 is 4.9%. The following are the criteria to define OF and classification as based on EASL-CLIF:
- *Liver failure:* Total bilirubin >12.0 mg/dL
- *Kidney failure*: Serum creatinine >2.0 mg/dL or the requirement of renal replacement therapy

- *Cerebral failure*: West-Haven HE grade 3 or 4
- *Coagulation failure:* International normalized ratio (INR) >2.5 or platelets are <20 × 10^9/L
- *Circulatory failure:* Vasopressor requirement (dopamine, dobutamine, epinephrine, or norepinephrine, terlipressin)
- *Respiratory failure:* Partial pressure of arterial oxygen to fraction of inspired oxygen (PaO_2/FiO_2) ratio is <200 or peripheral oxygen saturation (SpO_2)/FiO_2 ratio is <214.

Based on the OFs, ACLF is classified into the following grades:
- *ACLF-1:*
  - Single-organ kidney failure
  - A single failure of the liver, coagulation, circulation, or respiration with serum creatinine 1.5–1.9 mg/dL (kidney dysfunction) and/or mild-to-moderate HE
  - Single cerebral failure with kidney dysfunction
- ACLF-2 occurs in patients with two OFs.
- ACLF-3 occurs in patients with three or more OFs.

  The other factors that are incorporated in calculating the CLIF-C ACLF and are important in determining prognosis are *age and white blood cell count at presentation*.

  On the other hand, the AARC model incorporates five variables, bilirubin, creatinine, presence of encephalopathy, INR, and lactate and divides into three grades—*ACLF-1:* Score of 5–7, *ACLF-2:* Scores 8–10, and *ACLF grade 3:* Scores 11–15.

Coming back to our case, if we apply the individual scores, we would get the following results **(Table 1)**:
- *EASL-CLIF:* OFs two (liver, coagulation), Organ Failure Score: 10; CLIF-CACLF Score 46; 28-day estimated mortality: 20%
- *AARC:* AARC grade 2, AARC score 10; 28-day mortality 20%

STEP 4: UNDERSTANDING THE DYNAMICITY OF CHANGES IN ACLF

Once the baseline disease severity is assessed, it is imperative to closely assess the dynamicity of the disease daily with respect to the worsening of OFs or the development of new-onset OFs. The initial management centers around stoppage of the acute insult, hospitalization, and maintaining adequate nutritional support, as was done in our case. However, by day 4 our patient had progressive worsening of liver and coagulation failure as well as development of a new organ dysfunction as HE grade 2 in addition to an increasing trend of creatinine **(Table 1)**. Hence, in comparison to the baseline status the patient has worsening prognostic scores which drives further decisions on management.

STEP 5: PROVIDING HOLISTIC MANAGEMENT IN ACLF

The core goals of management in any case of ACLF include:
- *Nutrition:* A target of 1.5–2.0 g protein/kg/day and 35–40 kcal/kg/day with adjustments for diabetes.
- *Etiology-specific therapies:* This includes specific cases as in HBV-related ACLF, autoimmune hepatitis, and corticosteroids in alcoholic hepatitis.
- *Liver transplantation (LT):* The ultimate cornerstone of management in patients with ACLF remains LT. This mandates an early referral to facilities with hepatology services and LT. LT in ACLF has been shown to have good results in ACLF, with studies showing 1-year probability of survival after LT up to 81% [95% confidence interval (CI) 74–87].[8] However, some studies have shown a lower overall survival, specifically in

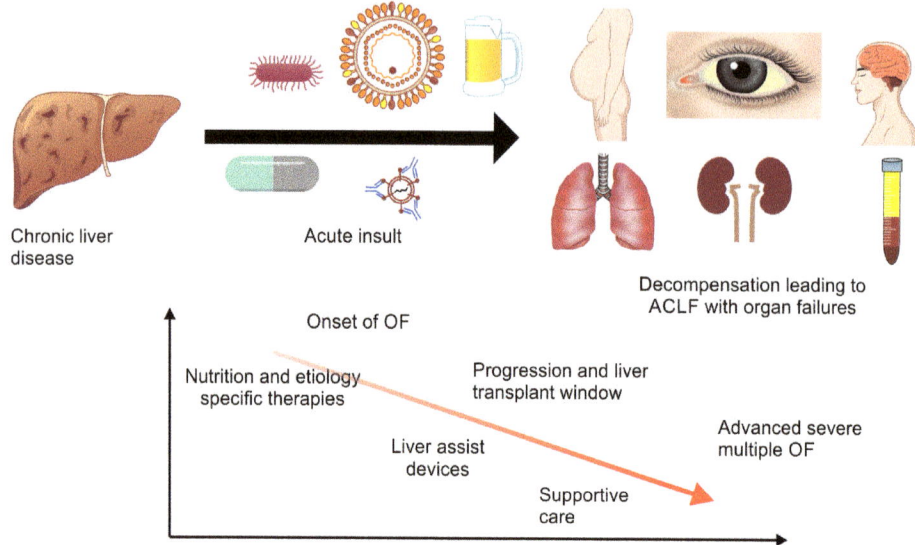

Fig. 1: Depicting the overall course in acute on chronic liver failure (ACLF) with options for therapy. (OF: organ failure)

patients in ACLF grade 3.[9] Hence, it is essential to identify patients in the correct "window" of opportunity for LT before the patient becomes too sick to transplant **(Fig. 1)**.[3] Some of the indicators toward the futility of transplant include active sepsis (persisting fever), PaO_2/FiO_2 ratio <150 mm Hg, a norepinephrine dose >1 μg/kg/min and a serum lactate level >9 mmol/L.[3]

- *Liver support therapies:* Multiple liver support therapies and devices have been attempted in the management of ACLF, including plasma exchange (PLEX), fecal microbiota transplantation (FMT), granulocyte-monocyte stimulating factors, extracorporeal albumin dialysis, molecular adsorbent recirculating system, hemodiafiltration techniques, and continuous renal replacement therapy either in presence or absence of renal failure.[10] The evidence regarding the timing, type of therapy as well as optimal duration is evolving. The objectives of these therapies are twofold, firstly, to act as a "bridge therapy" till the time LT can be done as well as in a subset provide support by acting as a detoxifying mechanism for to liver artificially which allows time for liver regeneration.[11] Of these PLEX has been most extensively utilized with a recent study with 131 patients showing improved systemic inflammation and lower development of OFs as well as survival benefit with PLEX compared to other liver assist devices.[12]

In view of overall deterioration at day 4, the patient was initiated on PLEX and continued on five sessions of PLEX over the next 5 days. The trajectories of the patients' parameters are shown in **Table 1**. Once we achieve a targeted number of sessions of PLEX, then we need to assess the serial dynamics of the patient. If parameters reworsens, then LT remains the best therapeutic modality of choice. In cases where LT is not an option, goals of care need to be discussed with caregivers, and options rotate around continuing PLEX sessions or alternate experimental modalities like FMT and G-CSF need to be explored. Fortunately, in the current case, the patient's parameters stabilized post-PLEX. He was continued on nutritional support with diuretics and anti-HE and, after a prolonged hospital stay of 23 days, he was discharged and did well on follow-up without any need for hospitalization over the next 3 months.

CONCLUSION

Acute on chronic liver failure is an important clinical syndrome, the recognition of which is key in initiating early goal-directed intensive care. Identifying acute precipitants, estimating prognostic scores in a dynamic manner and early therapeutic interventions are key to improved outcomes. However, mortality remains high even with the best care, and LT remains the best option in selected cases without absolute contraindications and must be timed at the appropriate therapeutic window.

REFERENCES

1. D'Amico G, Bernardi M, Angeli P. Towards a new definition of decompensated cirrhosis. J Hepatol. 2022;76(1):202-7.
2. Sen S, Williams R, Jalan R. The pathophysiological basis of acute-on-chronic liver failure. Liver Int. 2002;22(Suppl 2):5-13.
3. Sarin SK, Choudhury A, Sharma MK, Maiwall R, Al Mahtab M, Rahman S, et al; APASL ACLF Research Consortium (AARC) for APASL ACLF working Party. Acute-on-chronic liver failure: consensus recommendations of the Asian Pacific Association for the Study of the Liver (APASL): an update. Hepatol Int. 2019;13(4):353-90.
4. Moreau R, Jalan R, Gines P, Pavesi M, Angeli P, Cordoba J, et al; CANONIC Study Investigators of the EASL–CLIF Consortium. Acute-on-chronic liver failure is a distinct syndrome that develops in patients with acute decompensation of cirrhosis. Gastroenterology. 2013;144(7):1426-37, 1437.e1-9.
5. Chiang DJ, McCullough AJ. The impact of obesity and metabolic syndrome on alcoholic liver disease. Clin Liver Dis. 2014; 18(1):157-63.
6. European Foundation for the Study of Chronic Liver Failure. CLIF-C ACLF Calculator. [online] Available from https://www.efclif.com/scientific-activity/score-calculators/clif-c-aclf [Last accessed November 2023].
7. APASL ACLF Research Consortium. AARC Score and ACLF Grade. [online] Available from: http://www.aclf.in/?page=doctor_aarc_grade_cal [Last accessed November 2023].
8. Belli LS, Duvoux C, Artzner T, Bernal W, Conti S, Cortesi PA, et al; ELITA/EF-CLIF working group. Liver transplantation for patients with acute-on-chronic liver failure (ACLF) in Europe: Results of the ELITA/EF-CLIF collaborative study (ECLIS). J Hepatol. 2021; 75(3):610-22.
9. Sundaram V, Mahmud N, Perricone G, Katarey D, Wong RJ, Karvellas CJ, et al; Multi-Organ Dysfunction, Evaluation for Liver Transplantation (MODEL) Consortium. Long-term outcomes of patients undergoing liver transplantation for acute-on-chronic liver failure. Liver Transpl. 2020;26(12):1594-602.
10. Matar AJ, Subramanian R. Extracorporeal Liver Support: A Bridge to Somewhere. Clin Liver Dis (Hoboken). 2021;18(6):274-9.
11. Kanjo A, Ocskay K, Gede N, Kiss S, Szakács Z, Párniczky A, et al. Efficacy and safety of liver support devices in acute and hyperacute liver failure: a systematic review and network meta-analysis. Sci Rep. 2021;11(1):1-10.
12. Maiwall R, Bajpai M, Choudhury AK, Kumar A, Sharma MK, Duan Z, et al. Therapeutic plasma-exchange improves systemic inflammation and survival in acute-on-chronic liver failure: a propensity-score matched study from AARC. Liver Int. 2021;41(5):1083-96.

Chapter 16: Intrahepatic Cholestasis

Rajesh Upadhyay, VS Gaurav Narayan

■ INTRODUCTION

Cholestatic disorders of the liver can be due to both intra- and extrahepatic causes. Intrahepatic cholestasis classically presents as jaundice, pruritis, and pale stools, although there are exceptions to the norm. Cholestatic disorders of the liver have a wide range of etiology, including familial disorders like benign recurrent intrahepatic cholestasis and Alagille syndrome, gestational disorders like intrahepatic cholestasis of pregnancy, infections like acute viral hepatitis and sepsis, and drug-induced cholestasis **(Table 1)**. It is essential to differentiate extrahepatic from intrahepatic cholestasis in order to delineate the causes, as the line of management is diverse and predominantly cause-oriented. This chapter predominantly deals with the approach to and management of intrahepatic cholestasis.

■ CASE PRESENTATION

A 28-year-old male presented to our emergency department with sudden onset of vomiting, pruritis, abdominal pain, and jaundice. He did not exhibit any constitutional symptoms such as fever or malaise. He did not report any previous history of liver disease. He denied intake of alcohol or any drugs. The examination of the patient revealed a palpable, mildly tender liver, with a liver span of 16 cm. The pattern of jaundice was cholestatic [total bilirubin—58 mg/dL, direct bilirubin 50 mg/dL, aspartate transaminase (AST)—58 U/L, alanine transaminase (ALT)—60 U/L, alkaline phosphatase (ALP)—320 U/L, and gamma-glutamyl transpeptidase (GGT)—520 U/L]. Patient also had deranged renal parameters (creatinine—1.8 mg/dL, urea—58 mg/dL).

TABLE 1: Causes of intrahepatic cholestasis.

Category	Disorders
Drug-induced	• Refer to **Table 2**
Immune-mediated	• Primary biliary cholangitis • Primary sclerosing cholangitis
Infections	• Viral hepatitis A, E • HIV • Cytomegalovirus • Gram-negative bacterial sepsis
Pregnancy-related	Intrahepatic cholestasis of pregnancy
Systemic disorders	• Sarcoidosis • Amyloidosis
Inherited disorders	• Alagille syndrome • PFIC • RBIH • Cystic fibrosis • Dubin–Johnson syndrome

(HIV: human immunodeficiency virus; PFIC: progressive familial intrahepatic cholestasis; RBIH: recurrent benign intrahepatic cholestasis)

On initial investigation, the patient had a normal complete blood count, a negative viral panel [hepatitis A virus immunoglobulin M (HAV IgM), hepatitis E virus (HEV) IgM, hepatitis B surface antigen (HbsAg), hepatitis C virus (HCV) IgG], negative autoimmune hepatitis panel [ANA, ANCA, liver kidney microsomal antibody type 1 (LKM-1)], normal ceruloplasmin levels, and negative anti-mitochondrial antibodies (AMA). The abdominal ultrasonography (USG) revealed mild hepatomegaly with nephrolithiasis in the right kidney. Further, magnetic resonance cholangiopancreatography (MRCP) was done, which did not reveal any evidence of extrahepatic biliary obstruction, or intrahepatic ductal abnormalities. At this stage, the diagnosis was unclear. On further probing, the patient revealed that he regularly visited a gym wherein he was given multiple drugs (as off-label agents) for aesthetic muscle enhancement by the fitness trainer. These included syntropin (a growth hormone analog), testosterone propionate, trenbolone acetate, and drostanolone propionate (synthetic anabolic androgenic steroids). The patient was initiated on ursodeoxycholic acid and cholestyramine, in an attempt to improve the intrahepatic cholestasis. However, due to lack of improvement in pruritis and bilirubin, he was initiated on intravenous hydrocortisone. There was an initial improvement in the total bilirubin level (from 58 to 46 mg/dL) within a span of 72 hours. However, the patient's renal function continued to deteriorate, with the creatinine rising to 4.2 mg/dL in the same period. On consultation with the nephrology team, they initiated intravenous fluids suspecting a prerenal acute kidney injury. However, the renal function failed to improve. A noncontrast computed tomography (CT) of the kidney–ureter–bladder was performed, which showed a shrunken right kidney. This was followed by a DTPA (diethylenetriamine pentaacetate)) scan to assess kidney function which revealed grossly reduced function of the right kidney (32% function). This was an incidental finding, likely due to a previously untreated pyelonephritis. Over the next 5 days, the patients bilirubin reached a plateau, and did not reduce further, in spite of continuing steroid therapy.

A core biopsy of the liver was performed at this stage, which showed the presence of abundant bile plugs, with minimal infiltration of the portal tracts with eosinophils and neutrophils **(Figs. 1A and B)**. Literature suggests that recovery from androgen steroids-induced jaundice may take few weeks to 6 months.[1] The patient continues to be in our follow-up and his bilirubin is gradually improving.

This case is an example of the adverse impact of off-label androgenic steroids on the biliary flow, which could have potentially been life-threatening. It also helps to emphasizes on the importance of a detailed history in identifying the cause of intrahepatic cholestasis.

PATHOGENESIS OF CHOLESTASIS

Intrahepatic cholestasis is a relatively common finding, especially in patients who have sepsis or on antibiotic therapy. These cases are usually resolved upon eliminating the underlying cause. Multiple drugs have been implicated in cholestatic hepatic injury, out of which anabolic steroids have been well documented. There have been multiple advances in understanding the mechanism of biliary uptake and excretion. The hepatocytes are arranged in a plate-like formation, along the blood flow from the portal vein to the central vein. These hepatocytes

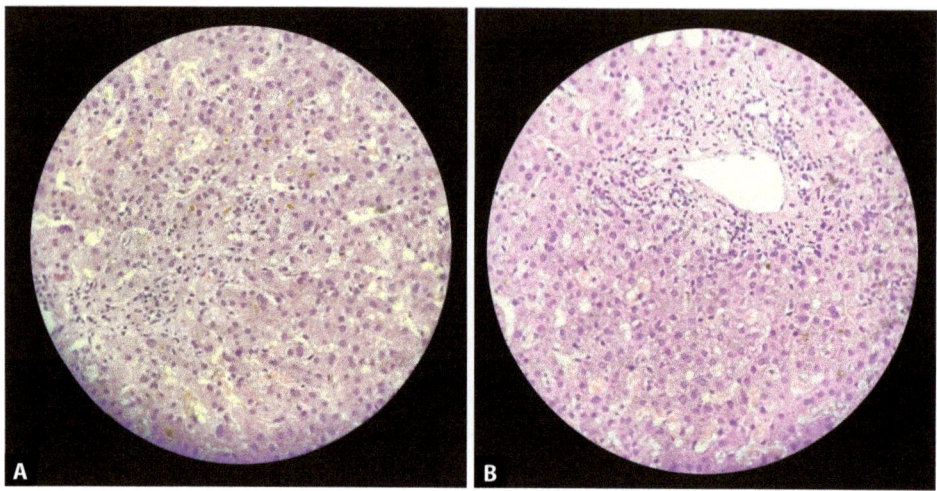

Figs. 1A and B: (A) The presence of multiple bile plugs; (B) Expanded portal tracts with mild increase in eosinophils and neutrophils.

contain intake and excretory systems, in the basolateral (sinusoidal) and apical (canalicular) membranes, respectively. Bile is secreted from the small to large bile ducts via osmosis through this system.[2] Bile acids enter via sodium taurocholate cotransporting polypeptide (NTCP), which helps in concentrating bile acids in the hepatocytes. Organic anion transporting polypeptides (OATP2/OATP1B1) located in the basolateral membranes of hepatocytes also help in entry of the bile acids into hepatocytes. Excretion of bile acids in to bile is facilitated by the canalicular proteins bile salt export pump (BSEP) and multidrug resistance associated protein 2 (MRP2). The MRP2 transporter (ABCC2) helps in secretion of bilirubin, glutathione, and antibiotics like ceftriaxone. Other canalicular membrane transporters are MDR1 (multidrug resistance 1), glycoprotein P (ABCB 1), and MDR3. Cholangiocytes contain another set of receptors that facilitate bile acid reabsorption through the apical membrane of the hepatocytes, namely apical sodium-dependent bile acid transporter (ASBT), and cystic fibrosis transmembrane conductance regulator (CFTR).[3] Cholestasis is caused by alteration in flow through bile ducts, due to mechanical causes or an aberration in the above-mentioned systems.

ETIOLOGY OF INTRAHEPATIC CHOLESTASIS

With advances in understanding the mechanisms of cholestasis, drugs are emerging as one of the primary causes of cholestatic liver injury. Many of these drugs cause a mixed patten of cholestatic and hepatocellular liver injury. These drugs may mimic other causes of intrahepatic and extrahepatic cholestatic disorders. Thus, it is important to identify the offending agent to prevent progression of hepatic injury. Drug-induced cholestasis can often present without jaundice, with merely an elevation of ALP levels. Between 17% and 50% of patients with drug-induced liver injury (DILI) can have features of cholestasis.[4,5] A wide variety of commonly used drugs can induce cholestatic liver injury, including nonsteroidal anti-inflammatory drugs, antihypertensives,

TABLE 2: Causes of drug-induced cholestasis.[11]

Cholestasis without hepatitis	Cholestasis with hepatitis	Cholestasis with bile duct injury	VBDS (ductopenia)	Sclerosing cholangitis-like cholestasis
Anabolic steroids	• INH, macrolides halothane, amoxicillin–clavulanic acid, NSAIDs chlorpromazine, captopril, carbamazepine, itraconazole, dextro-methorphan, atorvastatin, fenofibrate • Gabapentin	Carmustine, gold, amoxicillin–clavulanic acid, flucloxacillin, paraquat	Amitriptyline, amoxicillin–clavulanic acid, ampicillin, azathioprine, carbamazepine, chlorpromazine, clindamycin, diazepam, norandrosterone, phenytoin, tetracyclines, cotrimoxazole	Floxuridine, intralesional agents: hypertonic saline, absolute alcohol, iodine solution, aldehyde, silver nitrate
Estrogens				
Tamoxifen				
Cyclosporine, infliximab				
Nevirapine, glimepiride				
Cetirizine, metolazone				

(INH: isoniazid; NSAIDs: nonsteroidal anti-inflammatory drugs; VBDS: vanishing bile duct syndrome)

antidiabetic, anticonvulsants, lipid-lowering agents, and psychotropic drugs.[6-9] Many of these drugs target the biliary epithelium and can cause "drug-induced cholangiopathy" and vanishing bile duct syndrome (VBDS).[10] Individual drugs that induce drug-induced cholestasis tend to have a characteristic patterns of hepatic injury. However, a single drug can exhibit more than one specific pathological pattern of injury. **Table 2** shows the different kinds of cholestatic liver injury and the drugs that cause them.

Primary biliary cholangitis (PBC) and primary sclerosing cholangitis (PSC) are prototypical immune-mediated cholestatic disorders. PBC usually occurs in middle-aged women between 40 and 60 years of age, with prominent features of intrahepatic cholestasis, and positivity for AMA.[12] PSC predominantly affects men, with a median age of 40 years. Patients with PSC have typical multifocal strictures giving a "bead-like" appearance to the biliary tree on magnetic resonance imaging. Biopsies when taken may show an "onion-peel" pattern of fibrosis.[13,14] IgG4 disease-associated cholangiopathy has been identified relatively recently and may produce similar features.[15]

Pregnancy-generated cholestasis is associated with alteration of hepatic function, which may range from mild-to-severe hepatic injury. Hyperemesis gravidarum, which is present in the first trimester, can be associated with biochemical alteration of liver function tests. However, it does not usually lead to significant cholestasis.[16] Intrahepatic cholestasis of pregnancy, seen in the second and third trimesters, can cause severe cholestasis, associated with elevated bile acids (>40 mmol/L), which can result in poor pregnancy outcomes. It has been observed in up to 6% normal pregnancies.[17]

Total parenteral nutrition has often been associated with cholestasis. This is hypothesized due to lack of enteral feeding, which is necessary for bile secreting mechanisms to get activated. This also causes significant alterations in the entero-hepatic circulation.[18]

Sepsis is an important cause of intrahepatic cholestasis, especially in gram-negative bacterial infections. The endotoxins that are released by these pathogens, such as lipopolysaccharides, cause inhibition of the sodium taurocholate receptors on hepatocytes, causing reduced capture of bile acids. This phenomenon is mediated by inflammatory cytokines, mainly tumor necrosis factor alpha and interferon gamma. Bilirubin levels can exceed 20 mg/dL in sepsis, and other factors such as trauma, hemolysis, and hematoma formation can contribute to the derangement of hepatic parameters.[19-21]

Viral infections such as hepatitis A and E can present with cholestatic features. Cholestasis can be seen in 2–8% of patients with acute viral hepatitis A, which can also occur in a recurring pattern.[22] The incidence of cholestatic jaundice has been observed in up to 60% of patients with hepatitis E infection.[23] HIV (human immunodeficiency virus) cholangiopathy can be seen associated with cytomegalovirus and *Mycobacterium avium* complex infection, though the incidence of HIV-related complications have grossly diminished after the advent of HAART (highly active antiretroviral therapy).[24,25]

Systemic disorders like sarcoidosis can cause noncaseating granulomas in the liver, which can present with elevated ALP and angiotensin-converting enzyme (ACE) levels. This phenomenon may rarely be associated with cholestatic features.[26] Primary and secondary amyloidosis (due to plasm cell neoplasms, connective tissue disorders, tuberculosis) have also been known to cause cholestasis.[27,28]

There are multiple genetic disorders that cause intrahepatic cholestasis, which can present right from the neonatal period to early adulthood. Progressive familial intrahepatic cholestasis (PFIC) type 1 and type 2 are autosomal recessive disorders whose onset occurs during the neonatal period. Cholestatic features usually appear in the first month of life, together with high ALP levels but normal GGT levels. PFIC2 can have severe clinical manifestations, and result in cirrhosis, hepatocellular carcinoma, or cholangiocarcinoma. PRIC 3 occurs later in childhood and can be associated with elevated GGT levels.[29,30]

Recurrent benign intrahepatic cholestasis (RBIH) can present with episodic pruritis and elevated ALP levels, which can last few weeks to months, but the prognosis in usually benign. Alagille syndrome is multisystemic disorder caused due to *JAG1* mutation, that can present with jaundice and elevated ALP. Cystic fibrosis results due to mutation in the *CFTR* gene, causing impaired mucosal clearance. This can result in bronchiectasis, hepatic injury, and cirrhosis, and can often present with a cholestatic pattern of jaundice. Dubin–Johnson syndrome is a genetic form of conjugated hyperbilirubinemia, due to poor expression of the MRP2 transporter that results in altered excretion of bile.[31,32]

DIAGNOSIS

A detailed history, including a list of pharmacological agents and herbal medication that the patient is consuming, will help in narrowing down the etiology. Abdominal pain usually points toward an extrahepatic cause of cholestasis, but a vague abdominal pain can be present in certain cases of intrahepatic cholestasis, such as in DILI.[33] Fever and jaundice, with pain in the right upper abdomen can indicate cholangitis. Patients with malignancy of the gallbladder, pancreas, or cholangiocarcinoma may have associated features like weight loss and anorexia, and often present with painless progressive jaundice. Patients with intrahepatic cholestasis usually have pruritis, in combination with jaundice and/or clay-colored stools. However, many patients with intrahepatic cholestasis may be anicteric and have normal bilirubin levels.[34] In chronic cholestatic disorders, there may be features of fat-soluble vitamin deficiency such as xerosis, osteomalacia, and bleeding manifestations. On physical examination, a palpable lump (when associated with painless jaundice) may indicate a malignant extrahepatic biliary obstruction. Right hypochondrial tenderness may indicate cholangitis or choledocholithiasis. Hepatomegaly may be seen in some cases of intrahepatic cholestasis.

Alkaline phosphatase is the most sensitive test to identify cholestasis, although its specificity is low due to its multiple isoenzymes. Nearly half of the ALP in the body is produced from bones. Measurement of GGT, or ALP isoenzymes when available, helps in determining the hepatic origin of ALP. GGT levels may be elevated in alcoholics, thus limiting its use as supportive marker of cholestasis. It is important to consider the age, gender, and race of the patient in determining the normal limits of ALP. Infectious etiology, including viral hepatitis, should be ruled out in all cases of intrahepatic cholestasis. Additionally, markers of autoimmune hepatitis such as antinuclear antibody (ANA), anti-smooth muscle antibody (ASMA), and serum IgG levels should be measured in the event of clinical suspicion.

An USG of the abdomen is a useful initial investigative tool to exclude extrahepatic biliary obstruction. However, a USG can miss a biliary calculus in up to 60% of obese patients, and is user-dependent, which is a major drawback. A MRCP has far greater sensitivity and specificity for biliary disorders, and may show pathognomonic features in certain conditions like PSC.

A liver biopsy is not indicated in most cases of intrahepatic cholestasis. However, in the event of a diagnostic dilemma, it may be performed. However, pathological features may not be exclusive to a particular etiological agent.

MANAGEMENT

It is essential to identify the primary cause of intrahepatic cholestasis, as it responds well to treatment, or is self-limiting in the majority of the cases. Conventional therapy for mild pruritis includes warm water bath, and first-generation antihistamines like diphenhydramine and hydroxyzine, as their additional sedative effect is beneficial. Ursodeoxycholic acid has only been approved for use in PBC, but it has shown efficacy in other cholestatic disorders. It is hypothesized to work to by stimulating the detoxification of hydrophobic bile acids, by making them hydrophilic, and by stimulating the pregnane X receptor (PXR), facilitating bile excretion.[35] Bile acid sequestrants (BAS) can be used in more severe pruritis, especially if sleep is impaired. Agents such as cholestyramine and colestipol work by chloride anion exchange with bile acids, facilitating their excretion into the intestine. It is important to administer BAS 20 minutes before each meal, so that they act in conjunction with postmeal biliary secretion. It is also important to have a time interval of at least 2 hours before administering other drugs, so as to prevent drug interaction and preserve the sequestrant action. Cholestyramine can be administered up to 24 g/day, and Colestipol has a standard dose of 1 g thrice a day.[36,37]

Farsenoid X receptor agonists, such as obeticholic acid, are still under trial for cholestatic disorders, especially PBC.[38-40] Fibrates such as fenofibrate and bezafibrate are transcriptional modifiers of bile acids, which increases hepatocytic export of bile acids.[41] These are used off-label for the same. The value of steroids in treating cholestatic disorders is controversial. There have been multiple case reports of successful steroid therapy in viral hepatitis-associated cholestasis and drug-induced cholestasis. However, results with steroid use have been heterogeneous, and they may be considered on a case-to-case basis. Rifampicin (150-300 mg/day) can be used patient intolerant of bile acid resins, as it acts as a ligand for PXR and helps in detoxification of bile acids.[42] Phenobarbital (1-5 mg/kg/day divided in three doses) also induces hepatic microsomal enzymes and therefore may facilitate reduction of pruritogens.[43] However long-term administration of microsomal inducers may impair vitamin D metabolism.

CONCLUSION

Androgenic steroids have been extensively documented to cause cholestatic jaundice. However, their illicit use continues undeterred in the fitness industry. Recovery from jaundice caused by androgenic steroids can take several months, and no definitive therapy exists to hasten this process. Although most patients develop self-limiting cholestatic jaundice, few can develop severe vascular changes in the liver called "peliosis hepatitis".[44] On prolonged use, many patients can develop hepatic tumors like adenoma and hepatocellular carcinoma.[45] This should draw our attention to the ineffective regulation of multiple hepatotoxic drugs in the market.

Cholestatic disorders can range from seemingly benign and self-limiting conditions to chronic forms of cholestasis that can result in cirrhosis and portal hypertension. It is vital to identify and ameliorate the cause at an early stage to prevent ongoing hepatic injury. Drugs and infections, including viral etiology should be excluded in all cases of intrahepatic cholestasis as they form the majority of cases. Therapy should be targeted to facilitate bile flow, prevent injury due to bile acid accumulation, and potentiate enterohepatic circulation. Associated conditions, such as osteomalacia and other steatorrhea, should be identified and treated.

REFERENCES

1. LiverTox: Clinical and Research Information on Drug-Induced Liver Injury [Internet]. Bethesda (MD): National Institute of Diabetes and Digestive and Kidney Diseases; 2012.
2. Trauner M, Meier PJ, Boyer JL. Molecular pathogenesis of cholestasis. N Engl J Med. 1998;339(17):1217-27.
3. Elferink RO. Cholestasis. Gut. 2003;52 (Suppl 2): ii42-8.

4. Friis H, Andreasen PB. Drug-induced hepatic injury: an analysis of 1100 cases reported to the Danish Committee on Adverse Drug Reactions between 1978 and 1987. J Intern Med. 1992;232:133-8.
5. Björnsson E, Olsson R. Outcome and prognostic markers in severe drug-induced liver disease. Hepatology. 2005;42(2):481-9.
6. Chitturi S, George J. Hepatotoxicity of commonly used drugs: nonsteroidal anti-inflammatory drugs, antihypertensives, antidiabetic agents, anticonvulsants, lipid-lowering agents, psychotropic drugs. Semin Liver Dis. 2002;22:169-83.
7. Malchow-Møller A, Matzen P, Bjerregaard B, Hilden J, Holst-Christensen J, Staehr Johansen T, et al. Causes and characteristics of 500 consecutive causes of jaundice. Scand J Gastroenterol. 1981;16:1-6.
8. Bjørneboe M, Iversen O, Olsen S. Infective hepatitis and toxic jaundice in a municipal hospital during a five-year period. Incidence and prognosis. Acta Med Scand. 1967;182:491-501.
9. Whitehead MW, Hainsworth I, Kingham JGC. The causes of obvious jaundice in South West Wales: perceptions versus reality. 2000. Gut. 2001;48:409-13.
10. Pérez Fernández T, López Serrano P, Tomás E, Gutiérrez ML, Lledó JL, Cacho G, et al. Diagnostic and therapeutic approach to cholestatic liver disease. Rev Esp Enferm Dig. 2004;96(1):60-73.
11. Padda MS, Sanchez M, Akhtar AJ, Boyer JL. Drug-induced cholestasis. Hepatology. 2011; 53(4):1377-87.
12. Jansen PL, Ghallab A, Vartak N, Reif R, Schaap FG, Hampe J, et al. The ascending pathophysiology of cholestatic liver disease. Hepatology. 2017;65(2):722-38.
13. Williamson KD, Chapman RW. New Therapeutic Strategies for Primary Sclerosing Cholangitis. Semin Liver Dis. 2016;36(1): 5-14.
14. Lindor KD, Kowdley KV, Harrison ME; American College of Gastroenterology. ACG Clinical Guideline: Primary Sclerosing Cholangitis. Am J Gastroenterol. 2015;110(5): 646-59.
15. Zen Y, Harada K, Sasaki M, Sato Y, Tsuneyama K, Haratake J, et al. IgG4-related sclerosing cholangitis with and without hepatic inflammatory pseudotumor, and sclerosing pancreatitis-associated sclerosing cholangitis: do they belong to a spectrum of sclerosing pancreatitis? Am J Surg Pathol. 2004;28:1193-203.
16. Gaba N, Gaba S. Study of liver dysfunction in hyperemesis gravidarum. cureus. 2020; 12(6):e8709.
17. Gao XX, Ye MY, Liu Y Li JY, Li L, Chen W, et al. Prevalence and risk factors of intrahepatic cholestasis of pregnancy in a Chinese population. Sci Rep. 2020;10:16307.
18. Guglielmi FW, Regano N, Mazzuoli S, Fregnan S, Leogrande G, Guglielmi A, et al. Cholestasis induced by total parenteral nutrition. Clin Liver Dis. 2008;12(1):97-110, viii.
19. Geier A, Fickert P, Trauner M. Mechanisms of disease: mechanisms and clinical implications of cholestasis in sepsis. Nat Clin Pract Gastroenterol Hepatol. 2006;3:574-85.
20. Chand N, Sanyal AJ. Sepsis-induced cholestasis. Hepatology. 2007;45:230-41.
21. Geier A, Fickert P, Trauner M. Mechanisms of disease: mechanisms and clinical implications of cholestasis in sepsis. Nat Clin Pract Gastroenterol Hepatol. 2006;3:574-85.
22. Dubin IN, Sullivan BH, LeGolvan PC, Murphy LC. The cholestatic form of viral hepatitis. Am J Med. 1960;29(1):55-72.
23. Chau TN, Lai ST, Tse C, Ng TK, Leung VK, Lim W, et al. Epidemiology and clinical features of sporadic hepatitis E as compared with hepatitis A. Am J Gastroenterol. 2006;101(2):292.
24. Linz C, Ali M, Rotz S, Gholam P, Dumot J. AIDS Cholangiopathy: An Uncommon Presentation in the Antiretroviral Therapy Era: 960. Am J Gastroenterol. 2014;109: S286.
25. Naseer M, Dailey FE, Juboori AA, Samiullah S, Tahan V. Epidemiology, determinants, and management of AIDS cholangiopathy: a review. World J Gastroenterol. 2018;24(7): 767-74.

26. Bass NM, Burroughs AK, Scheuer PJ, James DG, Sherlock S. Chronic intrahepatic cholestasis due to sarcoidosis. Gut. 1982;23: 417-21.
27. Misiakos EP, Bagias G, Tiniakos D, Roditis K, Zavras N, Papanikolaou I, et al. Primary amyloidosis manifesting as cholestatic jaundice after laparoscopic cholecystectomy. Case Rep Surg. 2015;2015: 353818.
28. Kim HJ, Tomaszewski M, Lam EC, Xiong W, Moosavi S. Amyloidosis: A rare cause of severe cholestasis and acute liver failure. ACG Case Rep J. 2020;7(12):e00479.
29. Gunaydin M, Bozkurter Cil AT. Progressive familial intrahepatic cholestasis: diagnosis, management, and treatment. Hepat Med. 2018;10:95-104.
30. Davit-Spraul A, Gonzales E, Baussan C, Jacquemin E. Progressive familial intrahepatic cholestasis. Orphanet J Rare Dis. 2009;4:1.
31. Ermis F, Oncu K, Ozel M, Yazgan Y, Gurbuz AK, Demirturk L, et al. Benign recurrent intrahepatic cholestasis: Late initial diagnosis in adulthood. Ann Hepatol. 2010;9:207-10.
32. Lee YS, Kim MJ, Ki CS, Lee YM, Lee Y, Choe YH. Benign recurrent intrahepatic cholestasis with a single heterozygote mutation in the ATP8B1 gene. Pediatr Gastroenterol Hepatol Nutr. 2012;15:122-6.
33. Viteri AL, Greene JF Jr, Dyck WP. Erythromycin ethylsuccinate-induced cholestasis. Gastroenterology. 1979;76:1007-8.
34. Heathcote EJ. Diagnosis and management of cholestatic liver disease. Clin Gastroenterol Hepatol. 2007;5:776-82.
35. Beuers U. Drug insight: mechanisms and sites of action of ursodeoxycholic acid in cholestasis. Nat Rev Gastroenterol Hepatol. 2006;3:318-28.
36. Fuchs CD, Paumgartner G, Mlitz V, Kuncser V, Halilbasic E, Leditznig N, et al. Colesevelam attenuates cholestatic liver and bile duct injury in Mdr2(-/-) mice by modulating composition, signalling and excretion of faecal bile acids. Gut. 2018;67:1683-91.
37. Scaldaferri F, Pizzoferrato M, Ponziani FR, Gasbarrini G, Gasbarrini A. Use and indications of cholestyramine and bile acid sequestrants. Intern Emerg Med. 2013;8(3):205-10.
38. Brown RS Jr. Use of obeticholic acid in patients with primary biliary cholangitis. Gastroenterol Hepatol (NY). 2018;14(11): 654-7.
39. Manne V, Kowdley KV. Obeticholic acid in primary biliary cholangitis: where we stand. Curr Opin Gastroenterol. 2019;35(3):191-6.
40. Nevens F, Andreone P, Mazzella G, Strasser SI, Bowlus C, Invernizzi P, et al; POISE Study Group. A Placebo-Controlled Trial of Obeticholic Acid in Primary Biliary Cholangitis. N Engl J Med. 2016;375:631-43.
41. Post SM, Duez H, Gervois PP, Staels B, Kuipers F, Princen HM. Fibrates suppress bile acid synthesis via peroxisome proliferator-activated receptor-alpha-mediated downregulation of cholesterol 7alpha-hydroxylase and sterol 27-hydroxylase expression. Arterioscler Thromb Vasc Biol. 2001;21(11):1840-5.
42. Hofmann AF. Rifampicin and treatment of cholestatic pruritus. Gut. 2002;51(5):756-7.
43. Lewis T, Kuye S, Sherman A. Ursodeoxycholic acid versus phenobarbital for cholestasis in the neonatal intensive care unit. BMC Pediatr. 2018;18(1):197.
44. Tsirigotis P, Sella T, Shapira MY, Bitan M, Bloom A, Kiselgoff D, et al. Peliosis hepatis following treatment with androgen-steroids in patients with bone marrow failure syndromes. Haematologica. 2007;92(11): e106-10.
45. Martin NM, Abu Dayyeh BK, Chung RT. Anabolic steroid abuse causing recurrent hepatic adenomas and hemorrhage. World J Gastroenterol. 2008;14(28):4573-5.

Herb-induced Liver Injury

Bhabadev Goswami, Preeti Sarma

■ INTRODUCTION

People all around the world are turning more and more toward natural and organic options, be it food, be it day-to-day use commodities, or even medicines. It is a common understanding among the general population that natural products do not cause any harm and are "fully safe". Our country India has given the world the gift of Ayurveda. Used in correct ways as advised by a qualified ayurvedic practitioner, plant-based remedies help heal a number of illnesses. However, in the hands of quacks or unscrupulous persons, or if such remedies are incorrectly used, then it may lead to very distraughtful results. In this chapter, we will discuss some aspects of herb-induced liver injury (HILI).

Drug-induced liver injury (DILI) has a very high mortality of around 10%. It is a type of hepatic injury wherein the causal agent is usually known in full or part. The causative chemical may be a drug or food supplement or herbal product. Unlike the conventional drugs that we use in our day-to-day practice, herbal medicines/preparations are composed of multiple chemical compounds, many of whose actions or effects are not fully known. In HILI, the causative agent is usually an extract containing different chemical compounds of which one or more product is responsible for the hepatotoxicity. The causative agent in HILI may be a herb or natural product.[1] The liver is usually one of the chief organs responsible for drug metabolism and hence bears the brunt of the toxicity.

The World Health Organization (WHO) defines traditional medicine as theories, beliefs, experiments, knowledge, skills, and practices that are used by people in different cultures and communities to prevent, diagnose, treat, or maintain physical and/or mental health. For example, Ayurveda from India, Sowa Rigpa from Bhutan, Jamu from Indonesia, traditional Chinese medicine, Korean traditional medicine, Kampo from Japan, Unani from Persia and the Arab world, etc.[1] The different types of herbal products may be in the form of leaves, flowers, fruits, tree bark, seeds, roots or the aerial parts of plants. Since time immemorial, people have relied on these different systems of traditional medicine for their health. Proper research and study of these different systems in the near future can help mankind to advance further in the field of health.

■ CASE SCENARIO

When 32-year-old Mr X, a vegetable vendor by occupation, walked into the gastroenterology outpatient department (OPD), he presented with jaundice for more than a month, with itching all over the body and decreased urine output for the last 4 days. He had no history of ethanol intake and smoking. He gave a history of intake of some herbal medication in the form of unidentified dried roots and leaves that was provided to him by a local quack for his jaundice. He had taken the formulation for 5 consecutive days, about 20 days back. But there was no change in his jaundice. His past history did not reveal any significant illness. His general examination was suggestive of icterus, itch marks all over his body, a central patch of hair loss on the head about 3 cm in diameter (which he attributed to herbal medicine that was applied to that area to supposedly suck out his "jaundice"). His vitals were in the normal range. On systemic examination, there was mild hepatomegaly (around 2 cm from the right subcostal margin in the midclavicular line). On analyses of his blood reports, it was found that he had a total serum bilirubin of 43 mg/dL, majority of it being conjugated. His alkaline phosphatase (ALKP) was 465 U/L, AST—182 U/L, and alanine aminotransferase (ALT)—267 U/L. International normalized ratio (INR) was 1.5. He was carrying a report of viral markers suggestive of immunoglobulin M (IgM) anti-HAV positivity that was done in the initial part of his illness by a registered medical practitioner. Rest of the viral markers were negative. The patient had not followed the advice of the doctor and had instead approached the quack for remedy of his jaundice.

He was admitted, further investigations were done, RUCAM (Roussel Uclaf Causality Assessment Method) calculated (except rechallenge), and ultimately a diagnosis of HILI was made. Despite our best efforts, we lost the patient.

EPIDEMIOLOGY

It is very difficult to estimate the exact incidence and prevalence of HILI worldwide. Till a few years back, HILI prevalence was underestimated. Many a time, patients do not give the history of intake of herbal products, considering it to be unimportant and a lot of perseverance is needed on the part of the clinician to elicit that history. Countries where resources for pharmacovigilance is poor, countries where healthcare is costly or inaccessible to the economically backward have a higher incidence of HILI. Some epidemiological data suggest that incidence of HILI in hospital admitted patients in Korea stands at around 0.6%. Whereas, another study from Germany claims an incidence of about 0.12% amongst hospitalized patients. Spain reports an incidence of about 6% in the year 2016 via their DILI registry. In India, data has been limited and approximately 1.3% cases of HILI amongst DILI cases has been recorded. Whereas, many studies report the incidence of HILI to be higher in Asia, Sub-Saharan Africa, one study reported that European countries have 2.75-fold higher caseloads of HILI in comparison to Asia.[1-3]

HERB-INDUCED LIVER INJURY CLASSIFICATION

Intrinsic Type

This type of injury is dose-dependent and predictable. Hepatic injury is seen in overdose. It has a short latency period and is reproducible in animal models, e.g., injury caused by germander and bush tea.

Idiosyncratic

This type of injury is not dose-dependent. Hence, it is not predictable and cannot be reproduced in animal models. This kind of injury may be related to allergic or immunologic events, e.g., injury caused by greater celandine.

Another important classification from the clinical point of view is to divide the injury into *hepatocellular/mixed/cholestatic*. The CIOMS (Council for International Organizations of Medical Sciences) defines hepatotoxicity as rise in ALT and or ALKP more than or equal to two times the upper normal limit. Again another significant recommendation comes from the DILI Expert Working Group that suggests that the ALT be more than or equal to five times the upper normal limit or else more than or equal to three times the upper normal limit with serum bilirubin more than or equal to two times the upper normal limit. There are many other studies with slight variations in the reference values. In order to distinguish between the different types of hepatic injury, we first need to calculate the R ratio. This is done by serum ALT divided by its upper normal limit to be divided by serum ALKP divided by its upper normal limit. If the R ratio is >5, it is suggestive of hepatocellular type of injury. If it is <2, it is indicative of cholestatic injury. Between 2 and 5, the injury is a mixed type.[1,2,4]

■ RISK FACTORS

There have been plenty of variations in age- and gender-related risk factors in different studies from different parts of the world. Preexisting liver disease and alcohol consumption are definite risk factors. Along with that comes certain issues like place of harvesting the plant, soil quality, contamination, insecticides used, storage, and processing conditions, misidentification of the plant parts, etc. Many a time herbal products have been found to be adulterated with heavy metals like mercury, arsenic, lead, cadmium, etc., in an effort to increase the efficacy and to give consumers immediate results to satisfy their requirements. Again, many a time, unscrupulous persons may add synthetic agents to the herbal product without informing the consumer or the clinician so as to fortify the results.

Common agents that have been implicated in HILI from reports all around the world are greater celandine mostly reported from Germany (20.8%), germander reported mostly from France (18.9%), seeds of *Psoralea corylifolia*, chaparral leaf, *Camellia sinensis*, carp juice, arrowroot juice, bee pollen, ginseng, *Polygonum multiflorum* (contains anthraquinones), *Senecio scandens* (contains pyrrolizidine alkaloids), aloe, mistletoe, skullcap, and senna.[1,2,5]

■ CLINICAL PRESENTATION

The diagnosis of HILI is a diagnosis of exclusion. Most important part is the history-taking. The symptoms of HILI are nonspecific and differs according to the type of product used. For example, many patients who presented with HILI after taking Chinese traditional medications showed fatigue, jaundice, anorexia, nausea, fever, rash, pruritus, and pale stools. In India, common presentation was with pruritus, anorexia, fatigue, nausea, vomiting, dark urine, pale stools, and jaundice. HILI due to pyrrolizidine alkaloids presents with features of sinusoidal obstruction syndrome. Products with these type of alkaloids can cross the placenta and cause damage to the unborn fetus. There have been reports from some parts of the world that HILI may also lead on to acute kidney injury and also acute liver failure.[1,5] In another study, it was found that the most common feature was jaundice, followed by pain in abdomen, nausea, fatigue, and choluria.[6]

■ CAUSALITY ASSESSMENT

Diagnoses of HILI requires high degree of suspicion on the part of the clinician. Like many other diseases in medical science, HILI does not have any specific diagnostic test. Rather, there are some scales to measure the likelihood of HILI. These include RUCAM/CIOMS scale, scale of Maria and Victorino. Amongst these, the RUCAM/CIOMS scale is by far the most widely used and validated one. First developed in 1993 and then updated in 2016, it is a quantitative and objective scale.

The RUCAM scale is calculated for each suspected drug with eight separate factors—time to onset, course, risk factors, concomitant drugs, nondrug causes of liver injury, previously known information about hepatotoxicity related to the said drug and response to rechallenge. The individual points range from −3 to +3 whereas the total possible score stands between −9 and +14.[4]

MANAGEMENT

- The first and most important point is to stop usage of the suspected herbal product, in all possible ways.
- Close monitoring of symptoms and liver function
- Glycyrrhizin, ursodeoxycholic acid, N-acetyl cysteine, and corticosteroids have been used by some clinicians with mixed responses.[6]
- For hepatic sinusoidal obstruction syndrome, use of anticoagulation may be considered.
- However, in cases that develop acute liver failure, only liver transplant may be the saving grace.
- There have been case reports of HILI associated with acute kidney injury that have required hemodialysis too.
- All in all, it can be said that management differs from case to case according to the type of presentation.

Coming back to the case mentioned at the beginning of the chapter, the northeastern part of India has a unique problem related to treatment of jaundice by quacks with the usage of local herbs and their products. Many a time, patients come to us with severe jaundice, itching, and renal failure that ultimately portends a poor result.[7] This problem needs to be addressed scientifically and also with the aid of regulations.

CONCLUSION

It can be mentioned that plant and animal products, when used by a qualified practitioner and when the quality of the product can be assured to be safe, then it may definitely help in healing and maintenance of good health. What we need at the moment is research into these different systems of traditional medicine. Also, strict legislature and regulations are needed to ensure quality maintenance and safety.

REFERENCES

1. Nunes DRDCMA, Monteiro CSJ, Dos Santos JL. Herb-Induced Liver Injury—A Challenging Diagnosis. Healthcare (Basel). 2022;10(2):278.
2. Lin NH, Yang HW, Su YJ, Chang CW. Herb induced liver injury after using herbal medicine: a systemic review and case-control study. Medicine (Baltimore). 2019;98(13):e14992.
3. Bunchorntavakul C, Reddy KR. Review article: Herbal and dietary supplement hepatotoxicity. Aliment Pharmacol Ther. 2013;37:3-17.
4. Teschke R, Eickhoff A, Schulze J, Danan G. Herb-induced liver injury (HILI) with 12,068 worldwide cases published with causality assessments by Roussel Uclaf Causality Assessment Method (RUCAM): an overview. Transl Gastroenterol Hepatol. 2021;6:51.
5. Frenzel C, Teschke R. Herbal Hepatotoxicity: Clinical characteristics and listing compilation. Int J Mol Sci. 2016;17(5):588.
6. Ballotin VR, Bigarella LG, Brandão ABM, Balbinot RA, Balbinot SS, Soldera J. Herb-induced liver injury: Systematic review and meta-analysis. World J Clin Cases. 2021;9(20):5490-513.
7. Goswami B, Sharma P, Saikia S, Barooah P, Bhattacharyya M, Medhi S. Acute Toxic hepatitis Induced by Herbal Medicine in Assam: A Pilot Study. Am J Gastroenterol. 113(Supplement):S567.

Autoimmune Hepatitis

Reethesh SR, Manav Wadhawan

CLINICAL CASE SCENARIO

A 32-year-old female patient with hypothyroidism presented with history of painless progressive jaundice of 20 days' duration not preceded by viral prodrome followed by abdominal distension of 10 days' duration. There is no history of altered sensorium or gastrointestinal (GI) bleed. She had history of fatigue, malaise, and arthralgia preceding jaundice by several months. She denies alcohol intake. She has taken oral contraceptives (OCPs) daily for 1 year and there is no complementary and alternative medicine (CAM) intake. There is no history of liver disease in family, but her mother and sister have hypothyroidism. Her physical examination is remarkable for body mass index (BMI) of 31 kg/m^2, icterus, pedal edema, and ascites.

Notable lab parameters include neutrophilic leukocytosis [total leukocyte count (TLC) 14,200 N 80%], total bilirubin 5 g/dL, aspartate transaminase/alanine transaminase (AST/ALT) 353/393 U/L, ALP 136 U/L, albumin (Alb) 2.8 g/dL, and international normalized ratio (INR) 2.4. Renal parameters were normal. Ultrasonography (USG) abdomen showed coarsened echotexture with portal vein diameter of 13.5 mm and grade II ascites.

Question 1: What are the syndromic diagnosis and possible etiologies?
Answer: This young lady has marked elevation of bilirubin, with moderate-to-severe elevation of her serum transferase levels and coagulopathy complicated within 4 weeks by the development of ascites favoring a syndromic diagnosis of acute on chronic liver failure (ACLF) [according to APASL (Asian Pacific Association for the Study of the Liver) Criteria for ACLF].[1]

The possible etiologies of underlying *chronic liver disease* would include viral, nonalcoholic steatohepatitis (NASH), autoimmune and metabolic liver diseases (Wilson disease). Since the patient is a young female with history of arthralgia, malaise, and fatigue and history of hypothyroidism with family history of possible autoimmune disorder (thyroid disease), it would be compelling to place autoimmune hepatitis (AIH) as the first etiological diagnosis. Considering the age, Wilson also would be an important differential if viral causes are ruled out. At the young age of 32, NASH is an unlikely etiology (**Figure 1**).

Acute insult could be an AIH flare, hepatitis B virus (HBV) reactivation, or acute viral hepatitis.

Question 2: How do you investigate this patient further?
Answer: Viral serologies [hepatitis B surface antigen (HBsAg), anti-hepatitis C virus (HCV), immunoglobulin hepatitis A virus (IgM HAV), IgM hepatitis E virus (HEV)], autoimmune markers [antinuclear antibody (ANA), anti-smooth muscle antibody (ASMA), anti-liver kidney microsomal antibody (LKM)], IgG

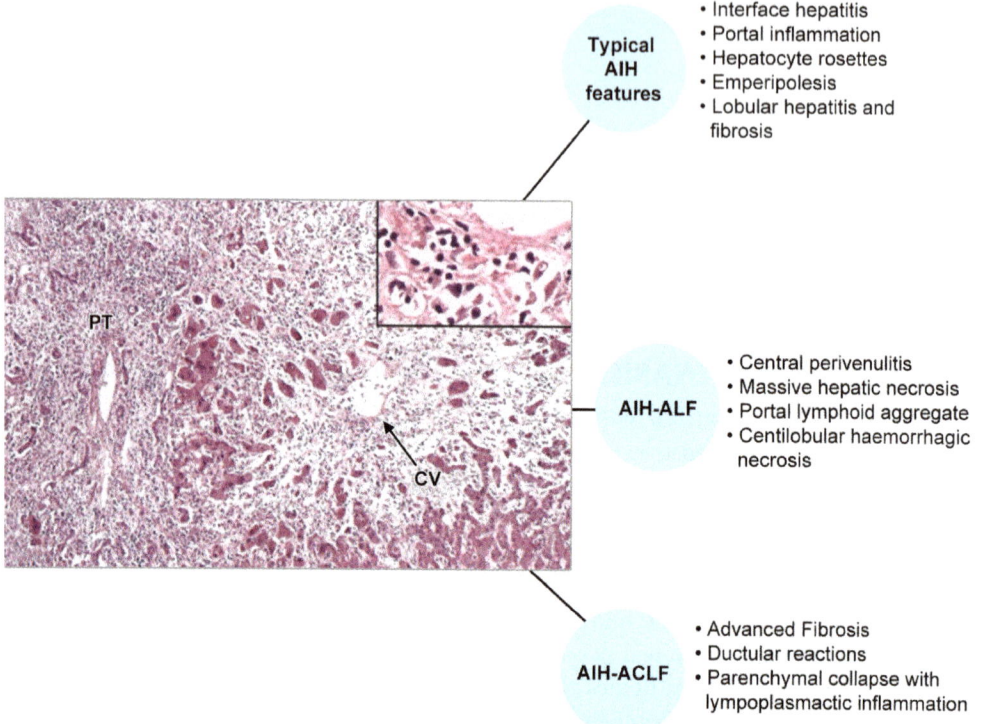

Fig. 1: Features of three types of AIH. (ACLF: acute on chronic liver failure; AIH: autoimmune hepatitis)

levels, and serum ceruloplasmin to establish acute and chronic insult.

In our case viral serologies were negative, autoimmune markers were negative with slightly raised IgG levels (1,800 mg/dL, n <1600) and normal serum ceruloplasmin levels.

It is imperative to note that similar to patients with fulminant AIH, nearly half of the patients with AIH-ACLF are seronegative with normal or mildly raised IgG levels. Hence in this clinical scenario (ACLF), if there is strong clinical suspicion of AIH, liver biopsy may be the only method for diagnosing AIH.[2]

Question 3: What are the indications of liver biopsy in ACLF?
Answer: Liver biopsy is considered essential when etiology is uncertain especially in the setting of negative autoantibodies and normal IgG levels with a high index of suspicion of autoimmunity (extrahepatic features of autoimmunity or family history of autoimmune disorder including vitiligo, thyroiditis, type I diabetes, etc.). Transjugular route is preferred in view of coagulopathy/ascites. The indications for liver biopsy in the setting of ACLF needs to be individualized and should be considered in alcoholic hepatitis, severe AIH, and flare of Wilson disease. Liver biopsy indicates the stage of fibrosis and guiding in prognostication and outcomes in patients with ACLF. On the other hand, in viral or NASH-related ACLF, liver biopsy may be of little help in planning treatment.

Question 4: What do you expect to find in liver biopsy of AIH-related ACLF?

Answer: The histological features seen in AIH-ACLF shows distinctive features that is quite different from those seen in AIH-ALF (acute liver failure). Stravitz et al.[3] identified massive hepatic necrosis with lymphoid aggregates and perivenular inflammation in patients with AIH-ALF. Lymphoid aggregates and perivenular inflammation are less marked in AIH-ACLF. F3–F4 fibrosis, ductular reactions, and areas of parenchymal collapse with lymphoplasmacytic infiltrates are seen in addition to classical autoimmune features in AIH-ACLF as shown in the multicentric AIH-ACLF data from AARC (APASL-ACLF Research Consortium) database.[4]

In our patient liver biopsy showed chronic interface hepatitis with lymphoplasmacytic inflammation of portal tracts with large areas of parenchymal collapse, modified Ishak histology activity index (HAI) score 8/18, and fibrosis stage: 3/6.

Question 5: What further investigation would you obtain for management?
Answer: The further investigation includes upper gastrointestinal endoscopy (UGIE) for variceal status and workup for infections (ascitic fluid for counts and cultures, blood and urine cultures, chest X-ray and serum procalcitonin)

Question 6: What are the indications of steroids in AIH related ACLF?
Answer: Conventional therapy with steroids and azathioprine has shown clinical and biochemical improvement in 68–75% of patients with acute presentations, and high-dose steroids is found to be effective in 20–100% of patients with fulminant presentation of AIH.[5]

Role of corticosteroids in AIH-ACLF has not been extensively evaluated. In a study conducted by Anand et al.[4] which evaluated the safety and efficacy of steroids in AIH-ACLF, it was observed that 3 months' survival and reduced intensive care unit (ICU) stay was significantly better in those receiving steroids. It also highlighted the relative safety of prednisolone treatment as there were no increased risk of infections.

With respect to corticosteroid responsiveness, it was seen that young patients and milder form of disease [Model for End-Stage Liver Disease (MELD) <27] had a favorable response whereas hepatic encephalopathy and advanced liver fibrosis (≥F3) had a negative impact on responsiveness to steroids.

In another retrospective study of AIH patients presenting with ACLF with no extrahepatic organ involvement,[6] they observed transplant-free survival rates of 55% at 3 months and 30% at 6 months with steroids. Extrahepatic organ failure was the principal event contributing to substantially increased risk of mortality, and steroids were unlikely to have a statistically significant impact on such an advanced disease. Such patients were better managed with supportive treatment. Infections were seen in approximately 40% of patients receiving steroids despite administration of prophylactic antibiotics.

The decision to treat AIH-ACLF with steroids should therefore be based on baseline disease severity as assessed by MELD score, extrahepatic organ involvement, and stage of fibrosis. Once started on steroids, they have to be closely monitored for changes in liver disease severity (ΔMELD) and infections. Poor responders can be identified as early as 1–2 weeks with a need to stop steroids and should be counseled for liver transplantation (LT).

Our patient had a MELD score of 22 and did not have extrahepatic organ failure and infection workup (ascitic fluid, cultures, chest X-ray, and serum procalcitonin) were negative. She was started on steroids at

40 mg/day under the cover of prophylactic antibiotic cover.

She responded rapidly with improvement in clinical and laboratory parameters over a period of 1 week and was discharged at 2 weeks after starting steroids (tapering of steroids was done on OPD basis).

Question 7: What are the emerging therapies in AIH-ACLF?

Answer: Plasmapheresis may be offered as a specific therapy for patients with acute severe AIH or AIH-ACLF and those deemed unsuitable for steroid therapy.[7] Plasma exchange has shown promising results and acts as an effective bridging therapy in patients with ACLF to LT or spontaneous regeneration. Plasma exchange can be safely undertaken in patients with ACLF in specialized liver units.

Question 8: Describe liver transplant for AIH-ACLF.

Answer: Post-transplant survival rates in AIH-related ACLF is comparable to other etiologies of ACLF. Post-transplant survival rates among patients with grade 1 and 2 ACLF are similar to those seen in patients without ACLF. One-year survival rate of patients with grade 3 ACLF varies among studies and ranges from 44% to 83%.[8] Recurrent AIH is common post-LT and seen to occur in 8–12% of transplanted patients at 1 year and 36–68% at 5 years.[9]

■ SUMMARY

- AIH-ACLF often has an atypical presentation, with almost half of the patients being seronegative with normal IgG levels, necessitating a lower threshold for transjugular liver biopsy (TJLB) to make a diagnosis.
- The complex interplay of ongoing inflammation, increased susceptibility to infections, and high propensity for extrahepatic organ involvement makes ACLF a distinct entity and a difficult one to manage

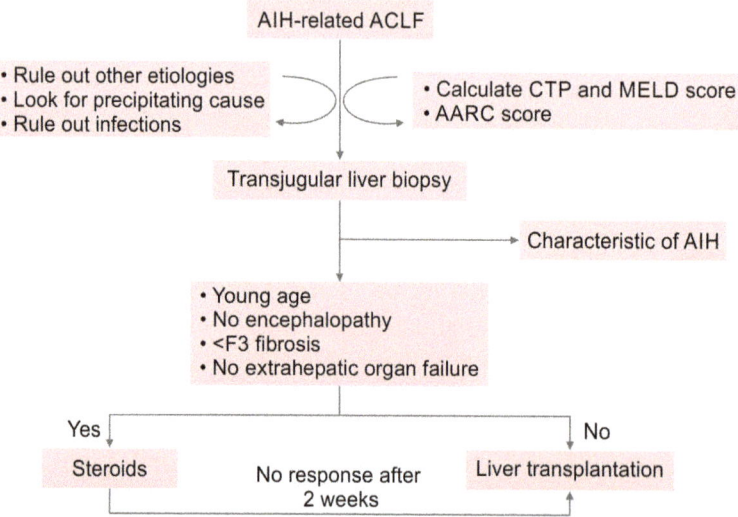

Flowchart 1: Treatment flow of AIH related ACLF.

(AARC: APASL-ACLF Research Consortium; ACLF: acute on chronic liver failure; AIH: autoimmune hepatitis; CTP: Child–Turcotte–Pugh; MELD: Model for End-Stage Liver Disease)

- The histological changes seen in AIH-ACLF are distinct from those found in AIH-ALF.
- Corticosteroids has shown a distinct benefit in management, especially in early and less severely ill patients.
- Patients with MELD ≤26 and no extrahepatic organ involvement may benefit with steroid treatment.
- Patients on steroids should be closely monitored for changes in MELD (ΔMELD) and infections over 1–2 weeks. Nonresponders should be offered LT and steroids stopped.
- MELD >26 can be offered liver transplant without steroid trial as survival with steroids is very poor in this subgroup **(Flowchart 1)**.

REFERENCES

1. Sarin SK, Choudhury A, Sharma MK, Maiwall R, Al Mahtab M, Rahman S, et al. APASL ACLF Research Consortium (AARC) for APASL ACLF working Party. Acute-on-chronic liver failure: consensus recommendations of the Asian Pacific association for the study of the liver (APASL): an update. Hepatol Int. 2019;13(4):353-90.
2. Czaja AJ, Carpenter HA, Santrach PJ, Moore SB, Homburger HA. The nature and prognosis of severe cryptogenic chronic active hepatitis. Gastroenterology. 1993;104(6):1755-61.
3. Stravitz RT, Lefkowitch JH, Fontana RJ, Gershwin ME, Leung PSC, Sterling RK, et al. Acute Liver Failure Study Group. Autoimmune acute liver failure: proposed clinical and histological criteria. Hepatology. 2011;53(2):517-26.
4. Anand L, Choudhury A, Bihari C, Sharma BC, Kumar M, Maiwall R, et al. APASL ACLF (APASL ACLF Research Consortium) Working Party. Flare of Autoimmune Hepatitis Causing Acute on Chronic Liver Failure: Diagnosis and Response to Corticosteroid Therapy. Hepatology. 2019;70(2):587-96.
5. Ichai P, Duclos-Vallée JC, Guettier C, Hamida SB, Antonini T, Delvart V, et al. Usefulness of corticosteroids for the treatment of severe and fulminant forms of autoimmune hepatitis. Liver Transpl. 2007;13(7):996-1003.
6. Sharma S, Agarwal S, Gopi S, Anand A, Mohta S, Gunjan D, et al. Determinants of Outcomes in Autoimmune Hepatitis Presenting as Acute on Chronic Liver Failure Without Extrahepatic Organ Dysfunction upon Treatment With Steroids. J Clin Exp Hepatol. 2021;11(2):171-80.
7. Tan EXX, Wang MX, Pang J, Lee GH. Plasma exchange in patients with acute and acute-on-chronic liver failure: a systematic review. World J Gastroenterol. 2020;26(2):219-45.
8. Levesque E, Winter A, Noorah Z, Daurès JP, Landais P, Feray C, et al. Impact of acute-on-chronic liver failure on 90-day mortality following a first liver transplantation. Liver Int. 2017;37(5):684-93.
9. Montano-Loza AJ, Mason AL, Ma M, Bastiampillai RJ, Bain VG, Tandon P. Risk factors for recurrence of autoimmune hepatitis after liver transplantation. Liver Transpl. 2009;15(10):1254-61.

19. Recompensation and Reversal of Cirrhosis: Myth or Reality?

Naveen Bhagat, Arka De, Ajay Duseja

■ CASE REPORT

A female child aged 13 years, diagnosed case of B-cell acute lymphoblastic leukemia in remission, presented to us in with abdominal distension for 3 months and pedal edema for 1 month. There was no history of jaundice, altered sensorium, bleeding, fever, sore throat, rash, frothy urine, respiratory distress, or growth failure. Physical examination revealed pedal edema and ascites with no organomegaly.

Routine investigations showed thrombocytopenia (14×10^9/L), hypoalbuminemia (2.9 g/dL), deranged liver functions [total bilirubin: 2.9 mg/dL, aspartate transaminase (AST): 292 U/L; alanine transaminase (ALT): 161 U/L; alkaline phosphatase (ALP): 250 U/L] and coagulopathy [international normalized ratio (INR): 1.9]. On ultrasound, liver was 10.9 cm in span with irregular outline and gross ascites was present. Etiological workup revealed seropositivity for hepatitis B surface antigen (HBsAg). She was hepatitis B e antigen (HBeAg) positive, anti-HBe negative, IgM anti-HBc negative with hepatitis B virus (HBV) DNA levels of 3.7×10^7 IU/mL. Diagnostic paracentesis revealed high-gradient [serum ascites albumin gradient (SAAG): 1.9], low-protein (0.9 g/dL) ascitic fluid without spontaneous bacterial peritonitis. Esophagogastroduodenoscopy showed mild portal hypertensive gastropathy and small, low-risk esophageal varices. Transjugular liver biopsy was done which showed marked bridging fibrosis with incomplete and complete nodule formation (METAVIR stage F4, histologic activity index—6) **(Fig. 1)**.

After the diagnosis, she was started on Tab entecavir 0.5 mg/day and within 3 months, there was normalization of liver function tests with resolution of ascites with no requirement of diuretics. She attained anti-HBe seroconversion with HBV negativity after 18 months of treatment. Liver stiffness measurement (LSM) using FibroScan done 2 years after the start of treatment was 7.8 kPa suggesting a reversal of cirrhosis. AST Platelet Ratio Index (APRI) score of 0.4 and Fibrosis-4 (FIB-4) score of 0.35 further corroborated the absence of advanced fibrosis. She continues to do well on follow-up with maintained

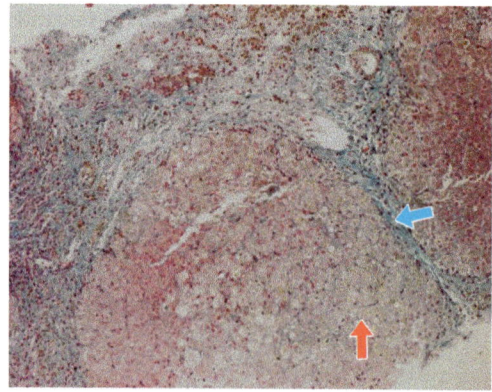

Fig. 1: Liver biopsy (Masson Trichrome stain) showing cirrhotic nodules (red arrow) surrounded by thin fibrous septa (blue arrow).

viral suppression and normal liver functions. Her LSM on last follow-up was 5.6 kPa suggesting continuing regression of fibrosis over time.

DISCUSSION

Cirrhosis has been traditionally considered to be relentlessly progressive ultimately culminating in end-stage liver disease. While most patients with compensated cirrhosis are asymptomatic, the onset of clinical decompensation including ascites, variceal bleed, and hepatic encephalopathy are landmark events in the natural history of cirrhosis and dramatically increases mortality. Indeed, while survival in compensated cirrhosis may well extend to more than a decade, the median survival after onset of ascites is only around 2 years.[1] Control of the etiologic driver of liver disease has been shown to alter the natural history of cirrhosis (including those with clinical decompensation) with increase in survival. In chronic hepatitis B (CHB), current guidelines recommend treatment with immunomodulatory agents, such as interferon alpha and pegylated interferon alpha, and oral nucleoside/nucleotide analogs (NAs), including lamivudine, adefovir, telbivudine, entecavir, and tenofovir. NAs with high barriers to resistance like tenofovir and entecavir are usually preferred drugs. Antivirals are recommended in compensated cirrhosis with detectable HBV DNA and in all patients of decompensated cirrhosis.[2,3]

In our patient who presented with decompensated cirrhosis, viral suppression with entecavir led to control of ascites even without the need of diuretics. Attainment of control of decompensation, i.e., recompensation following correction of underlying etiology has been clinically recognized for a long time. However, it is only

BOX 1: Criteria for recompensation as per Baveno VII consensus.

- Removal/suppression/cure of the primary etiology of cirrhosis (viral elimination for hepatitis C, sustained viral suppression for hepatitis B, sustained alcohol abstinence for alcohol-induced cirrhosis)
- Resolution of ascites (off diuretics), encephalopathy (off lactulose/rifaximin) and absence of recurrent variceal hemorrhage (for at least 12 months)
- Stable improvement of liver function tests (albumin, international normalized ratio, bilirubin)

recently that formal attempts have been made to define recompensation.[4] It is important to understand that recompensation should entail that there is at least a degree of regression of structural and functional changes of cirrhosis in addition to removal of the underlying etiologic driver. As per the recent Baveno VII consensus, definition of recompensation requires the fulfilment of three criteria as shown in **Box 1**.[5] In a recent multicentric study, entecavir treatment for 120 weeks was associated with recompensation (as per Baveno VII consensus) in 159 (56.2%) of 283 patients with decompensated (ascites) HBV-related cirrhosis.[6]

Classically cirrhosis has been considered to be an irreversible alteration of liver architecture. However, it is now recognized that reversal of cirrhosis is possible particularly if the etiology is treatable and the ongoing hepatic insult can be halted. Indeed, regression of fibrosis has been documented in etiologies where the necro-inflammatory injury can be arrested by therapy as in autoimmune hepatitis, chronic viral hepatitis, Wilson's disease and hemochromatosis.[7] Using paired-biopsies in 96 cirrhotic patients with HBV, Marcellin et al. observed reversal of cirrhosis with viral suppression

TABLE 1: Studies with paired biopsies documenting reversal of advanced fibrosis and cirrhosis in patients with chronic hepatitis B.

Studies	Number of patients with advanced fibrosis or cirrhosis at baseline	Nucleoside inhibitor	Time to second biopsy	Fibrosis regression at second biopsy in patients with advanced fibrosis or cirrhosis at baseline (%)
Dienstag et al.[13]	30	Lamivudine	3 years	67%
Rizzetto et al.[14]	24	Lamivudine	3 years	46%
Schiff et al.[15]	47	Lamivudine	1 year	41%
Hadziyannis et al.[16]	12	Adefovir	5 years	58%
Marcellin et al.[17]	15	Adefovir	5 years	60%
Yokosuka et al.[18]	13	Entecavir	3 years	85%
Chang et al.[19]	10	Entecavir	6 years	100%
Marcellin et al.[8]	348	Tenofovir	5 years	51%

in 74% patients over a follow-up period of 5 years.[8] Some of the other studies that have documented reversal of advanced fibrosis and cirrhosis with treatment of HBV are summarized in **Table 1**.

The baseline diagnosis of cirrhosis in our patient was established using the gold standard of liver biopsy. Repeat biopsy on follow-up was not feasible as the patient refused to consent for the same. Noninvasive tests for hepatic fibrosis like LSM, APRI, and FIB-4 have been consistently shown to have excellent negative predictive values for ruling out cirrhosis and advanced fibrosis.[9] Concordance between different noninvasive tests further increases the diagnostic certainty. In our patient, LSM, APRI, and FIB-4 on follow-up were all corroborative of the absence of advanced fibrosis thereby strongly suggesting the reversal of cirrhosis.

Apart from suppression of the etiologic driver, other key determinants of potential reversibility of cirrhosis are the width of the fibrous septa and size of the nodules on histology. Cirrhosis with large nodules and thin fibrous septa has high potential for reversibility while atrophic cirrhosis with small nodules and large fibrous septa are unlikely to reverse

TABLE 2: Laennec subclassification of cirrhosis (METAVIR stage 4).

Stage	Histology
A	Cirrhosis with large nodules and thin septa
B	Cirrhosis with smaller nodules and larger septa
C	Atrophic cirrhosis with small nodule and large fibrous septa

Potential for fibrosis regression even with control of etiology decreases with advancement of stage

after cessation of hepatic insult.[10,11] These histologic features have been incorporated in Laennec subclassification of cirrhosis **(Table 2)**.[12] In our patient, the presence of thin fibrous septa and incomplete nodules at baseline, the timely detection and treatment of HBV along with attainment of sustained viral suppression were key factors that led to the reversal of cirrhosis. The young age of the patient may have also helped in recovery.

■ CONCLUSION

Recompensation and even regression of cirrhosis may be possible if the underlying etiology is managed especially in a background of thin fibrous septa which may permit reestablishment of lobular architecture.

REFERENCES

1. European Association for the Study of the Liver. EASL Clinical Practice Guidelines for the management of patients with decompensated cirrhosis. J Hepatol. 2018; 69(2):406-60.
2. Terrault NA, Lok ASF, McMahon BJ, Chang KM, Hwang JP, Jonas MM, et al. Update on prevention, diagnosis, and treatment of chronic hepatitis B: AASLD 2018 hepatitis B guidance. Hepatology. 2018;67(4):1560-99.
3. European Association for the Study of the Liver. EASL 2017 Clinical Practice Guidelines on the management of hepatitis B virus infection. J Hepatol. 2017;67(2):370-98.
4. Zhao H, Wang Q, Luo C, Liu L, Xie W. Recompensation of Decompensated Hepatitis B Cirrhosis: Current Status and Challenges. Biomed Res Int. 2020 21;2020:9609731.
5. de Franchis R, Bosch J, Garcia-Tsao G, Reiberger T, Ripoll C; Baveno VII Faculty. Baveno VII - Renewing consensus in portal hypertension. J Hepatol. 2022;76(4):959-74.
6. Wang Q, Zhao H, Deng Y, Zheng H, Xiang H, Nan Y, et al. Validation of Baveno VII criteria for recompensation in entecavir-treated patients with hepatitis B-related decompensated cirrhosis. J Hepatol. 2022; 77(6):1564-72.
7. Sohrabpour AA, Mohamadnejad M, Malekzadeh R. Review article: the reversibility of cirrhosis. Aliment Pharmacol Ther. 2012;36:824-32.
8. Marcellin P, Gane E, Buti M, Afdhal N, Sievert W, Jacobson IM, et al. Regression of cirrhosis during treatment with tenofovir disoproxil fumarate for chronic hepatitis B: a 5-year open-label follow-up study. Lancet. 2013;381(9865):468-75.
9. European Association for the Study of the Liver. Electronic address: easloffice@easloffice.eu; Clinical Practice Guideline Panel; Chair: EASL Governing Board representative; Panel members. EASL Clinical Practice Guidelines on non-invasive tests for evaluation of liver disease severity and prognosis - 2021 update. J Hepatol. 2021; 75:659-89.
10. Bedossa P. Reversibility of hepatitis B virus cirrhosis after therapy: who and why? Liver Int. 2015;35 Suppl 1:78-81.
11. Rockey DC. Liver fibrosis reversion after suppression of hepatitis B virus. Clin Liver Dis. 2016;20:667-79.
12. Kim SU, Oh HJ, Wanless IR, Lee S, Han KH, Park YN. The Laennec staging system for histological sub-classification of cirrhosis is useful for stratification of prognosis in patients with liver cirrhosis. J Hepatol. 2012;57:556-63.
13. Dienstag JL, Goldin RD, Heathcote EJ, Hann HW, Woessner M, Stephenson SL, et al. Histological outcome during long-term lamivudine therapy. Gastroenterology. 2003; 124(1):105-17.
14. Rizzetto M, Tassopoulos NC, Goldin RD, Esteban R, Santantonio T, Heathcote EJ, et al. Extended lamivudine treatment in patients with HBeAg-negative chronic hepatitis B. J Hepatol. 2005;42(2):173-9.
15. Schiff E, Simsek H, Lee WM, Chao YC, Sette H Jr, Janssen HL, et al. Efficacy and safety of entecavir in patients with chronic hepatitis B and advanced hepatic fibrosis or cirrhosis. Am J Gastroenterol. 2008;103(11):2776-83.
16. Hadziyannis SJ, Tassopoulos NC, Heathcote EJ, Chang TT, Kitis G, Rizzetto M, et al. Long-term therapy with adefovir dipivoxil for HBeAg-negative chronic hepatitis B for up to 5 years. Gastroenterology. 2006;131(6): 1743-51.
17. Marcellin P, Chang TT, Lim SG, Sievert W, Tong M, Arterburn S, et al. Long-term efficacy and safety of adefovir dipivoxil for the treatment of hepatitis B e antigen-positive chronic hepatitis B. Hepatology. 2008;48(3):750-8.
18. Yokosuka O, Takaguchi K, Fujioka S, Shindo M, Chayama K, Kobashi H, et al. Long-term use of entecavir in nucleoside-naïve Japanese patients with chronic hepatitis B infection. J Hepatol. 2010;52(6):791-9.
19. Chang TT, Liaw YF, Wu SS, Schiff E, Han KH, Lai CL, et al. Long-term entecavir therapy results in the reversal of fibrosis/cirrhosis and continued histological improvement in patients with chronic hepatitis B. Hepatology. 2010;52(3):

Sickle Hepatopathy

AC Anand, Shivam Kalia, Dibyalochan Praharaj, Preetam Nath, Sarat Chandra Panigrahi, Bipadabhanjan Mallick, Saroj Kant Sahu

■ INTRODUCTION

Sickle cell disease (SCD) is one of the most common monogenetic disorders with an autosomal recessive inheritance that cause qualitative dysfunction of beta chain of hemoglobin.[1] The most frequently occurring form of SCD is sickle cell anemia (HbSS), followed by sickle hemoglobin C (HbSC) and sickle-beta (HbS/beta)-thalassemia. About 5–7% of the whole world population is the carrier of a hemoglobinopathy.[2] Prevalence in the Indian subcontinent is second only to Africa.[3] Early diagnosis and initiation of treatment is crucial, and without which, about 90% of children die in the first few years of life.[4]

Hepatic involvement can occur because of the complications of sickling process per se or hemolysis. In addition, these patients often receive multiple blood transfusions which leads to increased risk of viral hepatitis and iron overload (combined effect of chronic hemolysis and blood transfusion).[5]

Sickle cell hepatopathy or sickle hepatopathy (SH) encompasses a spectrum of liver diseases arising from a wide variety of these insults to the liver which include gall stone disease, hypoxic liver injury, hepatic sequestration, venous outflow obstruction, viral hepatitis, hepatic crisis, and sickle cell intrahepatic cholestasis (SCIC).[6] Predominantly, SH occurs in patients with homozygous HbSS, and less commonly in patients with HbSC disease or HbS/beta-thalassemia.[7]

Acute sickle hepatic crisis occurs in approximately 10% patients with SCD.[8] The classical presentation of patients is right upper quadrant (RUQ) abdominal pain, nausea, low-grade fever, tender hepatomegaly, and elevated bilirubin levels (predominantly the conjugated fraction). The pathogenesis of sickle hepatic crisis involves formation of sickle cell thrombi in sinusoidal space which leads to sinusoidal obstruction and ischemia.[8,9]

Sickle cell intrahepatic cholestasis represents a severe variant of acute sickle cell crisis which is characterized by a disseminated sinusoidal occlusion followed by hepatic ischemia and acute liver failure (ALF). Unless treated aggressively, these patients develop coagulopathy, encephalopathy and multiorgan failure (MOF).[10,11] Outcome is usually fatal without vigorous exchange transfusions or liver transplantation (LT). Here we describe a young girl who presented to us with progressive jaundice for 3 months.

■ CASE REPORT

Nine-year-old girl from western Odisha, with no prior comorbidities and sickle cell trait in father presented with complaints of jaundice for 3 months which was painful, progressive, with pruritus. Abdominal pain was localized to RUQ, dull aching type and was not related to position or food intake. One day prior to presentation, she developed lethargy, progressive drowsiness and altered behavior. On examination she was found to have pulse rate—120/min, blood pressure—70/40 mm Hg; respiratory rate—32 breaths/min, and was febrile (temperature—101 F). On general examination she was found to have Icterus, abdominal examination revealed palpable liver and spleen. Rest of the systemic examination were within normal limits.

Hematological examination done revealed hemoglobin of 8.6 g/dL. Total leukocyte counts and platelet counts were within normal limits. Corrected reticulocyte count was elevated to 10%. Peripheral smear showed presence of sickle cells. International normalized ratio (INR) was 2.8. Liver function showed hyperbilirubinemia (total serum bilirubin—26 mg/dL with the conjugated fraction being 22 mg/dL). Serum aspartate transaminase (AST) level was elevated to about three times upper limit of normal. Serum alkaline phosphatase (ALP) and gamma-glutamyl-transpeptidase (GGT) were also significantly elevated. She also had hypoalbuminemia with serum albumin level of 2.8 g/dL. Surprisingly, serum alanine transaminase (ALT) level was with in normal limits. Serum ceruloplasmin level was 43 mg/dL and 24-hour urinary copper was 80 µg/dL. Slit lamp bi-microscopic examination revealed absence of Kayser-Fleischer (KF) ring. Autoimmune markers (antinuclear antibody, anti-smooth muscle antibody and anti-liver–kidney–microsomal antibodies) were also negative. In view of presence of fever, jaundice, altered sensorium, and hepatosplenomegaly the patient was also worked up for malaria, enteric fever, scrub typhus, leptospirosis, and dengue fever. All these workup also came out negative. Serological markers for hepatitis A virus (IgM-HAV), hepatitis E virus (IgM-HEV), and hepatitis B virus [hepatitis B surface antigen (HBsAg) and IgM anti-hepatitis B core antigen (HBc)] were also negative. As she had family history of sickle cell trait in father and peripheral smear showed presence of sickle cells, hemoglobin electrophoresis was done to rule out HbSS. Surprisingly, about 70% of hemoglobin was found to be HbS and diagnosed to have HbSS. In presence of classical clinical symptoms (jaundice/encephalopathy) with conjugated hyperbilirubinemia and coagulopathy the syndromic diagnosis of ALF was done. In the presence of background SCD, the possibility of SCIC was considered.

She was started on intravenous (IV) fluid, IV antibiotics, N-acetyl cysteine (NAC) and anti-encephalopathy measures. In view of deteriorating sensorium, she was intubated and put on mechanical ventilation. Aggressive exchange transfusion using packed red blood cells (RBCs) and fresh frozen plasma (FFP) was initiated to tide over the sickle crisis. The target was to reduce HbS percentage to <30% so as to revert the episode. After three sessions of double-volume exchange transfusion, HbS level came down to 25%. Serum bilirubin level came down to 12 mg/dL and INR reduced to 1.7. She was extubated and did well for another 4 days. However, afterward she developed fever and drowsiness. On examination, she had deep icterus and INR was 2.5. Repeat hemoglobin electrophoresis revealed HbS level of 80%. In view of worsening sensorium, she was reintubated and put on mechanical ventilator. Injection NAC, antibiotics and anti-encephalopathy measures were continued. Chest roentogram showed patchy opacity on right side. Exchange transfusion was restarted. However, she continued to have high-grade fever, later developed shock, oliguria, and metabolic acidosis. Continuous renal replacement therapy was started. However, her condition continued to deteriorate and she died after 5 days. Postmortem liver biopsy was done which revealed sinusoidal obstruction, extensive centrilobular necrosis along with ductular and canalicular cholestasis suggestive of SCIC.

DISCUSSION

In the spectrum of sickle cell hepatopathy, SCIC is probably the most severe manifestation of acute hepatic manifestation of SCD and resembles ALF. It carries high mortality. It presents initially as acute hepatic crisis with fever, abdominal pain, and deep jaundice but can rapidly evolve into ALF with raised an INR and hepatic encephalopathy. Renal failure and MOF may also follow. Renal failure in this context may be due to circulatory disturbances secondary to liver failure or sickle cell nephropathy. Pathophysiology involves diffuse sickling of erythrocytes in hepatic sinusoids leading to widespread ischemia. This leads to ballooning of hepatocytes and intracanalicular cholestasis as seen in histology.[11]

The high level of hyperbilirubinemia seen in these patients is due to a combination of three factors which include (1) ongoing hemolysis, (2) cholestasis, and (3) associated acute kidney injury. Serum ALP levels are elevated because of intrahepatic cholestasis. Coagulopathy with elevated prothrombin time (PT) and INRs and decreased fibrinogen is also commonly observed.

Diagnosis of SCIC should be suspected in any patient with prior history of sickling crisis or family history of SCD who presents with deep jaundice, pain abdomen, hepatomegaly, coagulopathy, and encephalopathy. Other common causes of ALF including autoimmune hepatitis, Wilson's disease, and acute viral hepatitis must be ruled out in these patients.

Performing liver biopsy to diagnose SCIC in these sick patients is not without risks. Historically, performing percutaneous liver biopsy in patients with SCD has been noted to be associated with high risk of bleeding complications. In the series by Zakaria et al. 36% patients undergoing percutaneous liver biopsy developed bleeding complications out of which 28% patients died. Most of these bleeding complications occurred in patients in acute sickle cell crisis. In contrast, the patients who underwent biopsy procedure electively, bleeding complication was not observed. Increased risk of bleeding during acute episodes can be explained by the sinusoidal congestion that commonly occurs in these sick patients.[3,12] In contrast, performing a transjugular liver biopsy (TJLB) might be a safer option in these patients. Moreover, studies regarding use of TJLB in these patients is limited and ultimately liver biopsy may not provide any therapeutic benefit in these patients. Thus to conclude, liver biopsy may be done in patients with SCIC when one needs to rule out the other treatable causes of ALF (e.g., autoimmune hepatitis).

Though, simple blood transfusion and other supportive measures may reverse the condition. Reversal of liver failure by the aggressive exchange transfusion strategy with RBCs and FFPs have been the preferred treatment approach in most of these patients.[13] This treatment strategy involves maintaining HbS <20–30% and hemoglobin of 10 mg/dL to restore and maintain adequate tissue oxygenation. The role of LT in this context is controversial with variable outcomes.

Ahn et al. in a review of 22 cases, with acute intrahepatic cholestasis presenting as liver failure, showed good response in 8 of 9 patients with exchange transfusion. One patient who did not respond died after LT. Two of 8 patients had recurrence that responded to exchange transfusion. Of the 13 patients in this cohort who did not undergo exchange transfusion, 11 died during initial hospitalization. These data indicate that exchange transfusion may offer potential therapeutic benefit. Nonresponders to exchange transfusion may indicate poor prognosis.[14,15]

Hydroxyurea is commonly used in the patients with SCD, hydroxyurea increases the concentration of fetal hemoglobin thus reduces sickling and hemolysis. It also increases water content of red cells and increase their deformability. Hydroxyurea has been shown to reduce the frequency of painful crisis and hospital admission in these patients. In contrast, role of hydroxyurea to treat or prevent hepatic crises is unclear at present.

Performing LT in these sick patients may altogether change the natural course of illness and remains a matter of interest. However, the experience of performing a transplantation in these patients is very limited and only 20 cases have been described in literature. Most common indication of performing LT in these patients was SCIC presenting as ALF. Outcomes of LT is variable in these patients with high incidence of vascular and infectious complications. Long-term follow-up data is not available. The most comprehensive follow-up data included six adult patients who underwent LT (five for SCIC and one for ALF related to autoimmune hepatitis). One patient died in the immediate postoperative period because of severe rejection. In rest five patients, 1-year survival was 83% while 5-year survival was 44%.[13] Peritransplant hematologic management included aggressive exchange transfusion to maintain HbS <30% and hemoglobin 8-10 mg/dL up to 6 months of LT.[13] Our patient was also advised to undergo LT but it was not feasible because of financial constraints and unavailability of a suitable donor. Moreover, isolated LT may not be sufficient to treat the illness as sickle cells may damage the transplanted liver. Combined bone marrow and LT may be an interesting option in these patients.

A new ray of hope in treating these patients is drug voxelotor. Voxelotor is an oral inhibitor of hemoglobin S polymerase, an enzyme, which promotes aggregation of deoxygenated hemoglobin S. Recently, a phase 3 trial reported an increase in mean hemoglobin level from baseline for voxelotor compared with placebo (1.1 vs. −0.1 g/dL; p <0.001).[16]

CONCLUSION

Sickle cell intrahepatic cholestasis may be a life-threatening complication in patients of SCD. Any patient residing in a sickle cell endemic region or having family history of SCD or prior history of sickle cell crises who presents with jaundice, coagulopathy, and encephalopathy possibility of SCIC should be considered. Early diagnosis and institution of exchange transfusion may be useful to revert this fatal complication of SCD. Patients not responding to exchange transfusion may be considered for LT. Combined bone marrow and LT may be the definite treatment option but clinical data is limited at present.

REFERENCES

1. Forget BG, Bunn HF. Classification of the disorders of hemoglobin. Cold Spring Harb Perspect Med. 2013;3:a011684.
2. Shukla AK, Srivastava S, Verma G. Effect of maternal anemia on the status of iron

stores in infants: a cohort study. J Family Community Med. 2019;26:118-22.
3. Praharaj DL, Anand AC. Sickle hepatopathy. J Clin Exp Hepatol. 2021;11:82-96.
4. Grosse SD, Odame I, Atrash HK, Amendah DD, Piel FB, Williams TN. Sickle cell disease in Africa: a neglected cause of early childhood mortality. Am J Prev Med. 2011;41.
5. Banerjee S, Owen C, Chopra S. Sickle cell hepatopathy. Hepatology. 2001;33:1021-8.
6. Berry PA, Cross TJS, Thein SL, Portmann BC, Wendon JA, Karani JB, et al. Hepatic Dysfunction in sickle cell disease: a new system of classification based on global assessment. Clin Gastroenterol Hepatol. 2007;5:1469-76.
7. Vlachaki E, Andreadis P, Neokleous N, Agapidou A, Vetsiou E, Katsinelos P, et al. Successful Outcome of chronic intrahepatic cholestasis in an adult patient with sickle cell/β (+) thalassemia. Case Rep Hematol. 2014;2014:213631.
8. Ebert EC, Nagar M, Hagspiel KD. Gastrointestinal and hepatic complications of sickle cell disease. Clinical Gastroenterology and Hepatology 2010;8:483-9; quiz e70.
9. Shah R, Taborda C, Chawla S. Acute and chronic hepatobiliary manifestations of sickle cell disease: A review. World J Gastrointest Pathophysiol. 2017;8:108.
10. Malik A, Merchant C, Rao M, Fiore RP. Rare but lethal hepatopathy-sickle cell intrahepatic cholestasis and management strategies. Am J Case Rep. 2015;16:840-3.
11. Khan A, Nashed B, Issa M, Khan MZ. Sickle Cell Intrahepatic Cholestasis: Extremely Rare but Fatal Complication of Sickle Cell Disease. Cureus. 2022;14(2):e22050.
12. Ghosh K, Colah RB, Mukherjee MB. Haemoglobinopathies in tribal populations of India. Indian J Med Res. 2015;141(5):505-8.
13. Hurtova M, Bachir D, Lee K, Calderaro J, Decaens T, Kluger MD, et al. Transplantation for liver failure in patients with sickle cell disease: Challenging but feasible. Liver Transpl. 2011;17:381-92.
14. Costa DB, Miksad RA, Buff MS, Wang Y, Dezube BJ. Case of Fatal Sickle Cell Intrahepatic Cholestasis Despite Use of Exchange Transfusion in an African-American Patient. J Natl Med Assoc. 2006;98(7):1183-7.
15. Guimarães JA, Silva LCDS. Sickle cell intrahepatic cholestasis unresponsive to exchange blood transfusion: a case report. Rev Bras Hematol Hemoter. 2017;39:163-6.
16. Vichinsky E, Hoppe CC, Ataga KI, Ware RE, Nduba V, El-Beshlawy A, et al; HOPE Trial Investigators. A Phase 3 Randomized Trial of Voxelotor in Sickle Cell Disease. N Engl J Med. 2019;381:509-19.

Section 5

Diseases of the Gallbladder and Biliary Tract

21. **Choledocholithiasis**
    Nitin Jagtap, D Nageshwar Reddy

22. **Obstructive Jaundice**
    Deepanshu Khanna, Premashis Kar

23. **Spontaneous Rupture of Cystic Artery Pseudoaneurysm Presented as Hemobilia**
    VK Dixit, Mayank Bhusan Pateria, Vinod Kumar

24. **Immunoglobulin G4-related Gastrointestinal Diseases**
    TS Chandrasekar, BJ Gokul, S Sathiamoorthy, K Raja Yogesh, MS Prasad, TC Viveksandeep

Choledocholithiasis

Nitin Jagtap, D Nageshwar Reddy

CASE 1: PATIENT WITH INTERMEDIATE LIKELIHOOD OF CHOLEDOCHOLITHIASIS

A 55-year-old female, who is obese presented to emergency department with 2 days' history of right upper quadrant pain radiating to back, which increases with food intake without any fever. Her hemogram at presentation was normal, liver function test (LFT) showed bilirubin of 8.5 mg/dL, aspartate aminotransferase (AST) of 122 U/L, alanine aminotransferase (ALT) of 116 U/L, and alkaline phosphatase (ALP) of 234 U/L. Serum amylase and lipase were normal. Abdominal ultrasound (USG) showed distend gallbladder with multiple stones and dilated common bile duct (CBD) of 8 mm.

The above clinical presentation is typical of complicated gallstones. In majority cases, gallstones remain asymptomatic, 10–25% of them develop choledocholithiasis.[1] Choledocholithiasis is a common clinical problem and is associated with varied presentation which includes abdominal pain, jaundice, acute cholangitis, and acute pancreatitis.[2]

The recent guidelines published by American Society of Gastrointestinal Endoscopy (ASGE) and European Society of Gastrointestinal Endoscopy (ESGE) separately provided a risk stratification for evaluation and management of suspected choledocholithiasis **(Flowchart 1)**.[3,4]

The risk stratification criteria of ASGE and ESGE combines LFTs and abdominal USG along with clinical presentation to define the probability of having choledocholithiasis. Once probability of CBD stone is defined these guidelines recommend whether to proceed for directly cholecystectomy in low-likelihood group or preoperative endoscopic retrograde cholangiopancreatography (ERCP)/cholecystectomy with CBD exploration for high-likelihood group; for patients following into intermediate likelihood of CBD stone, both guidelines recommend either endoscopic ultrasound (EUS) or magnetic resonance cholangiopancreatography (MRCP) as confirmatory test before preoperative ERCP or cholecystectomy.[3,4]

As per ESGE risk stratification criteria, the above case is having intermediate likelihood of cholechodolithiasis and high likelihood according to ASGE criteria. In our study, we found that the ESGE risk stratification criteria appears more specific compared to ASGE criteria.[5]

The next question for intermediate likelihood patient is to perform confirmatory test which is either EUS or MRCP. In a randomized control study, we have shown that for intermediate likelihood criteria both

Flowchart 1: Risk stratification criteria of ASGE and ESGE guidelines.

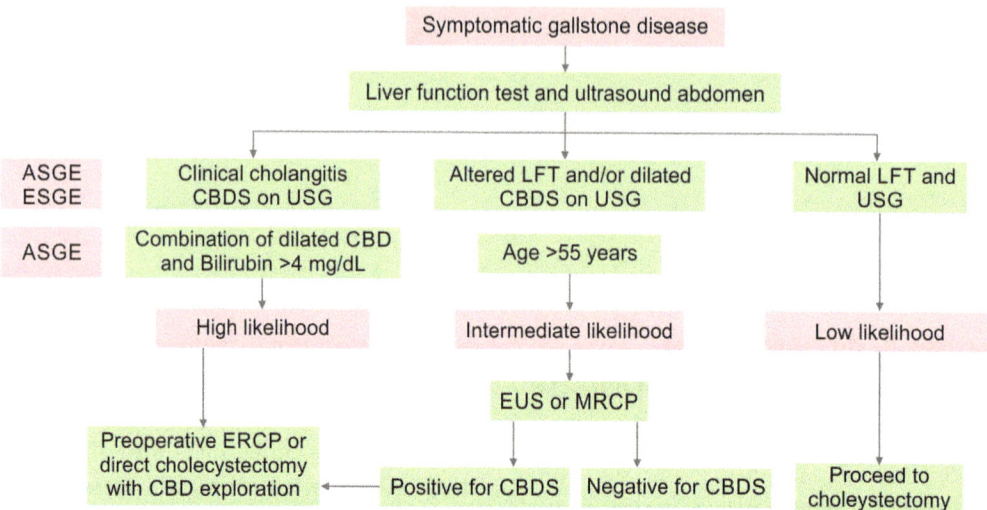

(ASGE: American Society of Gastrointestinal Endoscopy; CBD: common bile duct; CBDS: CBD stenosis; ERCP: endoscopic retrograde cholangiopancreatography; ESGE: European Society of Gastrointestinal Endoscopy; LFT: liver function test; MRCP: magnetic resonance cholangiopancreatography; USG: ultrasound)

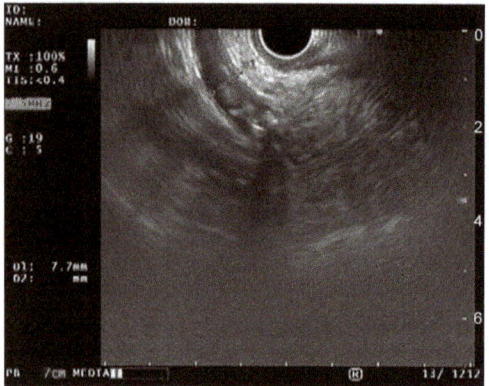

Fig. 1: Endoscopic ultrasound (EUS) showing dilated common bile duct (CBD) with calculi.

EUS and MRCP have similar sensitivity and specificity.[6] This patient underwent EUS which has shown gallstones with dilated CBD with calculi at lower end **(Fig. 1)**.

Both guidelines recommended CBD stone extraction in all patients, symptomatic or not, who are fit enough to tolerate intervention.[3,4] The conservative approach can only be considered in patients where the risk of surgical or endoscopic CBD stenosis (CBDS) extraction is higher than the risks of leaving stones in situ. Subsequently this patient underwent ERCP for CBS stone extraction with biliary sphincterotomy and balloon sweep. Patient underwent laparoscopic cholecystectomy within 1 week after ERCP.

There is option of laparoscopic cholecystectomy and CBD exploration after EUS has confirmed CBD stone; which might be more cost-effective strategy.[7] However, in recent survey ERCP prior to cholecystectomy is preferred treatment strategy for >97% physicians and surgeons in India.

The current guidelines defined intermediate likelihood category as altered LFT, and not defined what should be considered as altered LFT. We believe intermediate likelihood category is more heterogenous and unless altered LFT is defined appropriately there are chances that unnecessary use of EUS and/MRCP as confirmatory test.[8]

Male gender, presence of acute calculus cholecystitis (ACC) and raised bilirubin >1.8 mg/dL are independent risk factors for choledocholithiasis in patients with intermediate likelihood group. The presence of at least one of the above three parameters if considered for confirmatory test then need for EUS and MRCP can be decreased.[8] Those patients who do not have any one of the above parameters can be followed up for next 48 hours, if persistent clinical suspicion then EUS or MRCP can be considered before cholecystectomy.[8]

There are two different scenarios which can be associated with choledocholithiasis, namely, acute biliary pancreatitis (ABP) and ACC. ABP is a negative predictor of residual choledocholithiasis and should not be considered directly for ERCP.[9] In all patients with any severity of pancreatitis, indication for ERCP should be based on above risk stratification criteria.[10] Patients with ACC can have altered LFT independent of CBD stone and diagnostic performance of ASGE and ESGE risk stratification appears to be inadequate in patients with ACC. We proposed separate predictive model for coexisting choledocholithiasis in patients with ACC in which dilated CBD on USG and ALP level above the upper limit of normal are positive predictors while coexisting acute pancreatitis is a negative predictor of choledocholithiasis.[11] The predictive score was calculated by allotting +1 score for each positive predictor and –1 for each negative predictor, giving a range from –1 to +2. Patients with score 2 can undergo preoperative ERCP or intraoperative cholangiogram. Patients with score of 1 should undergo confirmatory test in the form of EUS or MRCP before ERCP or cholecystectomy. Remaining patients with score of 0 or –1 can be considered for cholecystectomy directly.[11]

CASE 2: PATIENT WITH DIFFICULT CBD STONE

A 60-year-old male patient presented with high-grade fever with jaundice since 3 days, along with right upper quadrant pain radiating to back. At presentation he was febrile (temperature 101°F) with tachycardia (heart rate 110 beats/min) and mild hypotension (blood pressure 100/70 mm Hg). His hemogram showed neutrophilic leukocytosis, LFT showed bilirubin on 9.8 mg/dL, ALT of 220 U/L, and ALP of 350 U/L. He underwent initial resuscitation and his blood pressure and tachycardia normalized. USG showed gallstones with dilated CBD with 15-mm calculi in CBD.

This patient's clinical presentation is of acute cholangitis; presence of pain, fever, and jaundice represent Charcot's triad of acute cholangitis.[12] Due to presence of clinical cholangitis, this patient can be stratified into high likelihood of CBD stone and can be considered for ERCP directly. As this patient is having mild/moderate acute cholangitis, we planned for ERCP with therapeutic intent to retrieve CBD stone. ERCP cholangiogram showed large CBD stones **(Fig. 2)**, which could not be retrieved after large balloon sphincterotomy, so temporary nasobiliary tube has placed till further therapy is planned.

Difficult biliary stones are defined according to their diameter (>15 mm), number, unusual shape (barrel-shaped) or location (intrahepatic, cystic duct) or because of anatomical factors (narrowing of the bile duct, distal to the stone, sigmoid-shaped CBD, stone impaction, shorter length of the distal CBD, or acute distal CBD angulation).[4] In such cases, there are two approaches either to perform biliary lithotripsy endoscopic/extracorporeal or to proceed with cholecystectomy and CBD exploration.

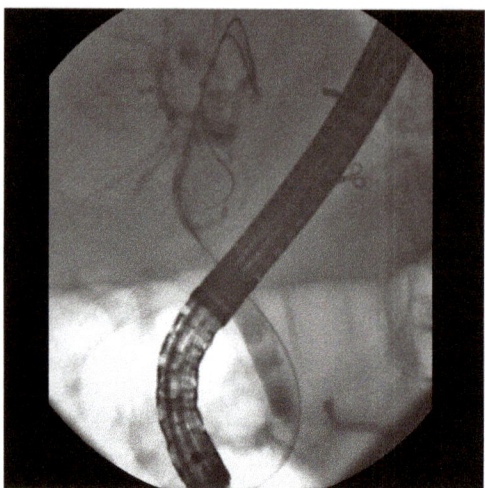

Fig. 2: Endoscopic retrograde cholangiopancreatography (ERCP) showing difficult common bile duct (CBD) stones.

Mechanical lithotripsy is the simplest available method of fragmenting CBD stones. It is reported as an effective and safe technique, but multiple sessions may be required. The most common and feared complication of mechanical lithotripsy is entrapment of the basket, broken basket, or traction wire fracture.[13] Intraductal shock wave lithotripsy represents an alternative method to fragment bile stones and allow their removal. There are two methods of generating shock waves in a fluid, using either a bipolar probe in case of electrohydraulic laser (EHL) or a pulsed dye laser system in the case of laser lithotripsy. Both EHL and laser lithotripsy are preferably performed under direct visualization with cholangioscopy. Cholangitis is the most frequently reported complication.[14]

Extracorporeal shock wave lithotripsy (ESWL) generate shock waves that travel through the soft tissue of the body to fragment CBD stones. A nasobiliary drain is inserted to allow fluoroscopic identification and targeting of CBD stones and to perform continuous irrigation of bile duct with saline during ESWL. Multiple ESWL sessions and subsequent ERCP procedures to extract stone fragment are required.[15] ESWL-related severe adverse events includes cholangitis and pancreatitis, minor adverse events includes pain, local hematoma, and microhematuria. In patients undergoing laparoscopic cholecystectomy, transcystic or transductal exploration of the CBD is a safe and effective technique for CBD stone clearance.[4]

After discussing various options for difficult CBD stone retrieval, patients underwent cholangioscopy-guided EHL followed by laparoscopic cholecystectomy. The decision about whether to perform advanced endoscopic lithotripsy or ESWL or surgical CBD exploration should depend on local availability, experience, and patients preference.

REFERENCES

1. Halldestam I, Enell EL, Kullman E, Borch K. Development of symptoms and complications in individuals with asymptomatic gallstones. Br J Surg. 2004;91:734-8.
2. Shabanzadeh DM, Sorensen LT, Jorgensen T. A Prediction Rule for Risk Stratification of Incidentally Discovered Gallstones: Results From a Large Cohort Study. Gastroenterology. 2016;150:156-167.e1.
3. ASGE Standards of Practice Committee; Buxbaum JL, Abbas Fehmi SM, Sultan S, Fishman DS, Qumseya BJ, Cortessis VK, et al. ASGE guideline on the role of endoscopy in the evaluation and management of choledocholithiasis. Gastrointest Endosc. 2019;89:1075-1105.e15.
4. Manes G, Paspatis G, Aabakken L, Anderloni A, Arvanitakis M, Ah-Soune P, et al. Endoscopic management of common bile duct stones: European Society of Gastrointestinal Endoscopy (ESGE) guideline. Endoscopy. 2019;51:472-91.
5. Jagtap N, Hs Y, Tandan M, Basha J, Chavan R, Nabi Z, et al. Clinical utility of ESGE and ASGE guidelines for prediction of

suspected choledocholithiasis in patients undergoing cholecystectomy. Endoscopy. 2020;52:569-73.
6. Jagtap N, Kumar JK, Chavan R, Basha J, Tandan M, Lakhtakia S, et al. EUS versus MRCP to perform ERCP in patients with intermediate likelihood of choledocholithiasis: a randomised controlled trial. Gut 2022.
7. Ali FS, DaVee T, Bernstam EV, Kao LS, Wandling M, Hussain MR, et al. Cost-effectiveness analysis of optimal diagnostic strategy for patients with symptomatic cholelithiasis with intermediate probability for choledocholithiasis. Gastrointest Endosc. 2022;95:327-38.
8. Jagtap N, Karyampudi A, Yashavanth HS, Ramchandani M, Lakhtakia S, Kalapala R, et al. Intermediate Likelihood of Choledocholithiasis: Do All Need EUS or MRCP? J Dig Endosc. 2021;12:019-023.
9. He H, Tan C, Wu J, Dai N, Hu W, Zhang Y, et al. Accuracy of ASGE high-risk criteria in evaluation of patients with suspected common bile duct stones. Gastrointest Endosc. 2017;86:525-32.
10. Schepers NJ, Hallensleben NDL, Besselink MG, Anten MGF, Bollen TL, da Costa DW, et al.; Dutch Pancreatitis Study Group. Urgent endoscopic retrograde cholangiopancreatography with sphincterotomy versus conservative treatment in predicted severe acute gallstone pancreatitis (APEC): a multicentre randomised controlled trial. Lancet. 2020;396:167-76.
11. Reddy S, Jagtap N, Kalapala R, Ramchandani M, Lakhtakia S, Basha J, et al. Choledocholithiasis in acute calculous cholecystitis: guidelines and beyond. Ann Gastroenterol. 2021;34:247-52.
12. Rumsey S, Winders J, MacCormick AD. Diagnostic accuracy of Charcot's triad: a systematic review. ANZ J Surg. 2017;87:232-8.
13. Garg PK, Tandon RK, Ahuja V, Makharia GK, Batra Y. Predictors of unsuccessful mechanical lithotripsy and endoscopic clearance of large bile duct stones. Gastrointest Endosc. 2004;59:601-5.
14. Buxbaum J, Sahakian A, Ko C, Jayaram P, Lane C, Yu CY, et al. Randomized trial of cholangioscopy-guided laser lithotripsy versus conventional therapy for large bile duct stones (with videos). Gastrointest Endosc. 2018;87:1050-60.
15. Tandan M, Reddy DN. Extracorporeal shock wave lithotripsy for pancreatic and large common bile duct stones. World J Gastroenterol. 2011;17:4365-71.

22
Obstructive Jaundice

Deepanshu Khanna, Premashis Kar

■ INTRODUCTION

A 73-year-old man arrived at the clinic with increasing jaundice, pale stools, dark urine, and itching that had been present for 4 weeks. He also complained of epigastric pain radiating to back. He gave a previous medical history of chronic pancreatitis, diabetes, hypertension, and hypothyroidism and he was taking regular medications for the same. The patient had been smoking 15 cigarettes a day and consumed 10 standard drinks a week of alcohol for last 50 years.

On examination, he was found to be afebrile, icterus was present, and he had a palpable liver edge 4 cm below the costal margin. Under the tip of the ninth rib, there was a globular bulge that extended forward and downward from just below the liver. Its upper border was continuous with the liver, and it could move slightly from side to side. The stigmata of chronic liver disease were not present. There were scratch marks on the chest and abdomen.

Question 1: What could this lump be?
Answer: This is a gallbladder swelling. In pathological conditions, the gallbladder can be felt just lateral to the right rectus abdominis muscle, close to the tip of the ninth costal cartilage. It is firm, smooth, and spherical to the touch. Its rounded boundaries and relative movement on respiration set it apart from a right kidney lump. Normally, gallbladder is not palpable.

Question 2: What are causes of palpable gallbladder?
Answer: The causes include:
- Mucocele/empyema of the gallbladder (firm and regular swelling): Not associated with jaundice
- Carcinoma of the head of pancreas (firm and globular swelling): Associated with jaundice
- Carcinoma of the gallbladder (stony, hard, irregular swelling): Associated with jaundice
- Carcinoma of the common bile duct (CBD) (firm and globular swelling): Associated with jaundice
- Calculus obstructing cystic duct (firm and globular swelling): Not associated with jaundice.

Question 3: What is Courvoisier's law?
Answer: Palpable, non-tender, smooth gallbladder is not due to an impacted stone in the CBD, but rather to neoplastic obstruction of the CBD in a patient with obstructive jaundice. Due to recurrent cholecystitis, the gallbladder in choledocholithiasis is frequently tiny, contracted, and non-palpable due to recurrent episodes of cholecystitis.

Question 4: What are exceptions to this law?
Answer: The exceptions include:
- Double impaction of stone—one in CBD and other in cystic duct

- Oriental cholangiohepatitis
- Pancreatic calculus obstructing ampulla of Vater
- Mucocele due to stone in cystic duct.

Question 5: What is the type of jaundice, extrahepatic (surgical) or intrahepatic (medical)?
Answer: This patient is likely having extrahepatic jaundice, since this is an old aged male, with gradually progressing jaundice, with history of abdominal pain, pale-colored stools and itching. On examination there is presence of a palpable gallbladder. All these features favor extrahepatic jaundice.

Question 6: What is your differential diagnosis based on history?
Answer: This is a case of obstructive jaundice. The site of obstruction is probably at (CBD, ampulla):
- Carcinoma of the head of the pancreas
- Ampullary carcinoma
- Cholangiocarcinoma
- Benign bile duct or pancreatic duct stricture.

Since patient is an elderly man who has come with gradually progressive obstructive jaundice associated with significant weight loss with past history of chronic pancreatitis, having risk factors of chronic alcohol abuse and smoking. Examination suggestive of palpable globular gallbladder, we kept differential diagnosis as carcinoma head of pancreas, periampullary carcinoma, and cholangiocarcinoma. It is important not to miss benign conditions in your differential diagnosis, since chronic pancreatitis can lead to stricture of lower end of bile duct leading to obstructive jaundice. Carcinoma gallbladder with porta hepatis block is unlikely in this case, as gallbladder is usually collapsed with this condition.

Investigations showed:
- Hemoglobin 11.4 g/dL, total leukocyte count (TLC) 11.9 × 10^9/L, platelets 757 × 10^9/L.
- Bilirubin total 6.9 mg/dL, bilirubin direct 6.1 mg/dL, alanine transaminase (ALT) 146 IU/L, aspartate transaminase (AST) 183 IU/L, alkaline phosphatase (ALP) 778 IU/L, gamma-glutamyl transferase (GGT) 702 IU/L, albumin 3.2 g/dL, globulin 2.9 g/dL.
- Na 126 mmol/L, K 4.5 mmol/L, urea 19 mg/dL, creatinine 0.5 mg/dL.
- Prothrombin time 14 seconds.
- Amylase 34 U/L, lipase 4 U/L, CA 19-9—8,536 U/mL.
- *Abdominal ultrasound:* Gallbladder is overdistended (measures 11.7 × 4.0 cm), pancreas is atrophic and shows ductal dilatation, measuring approximately 11.3 mm along with dilated intrahepatic biliary radicles with dilated CBD (20 mm) and MPD with abrupt cutoff secondary to a mass lesion in head of pancreas.
- Computed tomography (CT) scan of the abdomen (pancreatic protocol) showed findings suggestive of mitotic etiology involving the pancreatic head resulting in a mass which is causing ductal obstruction with moderate dilatation of biliary ductal system as well as the pancreatic duct. There is focal loss of fat planes with the confluence of the superior mesenteric vein (SMV) and splenic vein. There is hepatomegaly with no focal lesion noted in liver.

Question 7: What is double duct sign?
Answer: The double duct sign refers to the simultaneous dilatation of the pancreatic and bile ducts. Carcinoma of head of pancreas ampullary tumors (e.g., carcinoma of the ampulla of Vater) are the two most frequent

causes. Obstructive jaundice and weight loss are common symptoms of both diseases. The pancreatic and bile ducts may also enlarge simultaneously if there is cholelithiasis and a gallstone impaction in the ampullary region, however this is typically accompanied by biliary colic and is not associated with weight loss, which was present in our case. Double duct signs are unusual in cholangiocarcinoma, and benign bile duct stenosis typically results from iatrogenic injury; there was no history of previous surgery in this case, however there was a history of chronic pancreatitis which can lead to bile duct stenosis, and is also a risk factor for pancreatic carcinoma. Since we found a mass lesion in lead of pancreas with CA 19-9 levels of 8,536 U/L, carcinoma head of pancreas is the most likely diagnosis.

Question 8: What is the role of other radiologic modalities in this case?
Answer: Magnetic resonance imaging (MRI) is used only for individuals with severe contrast allergies, renal insufficiency, or contraindications to CT scan, in order to identify the cause of indeterminate liver lesions. Positron emission tomography (PET)-CT is useful for detecting occult metastatic lesions, especially when CA 19-9 levels are high. These two modalities are not required in our case, since mass is clearly seen in head of pancreas.

Question 9: What is the treatment of choice in this patient and what is the prognosis?
Answer: Pancreatoduodenectomy (Whipple's procedure) is the treatment of choice for patients with a pancreatic adenocarcinoma and ampullary carcinoma. Resectability rates approach 25% in pancreatic carcinoma, compared with 90% in ampullary carcinoma. Ampullary adenocarcinoma has a higher resectability rate, which could be explained with multiple reasons. Firstly because of the tumor's anatomic position, which causes jaundice at an early stage, secondly, it can be partially explained by earlier presentation, but it may also be explained by its distinct biological behavior from pancreatic cancer. The 5-year survival rate for pancreatic cancer after margin-negative (R0) pancreaticoduodenectomy is roughly 30% for lymph node negative disease and 10% for lymph node positive illness. 90% of tumors are discovered in the advanced stages, after they have left the pancreas and in >50% of cases have already developed systemic metastases. It is critical to note that while the overall 5-year survival rate for ampullary carcinoma is 40–50% following resection, this figure rises to 80% in the absence of nodal metastases.

Question 10: How will you stage this tumor?
Answer: Tumors are categorized and treatment choices are made using a four-category staging approach. They include resectable, borderline resectable, locally advanced, and metastatic disease. According to NCCN (National Comprehensive Cancer Network) criteria, resectable illness is defined as having no venous or arterial involvement and no distant spread. As long as the venous section is reconstructible, tumors with venous contact >180°, venous contour abnormality, or thrombosis are regarded as being borderline resectable. Locally advanced refers to SMV or portal vein involvement that cannot be repaired. Arterial contact that is <180° is seen to be borderline resectable, whereas contact that is >180° is thought to be locally advanced. Metastatic illness is characterized as distant spread.

Question 11: What is the approach to manage pancreatic cancer?
Answer: The approach to manage pancreatic cancer is shown in **Flowchart 1**.

Flowchart 1: Treatment algorithm for pancreatic cancer.

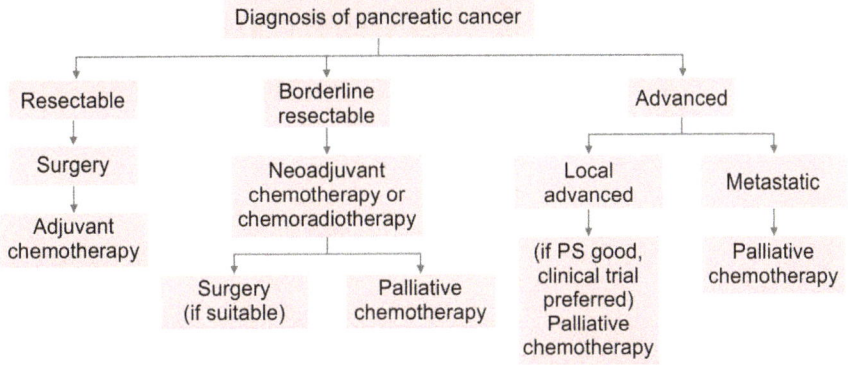

Question 12: What should be the next step in this case?
Answer: Since CT shows loss of fat planes between mass and SMV, and involvement is <180°, this disease becomes borderline resectable and will require neoadjuvant chemotherapy before surgery. Before starting any chemotherapy, a tissue diagnosis is required. So, next step in this case would be endoscopic ultrasound (EUS)-guided biopsy.
- Biopsy report symptomatic of pancreatic ductal adenocarcinoma

Question 13: What should be next step in this case?
Answer: Since this patient is planned for neoadjuvant chemotherapy, biliary drainage should be done to lower the bilirubin. Indications for biliary drainage are cholangitis/intractable pruritus, when surgery is delayed >2 weeks and when planned for neoadjuvant therapy.

Question 14: What should be the next step?
Answer: Endoscopic retrograde cholangiopancreatography (ERCP) was performed in this case for biliary drainage, however due to a stricture at lower end of CBD, cannulation could not be performed, and ERCP failed.

Question 15: What should be the next step?
Answer: Since ERCP has failed, next step should be percutaneous transhepatic biliary drainage (PTBD) to establish biliary drainage. Cholangiogram showed narrowing noted in distal CBD and ampullary region, stent was placed across the narrowing with proximal tip 2 cm distal to hilar region, a 10 F straight draining catheter was placed and kept for external drainage. Patient's bilirubin normalized and itching improved and he was planned for neoadjuvant chemotherapy.

Question 16: What drugs should be used for chemotherapy in this case?
Answer: FOLFIRONOX [5-fluorouracil (5-FU), leucovorin, irinotecan, and oxaliplatin] or gemcitabine plus albumin-bound (nab) paclitaxel are currently the accepted standard of care for first-line therapy.

Patient is currently undergoing chemotherapy and is planned for surgery after its completion.

Spontaneous Rupture of Cystic Artery Pseudoaneurysm Presented as Hemobilia

VK Dixit, Mayank Bhusan Pateria, Vinod Kumar

■ INTRODUCTION

Hemobilia is bleeding inside or from biliary tract. The classic presentation of hemobilia is formally known as Quincke's triad: jaundice, right upper quadrant abdominal pain, and upper gastrointestinal (UGI) hemorrhage, but the presentation of all three together only occur in 22–35% of cases.[1,2] As the incidence of hemobilia is around 2–5% in UGI hemorrhage[3] and only 25% of cases occurred from the gallbladder,[4] cystic artery pseudoaneurysm is undoubtedly rare. Hepatic artery aneurysms are rare lesions (20% of all visceral aneurysms[5]) and difficult to diagnose clinically. The common causes include surrounding inflammation, trauma, or atherosclerosis.[6] We present a case of gastrointestinal bleeding, jaundice, and colicky right upper quadrant abdominal pain (Quincke's clinical triad) as a result of a ruptured pseudoaneurysm of cystic artery.

■ CASE

A 56-year-old female without history of any previous comorbidity presented to our hospital with presenting complaint of right upper abdomen pain for 10 days; black tarry, foul-smelling sticky stool for 9 days, and yellowish discoloration of eyes and urine for 3 days. Character of her pain was biliary. She had history of orthostatic symptoms after passing melenic stools with significant drop of hemoglobin (up to 4.5 g/dL). She had history of 4 units of packed red blood cell (PRBC) transfusion before presentation to our hospital. Her ultrasonography (USG) abdomen suggestive of heterogenous mass lesion inside gallbladder. Contrast-enhanced computed tomography (CECT) abdomen suggestive of irregular-shaped endophytic soft tissue attenuation lesion of approximate size 4.3 × 3.0 cm in fundus/tumefactive sludge/mass **(Figs. 1A to D)**. USG + CECT were done before referral to our hospital). On examination she was pale with scleral icterus. Hepatomegaly (with liver span of 17 cm) and right hypochondrium tenderness was present on palpation. Her initial laboratory parameters were as follows: hemoglobin—9.9 g/dL, total leukocyte count (TLC)—15,180, differential leucocyte count (DLC)—N91L6, platelet count (PLT)—1.80 L, aspartate transaminase (AST)/alanine transaminase (ALT)—417/356, bilirubin (T/D)—6/4, and alkaline phosphatase (ALP)—810 (<310).

After achieving hemodynamic stability her UGI endoscopy was done which was suggestive active oozing of blood from papilla **(Fig. 2)**. With the possibility of tumoral bleed and cholangitis ERCP was done in the same setting. Biliary clearance done with retrieval of blood clots after balloon sweeping and deployment of two 10 Fr plastic stents was done to achieve tamponade effect. After 24 hours due to 3 g drop in her hemoglobin,

CHAPTER 23: Spontaneous Rupture of Cystic Artery Pseudoaneurysm Presented as Hemobilia

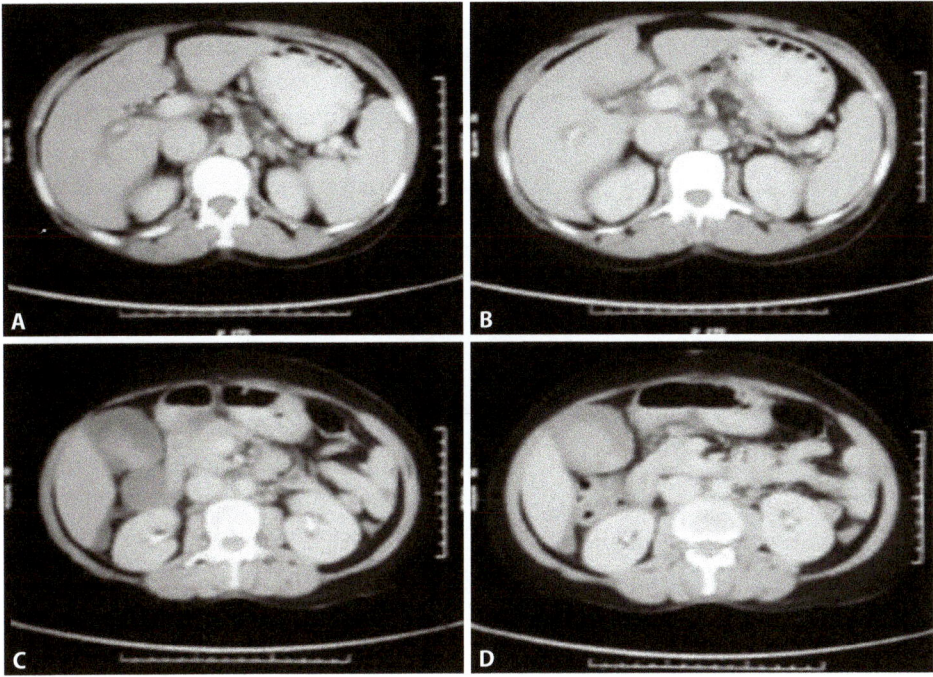

Figs. 1A to D: Hyperdense core surrounded peripheral hypodensity inside lumen of gallbladder tumefactive sludge/mass. There is no intrahepatic biliary dilatation (IHBRD).

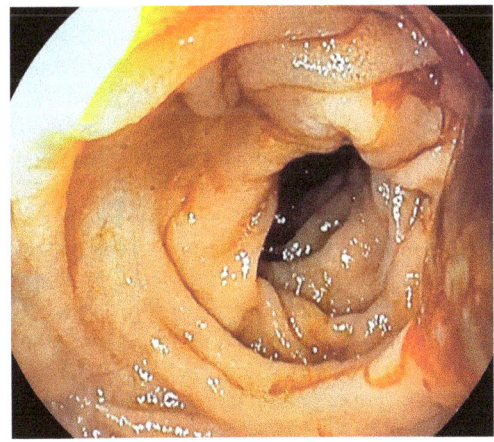

Fig. 2: Active oozing of blood from papilla.

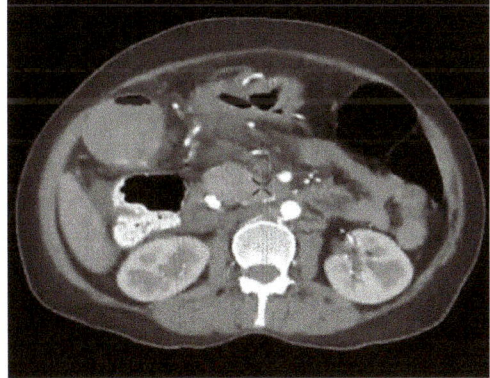

Fig. 3: Cystic artery pseudoaneurysm with active extravasation.

urgent CT angiography of abdomen was done which was suggestive of cystic artery pseudoaneurysm with active extravasation of contrast **(Fig. 3)**. For management of active bleeding options of cholecystectomy and interventional radiology were provided to relatives of the patient. With consent of her relative transcatheter coil embolization of the cystic artery was done with 2 mm × 2 cm hilal coil and hemostasis was achieved with

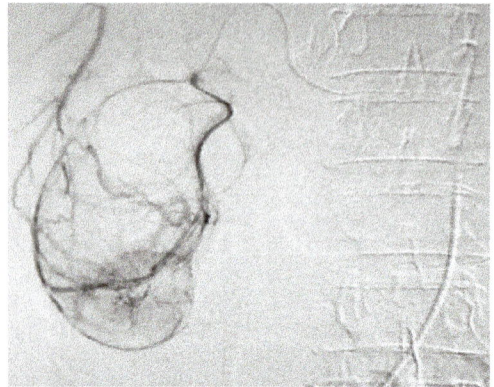

Fig. 4: Digital subtraction angiography (DSA) image after coil embolization of cystic artery.

no further drop in hemoglobin **(Fig. 4)**. Post procedure patient was stable and discharged after 4 days.

DISCUSSION

Hemobilia is an unusual cause of UGI bleeding. This could be either traumatic or nontraumatic. This could be due result of formation of a hepatic vessel pseudoaneurysm. This is a rare occurrence following laparoscopic or open cholecystectomy. The most important factor being direct iatrogenic injuries. The clinical presentation may be late and includes more frequently UGI bleed due to pseudoaneurysm dilatation, abdominal pain, and jaundice secondary to bilary compression.

The treatment includes transarterial embolization of feeding vessel. The surgery is reserved for refractory cases. This case also had presentation with abdominal pain, jaundice, and melena with significant drop in hemoglobin and required 4 units of blood before admission in this hospital. The gastroscopy revealed bleeding from papilla. ERCP was planned and fresh blood clots were removed with biliary stenting. But this did not help and CECT angiography was planned which showed the cystic duct pseudoaneurysm which was subsequently embolized with coiling. This led to stoppage of gastrointestinal bleed and patient was discharged in good condition.

The case is relatively uncommon presenting as hemobilia which is ultimately turned out to cystic duct artery aneurysm which was managed successfully will selective embolization at tertiary care center. This also highlights that if good interventional radiological facilities exist, surgery may be avoided.

REFERENCES

1. Green MH, Duell RM, Johnson CD, Jamieson NV. Haemobilia. Br J Surg. 2001;88: 773e786.
2. Murugesan SD, Sathyanesan J, Lakshmanan A, Ramaswami S, Perumal S, Perumal SU, et al. Massive hemobilia: a diagnostic and therapeutic challenge. World J Surg. 2014;38: 1755e1762.
3. Sandblom P. Hemorrhage into the biliary tract following trauma; traumatic hemobilia. Surgery. 1948;24(3):571-86.
4. Kerr HH, Mensh M, Gould EA. Biliary tract hemorrhage; a source of massive gastrointestinal bleeding. Ann Surg. 1950;131(5): 790-800.
5. Abbas MA, Fowl RJ, Stone WM, Panneton JM, Oldenburg WA, Bower TC, et al. Hepatic artery aneurysm: factors that predict complications. J Vasc Surg. 2003;38:41-5.
6. Parmar H, Shah J, Shah B, Patkar D, Varma R. Imaging findings in a giant hepatic artery aneurysm. J Postgrad Med. 2000;46:104-5.

Immunoglobulin G4-related Gastrointestinal Diseases

TS Chandrasekar, BJ Gokul, S Sathiamoorthy, K Raja Yogesh, MS Prasad, TC Viveksandeep

INTRODUCTION

Immunoglobulin G4-related disease (IgG4-RD) is a less common, long-standing, systemic, autoimmune disease. It may affect more than one organ in the body **(Fig. 1)**. The pancreas and biliary tract are most commonly affected. It is often easy to underdiagnose or completely not thought off. In view of rarity and low index of suspicion, it is challenging to diagnose IgG4 RD. But once diagnosed **(Box 1)**, it is gratifying because treatment is highly rewarding. Hence this topic assumes great importance in clinical practice and emphasizes a high index of suspicion for diagnosing such disorders. This chapter reports two interesting cases of IgG4-related obstructive jaundice, which otherwise would have led to a major surgery like Whipple's procedure but were successfully treated with medical treatment. The relevant information about when to suspect such disorders, the diagnostic and exclusion criteria, and the management algorithm have been highlighted in this chapter.

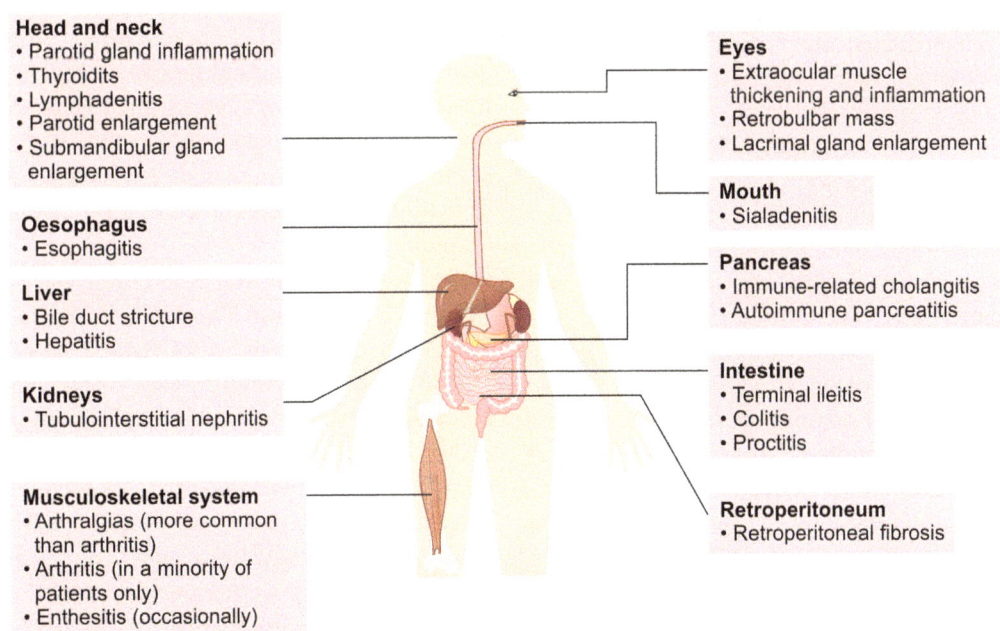

Fig. 1: Spectrum of immunoglobulin G4-related diseases (IgG4-RD).

> **BOX 1:** Indications for diagnostic evaluation.

- Patients with one of the characteristic patterns of organ or tissue involvement
- Patients at high risk for having immunoglobulin G4-related disease (IgG4-RD) are those with any of the following:
  - Pancreatitis of unknown origin
  - Sclerosing cholangitis
  - Bilateral salivary and/or lacrimal gland enlargement

TABLE 1: Diagnostic criteria.

Tests	Sample
Clinical (and radiologic)	Mass lesion in one or more organs
Histopathologic	Fibrosis and lymphoplasma-cytic infiltrate IgG4+ plasma cells >10/hpf Or IgG4: IgG >40%
Serologic	Serum IgG4 >1.35 g/L

TABLE 2: Diagnosis of IgG4-related disease.

Definite diagnosis	• Clinical (and radiologic) • Histopathologic • Serologic
Probable diagnosis	• Clinical (and radiologic) • Histopathologic
Possible diagnosis	• Clinical (and radiologic) • Serologic

■ CASE 1

A 72-year-old man presented with history of loss of appetite and weight and dark urine and pale stool for 3 months. There was no fever, abdominal pain, and no past history of surgery.

The patient was a teetotaller with no recent history of drug intake. On examination, he was icteric, and no mass was palpable per abdomen. He was anemic, and total blood counts were normal. His liver function tests showed elevated serum bilirubin two times and liver enzymes four times that of normal. An ultrasound (US) examination of abdomen revealed dilated common bile duct (CBD) and intrahepatic radicles and magnetic resonance cholangiopancreatography (MRCP) showed abnormal thickening of the bile duct wall with luminal obstruction of the common hepatic duct at the level of hepatic confluence suggestive of hilar cholangiocarcinoma—type 4. At this stage, in view of his age, malignant biliary obstruction was seriously considered and various diagnostic modalities like ERCP with the brush cytology, cholangioscopic biopsy, and endo ultrasonography (EUS)-guided biopsy were contemplated. But CA 19-9 was within normal limits, and other tumor markers were not positive. Further investigations revealed raised C-reactive protein (CRP), polyclonal hypergammaglobulinemia, and highly elevated IgG4 subclass. A PET CT (positron emission tomography–computed tomography) scan study revealed diffuse hypermetabolic circumferential thickening of the confluence of hepatic duct, and hypermetabolic activity over both kidneys, right parotid, ethmoidal sinuses, over the aortic arch and hilar, mediastinal para-aortic, iliac and inguinal lymph nodes. The above features were suggestive of IgG4-RD involving multiple organs. EUS-guided biopsy of the mediastinal lymph node revealed small- to medium-size lymphoid cells and negative for malignancy.

As per the diagnostic criteria of IgG4-RD **(Tables 1 and 2 and Fig. 2)**, IgG4-related sclerosing cholangitis (IgG4-RDSC) type 4 **(Fig. 3)** was considered in view of elevated serum IgG4 levels, coexistence of inflammatory activity in multiple organs as revealed by PET CT scan and negative tumor markers assay. He was started on oral prednisolone at 0.6 mg/kg/day, which was gradually tapered. He showed a remarkable improvement with a reduction in liver function abnormalities. His MRCP study **(Fig. 4)** showed a significant reduction

CHAPTER 24: Immunoglobulin G4-related Gastrointestinal Diseases

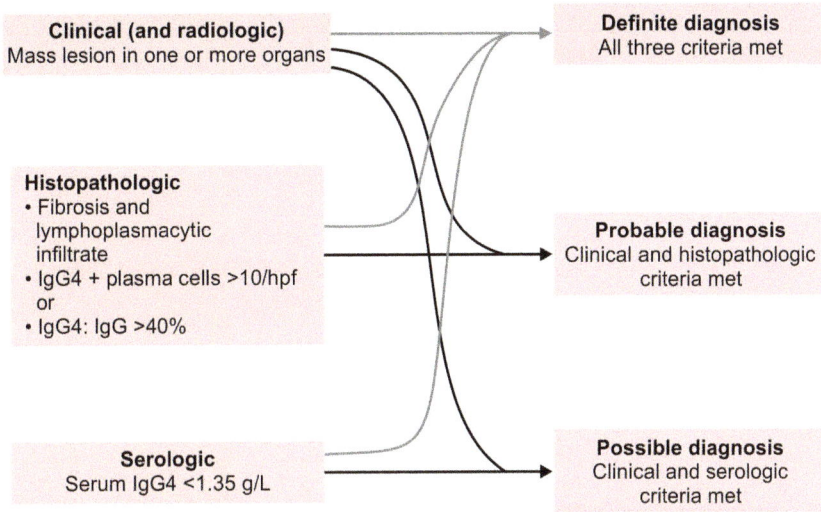

Fig. 2: Diagnostic criteria of immunoglobulin G4-related disease.

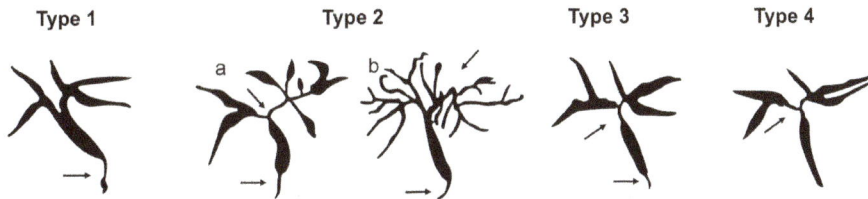

Fig. 3: Types of immunoglobulin G4 (IgG4)-sclerosing cholangitis. Arrows point to the site of involvement.

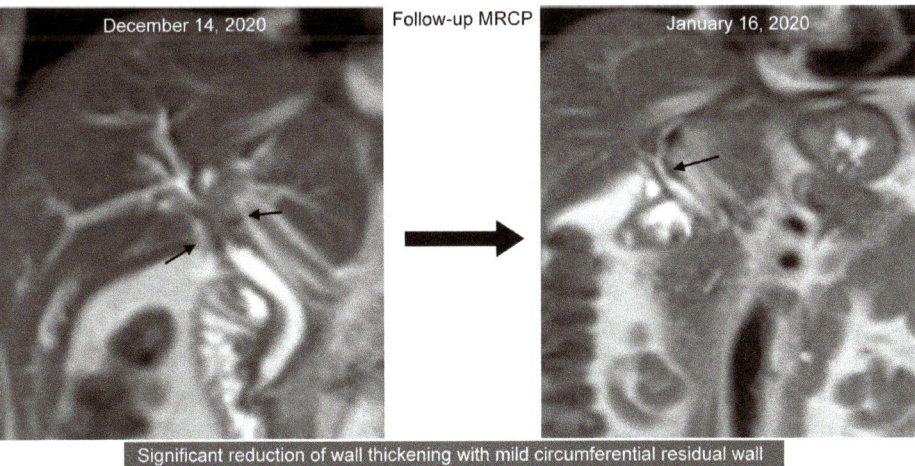

Fig. 4: Comparative MRCP (magnetic resonance cholangiopancreatography) images (case 1) showing marked improvement after steroid treatment *(arrow)*. (CHD: common hepatic duct LHD: left hepatic duct RHD: right hepatic duct)

TABLE 3: Exclusion criteria.

Types of tests	Exclusion criteria
Clinical	• Fever • Leukopenia/thrombocytopenia • Eosinophilia • Absence of respose to steroids • Splenomegaly
Serology	• Positive ANCA • High titers of Ro, La, ds-DNA, RNP OR sm cryoglobulins
Radiologic	• Findings suggestive of malignancy • Rapid progression • Long bone abnormalities consistent with ECD • Splenomegaly
Pathologic	• Inflammatory myofibroblastic tumor • Neutrophilic infiltrates • Necrotizing vasculitis • Primary granulomatous lesion • Features of macrophage/histocytic disorder

(ANCA: antineutrophil cytoplasmic antibodies; ECD: Erdheim–Chester disease)

of wall thickening of CBD with resolution of bilobar intrahepatic biliary dilatation. And a repeat PET CT scan also showed an excellent response to therapy. He was further managed with maintenance therapy with prednisolone 10 mg and azathioprine 50 mg and he is on follow-up since then. So what was thought initially a malignant lesion **(Table 3)** finally turned out to be a benign lesion and responded well to steroid.

■ CASE 2

A 60-year-old male presented with a short history of jaundice, pale stools, and itching. There was no cholangitis, and he had significant weight loss. The hemoglobin was 10.6 g/dL, and the liver functions were deranged with raised serum bilirubin, liver enzymes, and alkaline phosphatase. The USG abdomen revealed a dilated CBD, intrahepatic biliary radicals, and a distended gallbladder. The MRCP revealed a short stricture at the distal end of CBD with the dilated proximal biliary system. With a clinical diagnosis

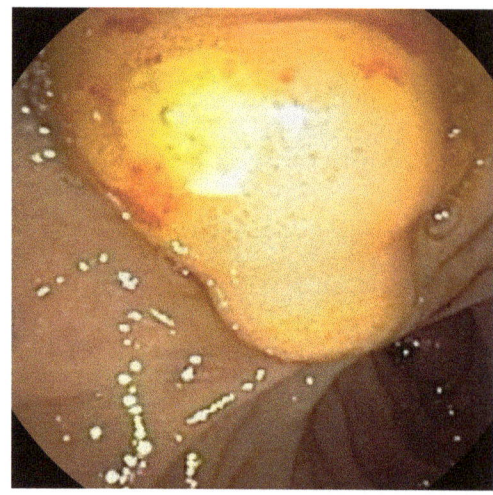

Fig. 5: Duodenoscopy showing a prominent duodenal papilla in the second part of the duodenum (case 2).

of obstructive jaundice, he was further investigated. A side viewing duodenoscopy showed a very prominent ampulla **(Fig. 5)** and an EUS examination revealed a mass engulfing the distal CBD. The biopsy of the ampulla revealed fragments of tissue which revealed

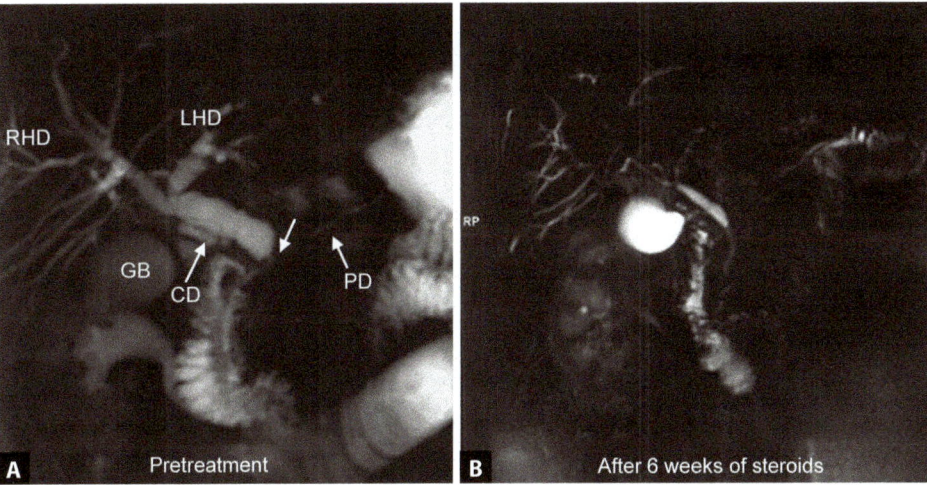

Figs. 6A and B: Comparative MRCP (magnetic resonance cholangiopancreatography) images (case 2) showing marked improvement after steroid treatment—remarkable reduction of the size of dilated common bile duct to normalcy. (CD: cystic duct; GB: gallbladder; LHD: left hepatic duct; PD: pancreatic duct; RHD: right hepatic duct)

necrosis, storiform fibrosis, and glandular structures surrounded by lymphocytes and plasma cells. A special immunohistochemistry study revealed that most of the plasma cells were positive for IgG4 and consistent with the diagnosis of IgG4-related type 1 sclerosing cholangitis. He was started on prednisolone at 0.6 mg/kg/day and was tapered over 2 weeks. His CA 19-9 level came down drastically from the pretreatment level. Six weeks after steroid treatment, an MRCP study **(Figs. 6A and B)** revealed resolution of the biliary dilatation. This is yet another patient who would have undergone Whipple's procedure for obstructive jaundice but finally diagnosed to be a benign IgG4-related obstructive jaundice and was successfully treated.

■ DISCUSSION

Pathogenesis

Human serum contains several types of Ig, the predominant being IgG. It is the major immunoglobulin in blood and other body fluids and responsible for the humoral immune response. Four IgG subclasses are described in humans, namely, IgG1, IgG2, IgG3, and IgG4. Recent studies have shown that elevated serum IgG4 levels are seen in patients suffering from cholangitis, sclerosing pancreatitis, and interstitial pneumonia. Infiltration of IgG4-positive plasma cells have been noticed. The exact role played by IgG4 is still unknown. IgG4 is involved in immune responses in both beneficial and detrimental paths, meaning a protective role in hypersensitivity reactions and allergen-specific immunotherapy and pathogenic one in autoimmune diseases.

IgG4 levels are elevated in some immune diseases and positively correlate with severity.

T helper 2 (Th2) immune response plays an important role in IgG4-RD. Th2 cytokines [interleukin 4 (IL-4), IL-10, IL-13] are highly expressed in affected tissue and peripheral monocytes. IL-4 and IL-13 seem to be promoting the conversion of IgG1 to IgG4. This process requires the recognition of

T and B cells. So, the cytokines of CD4+ T cells and follicular helper T cells (Tfhs) also play an important role in IgG4-RD.

Clinical Manifestations

Immunoglobulin G4-related disease manifests in several ways, such as jaundice, fatigue, joint pain, and enlarged glands. The disease may affect various organs, like the pancreas, biliary gland, lymph node, eye, thyroid, lung, kidney, prostate, and skin. One of the most commonly involved organs in IgG4-RD is biliary tract. But IgG4 rarely affects the intestinal tract, and most cases of IgG4-related gastric disease show a tumor endoscopically and are confirmed only after surgery.

Diagnosis of Immunoglobulin G4-Related Disease

Serum IgG4 Levels

The level of serum IgG4 is significantly increased in IgG4-RD. Yang et al. showed that 22.2% of non-IgG4-RD patients with rheumatic ailments had rise in IgG4 levels. Elevation of IgG4 can also be seen in infection-related diseases, allergy, and maligancies. Even though serum IgG4 elevation can occur in many other disorders, such as autoimmune liver disease, tumors, and viral hepatitis, IgG4-RD is the most common cause of serum IgG4 elevation. Normal serum IgG4 is typically <140 mg/dL, and values ≥280 mg/dL, or twice the upper limit of normal, is highly specific to autoimmune pancreatitis (AIP).

Imaging

Contrast-enhanced CT scan reveals several features characteristic of AIP such as diffuse pancreatic enlargement (i.e., sausage pancreas) **(Figs. 7A and B)** with featureless border and a capsule-like rim. EUS-guided biopsy will help rule out pancreatic malignancy and establish AIP.

MRCP study, ERCP with brush cytology, and cholangioscopic biopsy will be greatly beneficial to rule out cholangiocarcinoma before IgG4-RDSC is diagnosed. PET CT scan will reveal multiorgan involvement and direct further modalities for fixing the diagnosis.

Biopsy

The affected organs are infiltrated by many lymphocytes that form germinal centers, particularly IgG4-positive plasma cells. IgG4 immunostaining of the duodenal

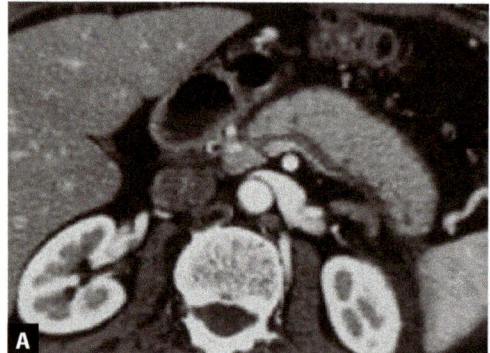 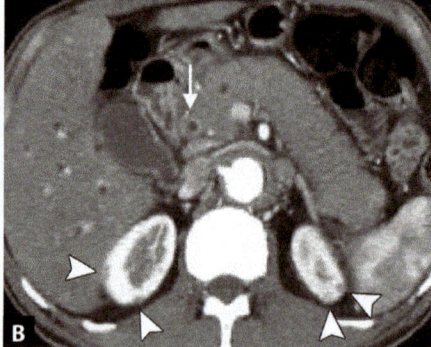

Figs. 7A and B: Computed tomography (CT) scan abdomen showing sausage-shaped pancreas suggestive of immunoglobulin G4-related pancreatitis.

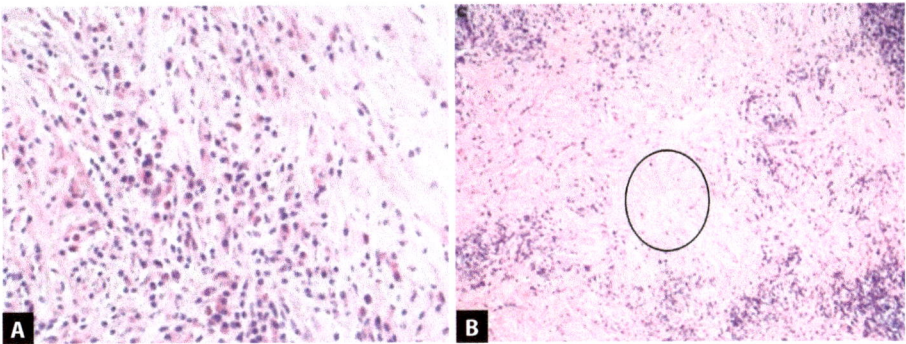

Figs. 8A and B: Histopathology. (A) Lymphoplasmacytic infiltration; (B) Storiform fibrosis.

papillary mucosa obtained from biopsy specimens is another helpful diagnostic tool **(Figs. 8A and B)**. In patients with type 1 AIP, swelling of the major duodenal papilla was first reported in 2002 by Ueno et al. Yoon SB et al. in his systematic reviews and meta-analyses, reported the availability of immunohistochemical staining for IgG4 in diagnosing AIP **(Fig. 9)** IgG4 staining from the biopsy specimens of the major duodenal papilla has a high specificity of the diagnosis of AIP.

Common Immunoglobulin G4-related Diseases

IgG4-related Bile Duct Disease— Sclerosing Cholangitis

Bile duct involvement in IgG4-RD is called IgG4-related sclerosing cholangitis (IgG4-RSC). It is often associated with AIP. A high serum IgG4 concentration in combination with bile duct stenosis on imaging can help to diagnose IgG4 RSC. It is divided into four types as described below according to the location of the bile duct stricture. Type 1: lower CBD stenosis; type 2: diffuse stenosis of the intrahepatic and extrahepatic bile ducts; type 3: hilar bile duct and lower CBD stenosis; and type 4: bile duct stenosis in the hilar area. The most difficult aspect is

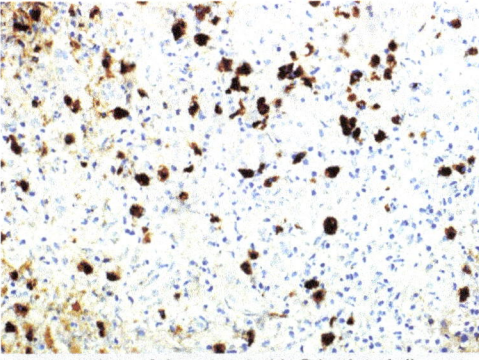

At most sites of documented IgG4-related disease, the IgG4*/IgG* plasma cell ratio is >40%

Fig. 9: Immunoglobulin G4 (IgG4) immunohistochemistry.
Source: Cheuk W Chan JK. IgG4-related sclerosing disease: a critical appraisal of an evolving clinicopathologic entity. Adv Anat Pathol. 2010;17(5):303-32.

distinguishing cholangiocarcinoma from IgG4-RSC. However, there are still significant differences between IgG4-RSC and cholangiocarcinoma. The obvious rise in tumor markers is valuable toward diagnosing cholangiocarcinoma. Apart from the clinical manifestations, the imaging details and pathology findings in support of IgG4, a therapeutic trial of steroids may be useful, particularly when the tumor markers are not positive and the histology is inconclusive for cholangiocarcinoma.

TABLE 4: Comparison of important characteristics of the two distinct types of autoimmune pancreatitis (AIP).

	Type 1 AIP	Type 2 AIP
Age of symptoms appearance	>50 years	30–50 years
Sex	Males more affected	Equally affects males and females
Geographical occurrence	More in Asia	More in the USA and Europe
Histology	Infiltration with lymphoplasmacytic; granulocytic epithelial lesions absent	Duct-centric pancreatitis; granulocytic epithelial lesions present
Serum IgG4 level	Raised	Normal
Extrapancreatic involvement	Biliary tract, retroperitoneum, renal, salivary gland, lung	None
Relationship with inflammatory bowel disease	Rare	Common
Confirmation	May be established clinically	Pancreatic biopsy required
Steroid efficacy	High	High
Recurrence rates	High	Low

IgG4-related Pancreatitis (Autoimmune Pancreatitis)

Pancreas is the most frequently affected organ in IgG4-RD. It is called as IgG4-related pancreatitis or AIP. The characteristic sausage-shaped image in the CT scan of abdomen and laboratory findings of elevated IgG4 level are highly suggestive of AIP. It has varied clinical manifestations, thus it is challenging to diagnose particularly considering symptoms alone. Obstructive jaundice nature is the most common presentation. The biliary tract involvement is the most common extra-pancreatic manifestation in AIP, seen in 65.9% of patients. Mild abdominal or back pain, fatigue, weight loss, pancreatic mass, or chronic pancreatitis are other less common symptoms. Two major types of AIP have been characterized by unique features **(Table 4)**.

Type 1 AIP, is typically present in late adulthood and also known as lymphoplasmacytic sclerosing pancreatitis (LPSP). Type 2 AIP, affects males and females equally and has a younger mean age of diagnosis. It is also known as idiopathic duct-centric pancreatitis (IDCP).

■ CONCLUSION

A gradual increase in the incidence of IgG4 disease has been noticed. It presents with varied clinical manifestations and it affects several organs throughout the body. Hence a high index of suspicion and appropriate screening of various organs are mandatory **(Fig. 10)**. In cases of biliary stricture and focal head mass in the pancreas, IgG4-RD should be considered. Chronic inflammation with fibrosis with tendency to form tumorous lesion with abundant infiltration of IgG4 plasma cells, are characteristic of IgG4-RD. Biopsy of the affected organs revealing storiform fibrosis is unique. Elevated serum IgG4 levels is seen frequently but not invariably. A quick initial improvement to glucocorticoids is characteristic, if tissue fibrosis has not settled **(Flowchart 1)**.

CHAPTER 24: Immunoglobulin G4-related Gastrointestinal Diseases

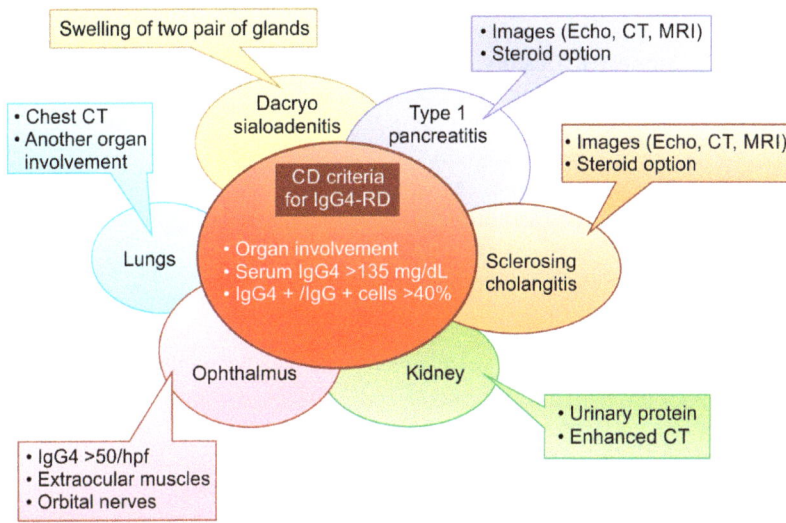

Fig. 10: Overview of immunoglobulin G4 (IgG4)-related diseases. (CD: comprehensive diagnostic; CT: computed tomography; MRI: magnetic resonance imaging)

Flowchart 1: Management algorithm of immunoglobulin G4-related diseases (IgG4-RD).

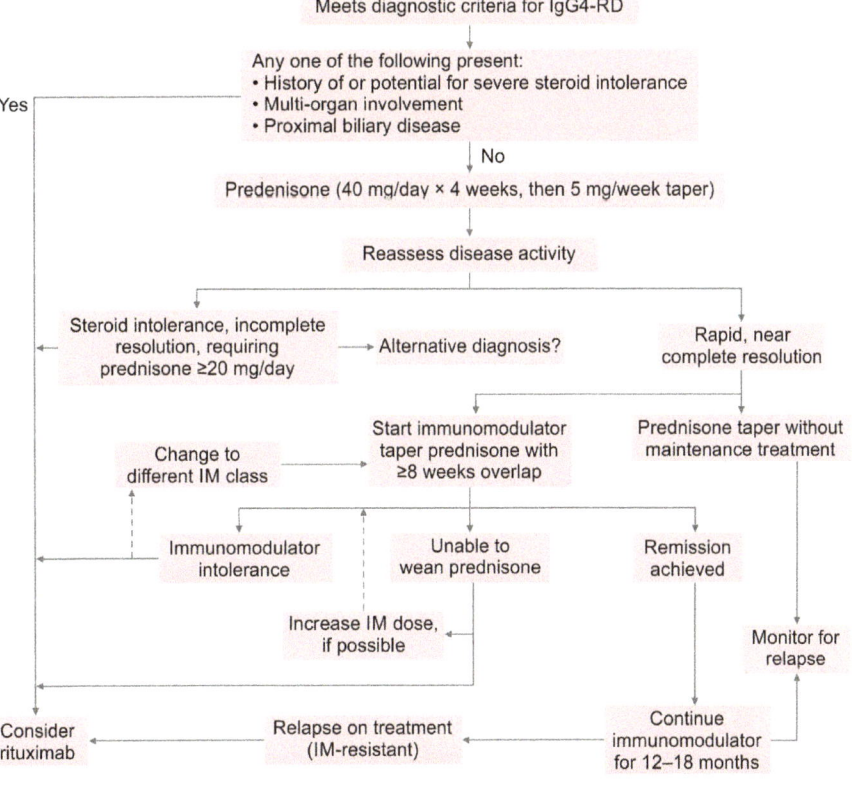

(IM: immunosuppressor)

SUGGESTED READING

1. Carruthers MN, Stone JH, Deshpande V, Khosroshahi A. Development of an IgG4-RD Responder Index. Int J Rheumatol. 2012;2012: 259408.
2. Kamisawa T, Nakazawa T, Tazuma S, Zen Y, Tanaka A, Ohara H, et al. Clinical practice guidelines for IgG4-related sclerosing cholangitis. J Hepatobiliary Pancreat Sci. 2019;26:9-42.
3. Kamisawa T, Okazaki K. Diagnosis and Treatment of IgG4-Related Disease. Curr Top Microbiol Immunol. 2017;401:19-33.
4. Madhusudhan KS, Das P, Gunjan D, Srivastava DN, Garg PK. IgG4-Related Sclerosing Cholangitis: A Clinical and Imaging Review. AJR Am J Roentgenol. 2019; 213(6):1221-31.
5. Mittelstaedt A, Meier PN, Dankoweit-Timpe E, Christ B, Jaehne J. IgG4-related sclerosing cholangitis mimicking hilar cholangiocarcinoma (Klatskin tumor): a case report of a challenging disease and review of the literature. Innov Surg Sci. 2018;3(2):157-63.
6. Nakazawa T, Naitoh I, Hayashi K, Miyabe K, Simizu S, Joh T. Diagnosis of IgG4-related sclerosing cholangitis. World J Gastroenterol. 2013;19(43):7661-70.
7. Ohara H, Okazaki K, Tsubouchi H, Inui K, Kawa S, Kamisawa T, et al. Research Committee of IgG4-related Diseases; Research Committee of Intractable Diseases of Liver and Biliary Tract; Ministry of Health, Labor and Welfare, Japan; Japan Biliary Association. J Hepatobiliary Pancreat Sci. 2012;19:536-42.
8. Zaydfudim VM, Wang AY, de Lange EE, Zhao Z, Moskaluk CA, Bauer TW, et al. IgG4-Associated Cholangitis Can Mimic Hilar Cholangiocarcinoma. Gut Liver. 2015;9(4):556-60.

Section 6

Diseases of the Pancreas

25. **Management of Acute Pancreatitis**
    Goutham Reddy Katukuri, Rupjyoti Talukdar

26. **Autoimmune Pancreatitis**
    Nitin Gupta

27. **Pancreatic Mass Lesion—A Diagnostic Dilemma**
    VK Gupta

25
Management of Acute Pancreatitis

Goutham Reddy Katukuri, Rupjyoti Talukdar

INTRODUCTION

Acute pancreatitis (AP) is characterized by inflammation of the exocrine pancreas and is associated with acinar cell injury and both a local and systemic inflammatory response.

DIAGNOSIS OF ACUTE PANCREATITIS

The diagnosis of acute pancreatitis is made if two of the following three features are noted:[1]
1. Pain abdomen consistent with AP (sudden onset of a severe, epigastric pain, radiating to the back);
2. Serum lipase levels (or amylase) at least three times the normal upper limit; and
3. Distinctive findings of acute pancreatitis on imaging.

The onset of AP is identified as the time of onset of pain abdomen (not the time of hospitalization).

HISTORY AND PHYSICAL EXAMINATION

A 29-year-old male presented to a tertiary care center with acute-onset severe pain in the epigastric region, radiating to back and associated with vomiting and postprandial worsening. Patient gives history of significant consumption of alcohol few days prior to the onset of pain. Examination of the patient showed tachycardia, tachypnea, and tenderness over the epigastric region. Rest of the systemic examination was normal.

A detailed history is needed to ascertain the nature of the pain abdomen, and for the existence of risk factors for pancreatic disorders such as history of heavy drinking and/or smoking, presence of gallstones, recent intake of new medication, history of dyslipidemia, long-standing diabetes, and family history of pancreatitis. Mass lesion needs to be considered in elderly patients **(Table 1)**.[2]

Patients may have diaphoresis with tachycardia which suggest hypovolemia. This may frequently be associated with tachypnea. Fever in the early stage of the disease may occur as a component of systemic inflammation due to cytokine release as part of the inflammatory response. Examination may reveal a tender and distended abdomen with guarding and bowel sounds may be reduced if there is a concomitant ileus.

LABORATORY INVESTIGATIONS AND IMAGING

On the day of presentation, the patient's hemogram revealed a hemoglobin of 17.2 g/dL with a leukocyte count of 16,400 cells/cumm. Serum lipase and amylase levels were elevated above three times the upper normal limit. Renal function and liver function tests were within normal limits.

TABLE 1: Etiology and pathogenesis of acute pancreatitis.

Pathophysiology	Etiology
Ductal obstruction	• Gallstones • Alcohol • Post-ERCP (endoscopic retrograde cholangiopancreatography) pancreatitis • Malignancy • Mucinous tumors • Pancreas divisum • Sphincter of Oddi dysfunction
Acinar cell injury	• Alcohol • Trauma • Ischemia • Drugs (thiazides, azathioprine, steroids, etc.) • Viruses
Defective intracellular transport	• Alcohol • Hereditary • Hypercalcemia • Hypertriglyceridemia • Autoimmune

Ultrasonography of abdomen revealed bulky pancreas with peripancreatic fat stranding suggestive of acute pancreatitis. Chest roentogram was normal.

Hemoconcentration may be associated with an increased risk of developing pancreatic necrosis. Elevated creatinine and urea represent acute kidney injury due to third space fluid loss. However, an elevated alanine aminotransferase (ALT) of >1.5-2 times at presentation and that falls over the next few days suggests a likely biliary etiology.[3]

A chest radiograph may show pleural effusion. Abdominal radiograph may demonstrate dilated bowel loops due to ileus. Transabdominal ultrasonography is the preferred initial study. The sensitivity of conventional ultrasound in detecting AP is up to 75% but is restricted by overlying bowel gas in 25-30% of subjects. Contrast-enhanced computed tomography (CECT) is the investigation of choice but not advisable in the first 48-72 hours of admission (unless due to diagnostic uncertainty) as this has been associated with increased length of stay, underestimation of the degree of pancreatic necrosis and with no improvement in patient outcomes.[4] Endoscopic ultrasound (EUS) needs to be considered to detect microlithiasis and pancreas protocol CT should be planned to rule out pancreatic neoplasm, especially in elderly patients. Magnetic resonance cholangiopancreatography (MRCP) may be suggested in patients with suspected ductal abnormalities especially in children and young patients when the etiology is not clear.

PROGNOSTICATION/PREDICTION OF SEVERITY

The patient had systemic inflammatory response syndrome (SIRS) at admission, which was persistent even at day 3 of hospital admission. Patient underwent a CECT abdomen on day 3 which showed evidence of necrotizing pancreatitis with extensive peripancreatic fast stranding with a CT severity index of 6/10. However, patient did not develop organ failure.

Severe AP may be predicted by presence of SIRS at admission and persistent SIRS at 48 hours. The criteria for SIRS is as follows (at least 2 out of 4):

- Body temperature of >38°C or <36°C
- Pulse rate >90 beats/min
- Tachypnea (>20 breaths/min or partial pressure of CO_2 <32 mm Hg)
- White cell count >12,000 or <4,000/mL or over 10% bands.

Various scores such as APACHE II (Accuracy of Acute Physiology and Chronic Health Evaluation II), Ranson, and modified Glasgow score have been used but none of these were found to be superior or inferior to (persistent) SIRS at predicting death.[5] Severity of pancreatitis is graded based on organ failure and presence of local or systemic complications of pancreatitis **(Table 2)**.[1] Organ failure is diagnosed based on Modified Marshall scoring system for organ dysfunction **(Table 3)**.

The treatment of severe pancreatitis should be delivered in an intensive care setting. A specialist center in the management of acute pancreatitis is one which is a high-volume center with intensive care unit including facility for organ replacement therapy, and with 24/7 access to interventional radiology, interventional endoscopy [EUS and ERCP (endoscopic retrograde cholangiopancreatography)] as well as surgical expertise in treating necrotizing pancreatitis.[6]

■ INITIAL MANAGEMENT

Patient was started on intravenous (IV) Ringer lactate at 175 mL/h initially and later titrated according to heart rate, mean arterial pressure, urine output, and hematocrit levels. Even though the leukocyte count was high, as the blood and urine cultures were negative, antibiotics were not administered. Patient was given enteral feeds initially via a nasojejunal feeding tube for few days followed by oral feeds as soon as patient could tolerate. Patient was discharged on day 7 after resolution of SIRS and normalization of hematocrit and total leukocyte count.

Fluid Therapy

Moderate fluid resuscitation using Ringer's lactate solution with a bolus of 10 mL/kg in patients with hypovolemia or no bolus in patients with normovolemia, followed by 1.5 mL/kg/h (goal-directed) has been shown noninferior to the previously practiced aggressive hydration therapy with fewer complications.[7] The most recently published

TABLE 2: Revised Atlanta Classification of severity of pancreatitis.

Grades of severity of acute pancreatitis

Mild acute pancreatitis	No organ failure/no local or systemic complications
Moderately severe acute pancreatitis	Organ failure that resolves within 48 hours (transient organ failure) and/or local or systemic complications without persistent organ failure
Severe acute pancreatitis	Persistent organ failure (>48 hours)

TABLE 3: Modified Marshall Organ Failure Score.

Organ system	Score 0	Score 1	Score 2	Score 3	Score 4
Cardiovascular (SBP)	>90 mm Hg	<90 mm Hg (fluid responsive)	<90 mm Hg (not fluid responsive)	<90 mm Hg (pH <7.3)	<90 mm Hg (pH <7.2)
Respiratory (PaO_2/FiO_2)	>400 mm Hg	301–400 mm Hg	201–300 mm Hg	101–200 mm Hg	<100 mm Hg
Renal	<1.4 mg/dL	1.4–1.8 mg/dL	1.9–3.6 mg/dL	3.6–4.9 mg/dL	>4.9 mg/dL

A score of 2 or more in any organ system indicates organ failure.

(FiO_2: fraction of inspired oxygen; PaO_2: partial pressure of arterial oxygen; SBP: systolic blood pressure)

Waterfall trial, an international multicenter RCT demonstrated that aggressive fluid therapy resulted in more harm compared to moderate fluid therapy. The trial was stopped after the first interim analyses.

Prophylactic Antibiotics

Using antibiotics prophylactically have not been shown to reduce the incidence of mortality, extrapancreatic infections or the need for surgical intervention and carry the risk of development of drug resistant organisms.[8]

Nutritional Support

Oral feeding in mild pancreatitis can be restarted once the pain is improving. In predicted severe acute pancreatitis, if the patient cannot tolerate oral feeding, enteral tube feeding should be the mainstay. Patients who can eat do not require further enteral nutrition via nasojejunal tube. Compared to enteral nutrition, parenteral nutrition increases the risk of infection, multi-organ failure, need for surgical intervention, and mortality.[9]

PERIPANCREATIC FLUID COLLECTIONS

The patient again presented 6 weeks later with pain abdomen and fever. Examination revealed tachycardia, tachypnea, and tenderness over the epigastric region. Laboratories showed elevated total leukocyte count and inflammatory markers (IL-6) and a high procalcitonin. Patient was started on imipenem. There was a transient improvement in symptoms, however SIRS was persistent and a CECT abdomen showed a large, thick-walled necrotic collection replacing nearly the entire body and tail of pancreas **(Fig. 1)**.

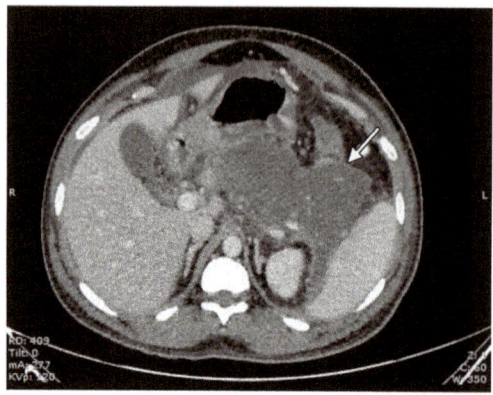

Fig. 1: Contrast-enhanced computed tomography (CECT) abdomen shows a thick-walled walled-off necrosis (WON) replacing the pancreatic body and tail (white arrow).

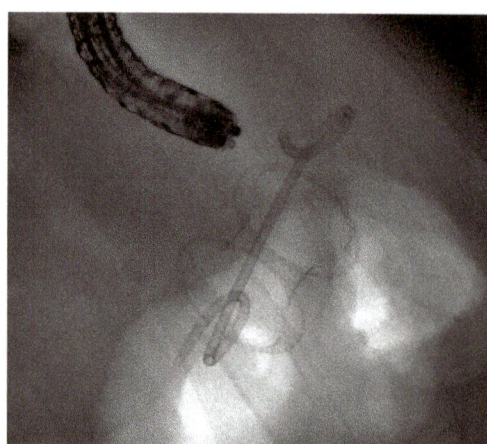

Fig. 2: Fluoroscopy image showing EUS-guided lumen-apposing metal stent (LAMS) and double pigtail stent (DPT) placement.

Since initial response to antibiotic was transient and the patient again started getting fever spikes, EUS was performed and endoscopic drainage of the WON (walled-off necrosis) was performed using a LAMS (lumen apposing metal stent) along with a double pigtail plastic stent **(Fig. 2)**. As patient had significant necrosum (>30 %) prior to drainage and persistent SIRS 48 hours after drainage, patient subsequently underwent

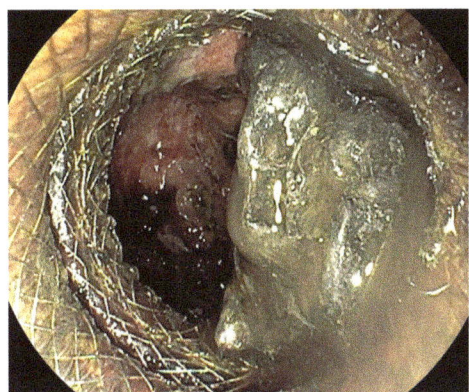 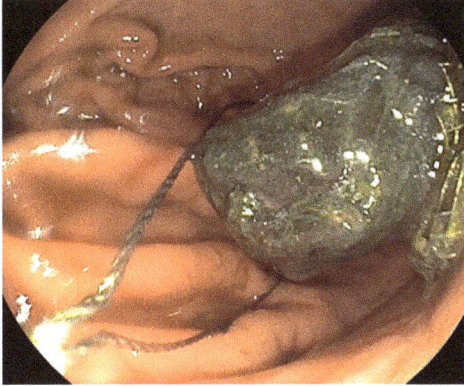

Fig. 3: Endoscopy image of direct endoscopy necrosectomy (DEN).

direct endoscopic necrotomy **(Fig. 3)**. There was substantial clinical improvement and SIRS resolved. Patient was discharged couple of days later.

The patient was reviewed 3 weeks later. MRCP was performed to rule out pancreatic ductal disruption and evaluate the morphology of the WON. The was a small residual WON without any evidence of ductal disruption. The LAMS was removed and a single plastic stent was placed inside the WON cavity to prevent recurrence. Patient was asymptomatic at 6 months of follow-up.

The 2012 Revised Atlanta Classification discerns four categories of peripancreatic fluid collections (PPFC) in acute pancreatitis depending on the content, degree of encapsulation, and time **(Table 4 and Flowchart 1)**.[1]

Indications for intervention (either radiological, endoscopic or surgical) for PPFC are:[6]
- Clinical suspicion or documented infected necrotizing pancreatitis with clinical worsening, if possible when the necrosis has become walled-off (after 4 weeks)
- In the absence of documented infection, ongoing organ failure for several weeks after the onset of acute pancreatitis

TABLE 4: Nomenclature of peripancreatic fluid collections according to Revised Atlanta Classification.

Acute peripancreatic fluid collection	Acute necrotic collection
• <4 weeks • Interstitial pancreatitis • Homogenous fluid density • No fully definable wall	• <4 weeks • Necrotizing pancreatitis • Heterogenous collection • No fully definable wall
Pseudocyst	**Walled-off necrosis**
• >4 weeks • Interstitial pancreatitis • Homogenous fluid density • Well-defined wall	• >4 weeks • Necrotizing pancreatitis • Heterogenous collection • Well-defined wall

Minimally invasive step-up approach reduces the rate of major complications and death as compared with open necrosectomy.[10,11]

SPECIFIC ADDITIONAL TREATMENT FOR SELECT CASES

Alcohol-related Pancreatitis

Patients with alcohol-related pancreatitis need management for alcohol-withdrawal.

Flowchart 1: Approach to the management of pancreatic fluid collections.[11]

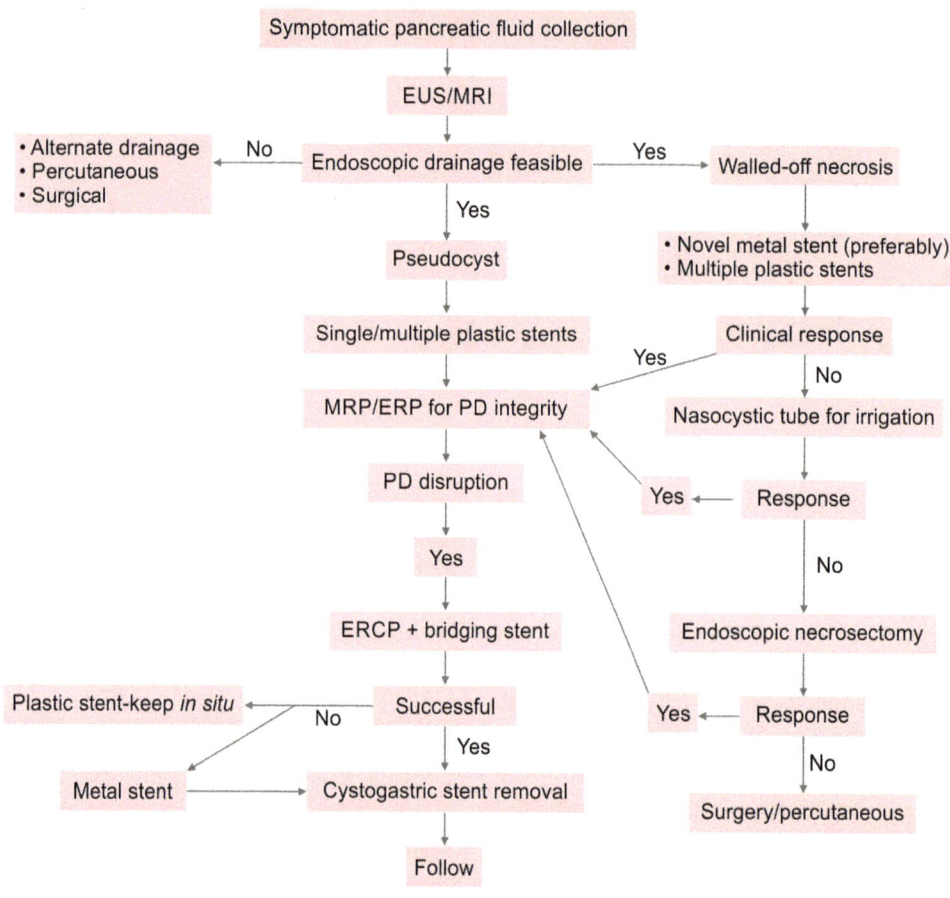

(ERCP: endoscopic retrograde cholangiopancreatography; ERP: endoscopic retrograde pancreatography; EUS: endoscopic ultrasound; MRI: magnetic resonance imaging; MRP: magnetic resonance pancreatography; PD: pancreatic duct)

Benzodiazepines, thiamine, folic acid and multivitamins need to be administered. Patient needs to be subjected to deaddiction therapy whenever necessary.

Gallstone Pancreatitis

All patients with gallstone pancreatitis should be offered cholecystectomy. In cases with mild biliary pancreatitis, cholecystectomy should be performed during the index admission if possible or within 2 weeks of discharge. In patients of severe gallstone pancreatitis, surgery may need to be deferred until collections have been managed or after 6 weeks.[6]

REFERENCES

1. Banks PA, Bollen TL, Dervenis C, Gooszen HG, Johnson CD, Sarr MG, et al. Acute Pancreatitis Classification Working Group. Classification of acute pancreatitis—2012: revision of the Atlanta classification and definitions by international consensus. Gut. 2013;62:102-11.

2. Goodchild G, Chouhan M, Johnson GJ. Practical guide to the management of acute pancreatitis. Frontline Gastroenterol. 201910(3):292-9.
3. Tenner S, Dubner H, Steinberg W. Predicting gallstone pancreatitis with laboratory parameters: a meta-analysis. Am J Gastroenterol. 1994;89:1863-6.
4. Spanier BWM, Nio Y, van der Hulst RW, Tuynman HA, Dijkgraaf MG, Bruno MJ. Practice and yield of early CT Scan in acute pancreatitis: a dutch observational multicenter study. Pancreatology. 2010;10(2-3):222-8.
5. Papachristou GI, Muddana V, Yadav D, O'Connell M, Sanders MK, Slivka A, et al. Comparison of BISAP, Ranson's, APACHE-II, and CTSI scores in predicting organ failure, complications, and mortality in acute pancreatitis. Am J Gastroenterol. 2010;105:435-41.
6. Working Group IAP/APA Acute Pancreatitis Guidelines. IAP/APA evidence-based guidelines for the management of acute pancreatitis. Pancreatology. 2013;13:e1-15.
7. De-Madaria E, Buxbaum JL, Maisonneuve P, García García de Paredes A, Zapater P, Guilabert L, et al; ERICA Consortium. Aggressive or Moderate Fluid Resuscitation in Acute Pancreatitis. N Engl J Med. 2022;387:989-1000.
8. Wittau M, Mayer B, Scheele J, Henne-Bruns D, Dellinger EP, Isenmann R. Systematic review and meta-analysis of antibiotic prophylaxis in severe acute pancreatitis. Scand J Gastroenterol. 2011;46:261-70.
9. Al-Omran M, Albalawi ZH, Tashkandi MF, Al-Ansary LA. Enteral versus parenteral nutrition for acute pancreatitis. Cochrane Database Syst Rev. 2010;2010:CD002837.
10. Van Santvoort HC, Besselink MG, Bakker OJ, Hofker HS, Boermeester MA, Dejong CH, et al; Dutch Pancreatitis Study Group. A step-up approach or open necrosectomy for necrotizing pancreatitis. N Engl J Med. 2010;362:1491-502.
11. Nabi Z, Basha J, Reddy DN. Endoscopic management of pancreatic fluid collections-revisited. World J Gastroenterol. 2017;23(15):2660-72.

Autoimmune Pancreatitis

Nitin Gupta

INTRODUCTION

A 51-year-old lady presented with painless progressive jaundice of 2 weeks duration. At the time of presentation, her total bilirubin 14 g%. Ultrasound abdomen **(Fig. 1)** revealed dilated common bile duct (CBD) till lower end with dilated intrahepatic biliary radicals (IHBR). No gallstones were present. Contrast-enhanced computed tomography (CECT) abdomen was performed, which showed dilated CBD till lower end with abrupt cutoff in the terminal CBD. Pancreas was bulky; however, no focal mass lesion was seen and the main pancreatic duct (MPD) was not dilated. No significant regional lymphadenopathy was found. Endoscopic ultrasound (EUS) was done, which also revealed dilated CBD with abrupt cutoff in the intrapancreatic portion. Pancreas was diffusely bulky and showed coarse echotexture with specks of calcification. The MPD was thin, being obliterated at places **(Fig. 1)**. A working diagnosis of autoimmune pancreatitis (AIP) was considered. EUS-guided biopsy was taken from the head and body of pancreas. Serum immunoglobulin G4 (IgG4) levels were 4.01 g/L. Biopsy showed chronic lymphoplasmacytic infiltrate with storiform fibrosis. IgG4 staining revealed increased IgG4 positive cells.

Patient was started on a tapering course of steroids starting with 40 mg/day, then

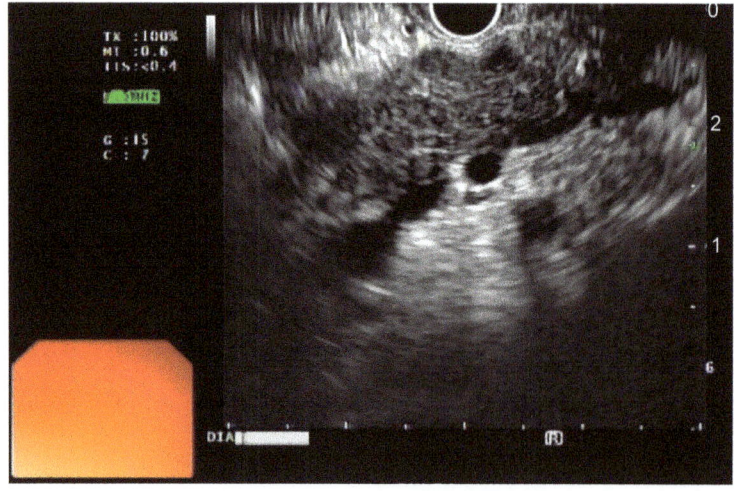

Fig. 1: Ultrasound of the abdomen.

tapered over next 3 months. She improved dramatically with reduction in bilirubin and improvement in appetite within 2 weeks. IgG4 levels returned to normal. CECT abdomen repeated after steroid treatment shows resolution of findings. Patient is 16-month follow-up and is presently asymptomatic. .

■ DISCUSSION

Autoimmune pancreatitis is an immune-mediated disease characterized by chronic inflammatory changes in the form of lymphoplasmacytic infiltrate and fibrosis, clinically manifesting as obstructive jaundice, radiologically presenting as bulky sausage-shaped pancreas with or without mass formation and showing a marked response to steroids.[1] There are two different types of AIP:[2]

- *Type 1 AIP:* It is a pancreatic involvement of systemic inflammation related to IgG4. Other organs commonly involved in systemic inflammation are liver, kidneys, and salivary glands.
- *Type 2 AIP:* It is pancreatic predominant disease and is not a part of systemic inflammation related to IgG4.

All these abovementioned features, i.e., clinical, radiological, pathological, serological features along with response to treatment (steroids) are used to make a diagnosis of AIP. Mayo Clinic has proposed a diagnostic criterion known by acronym (HISORt criteria) for making a diagnosis of AIP which involves five main features: *H*istology, *I*maging, *S*erology, involvement of other *O*rgans, and *R*esponse to steroid *t*herapy.[3] Recently, International Consensus Diagnostic Criteria (ICDC) have been published, which are now considered the standard criteria for diagnosis of AIP.[4] These criteria though more effective in making a correct diagnosis and are more difficult to use in clinical practice.

- *Histology:* As discussed above, type 1 AIP is a pancreatic manifestation of systemic inflammation related to IgG4, and is characterized histologically by lymphoplasmacytic infiltrates with >10 IgG4 positive plasma cells/high power field, storiform fibrosis and obliterative phlebitis.[5] In contrast, type 2 AIP does not involve inflammation IgG4-related inflammation but is characterized by the presence of granulocytic epithelial lesions (GELs) in the acini and ductular cells.[6] Biopsy samples for histopathological analysis can be easily obtained using EUS-guided fine needle aspiration biopsy (FNAB).
- *Imaging:* CT scan is commonly used in the diagnosis of AIP. Pancreas usually appears homogenously bulky, giving a sausage-shaped appearance. Sometimes, there can be a mass-like lesion in the head of pancreas, mimicking a pancreatic malignancy.[7] One differentiating feature from malignancy is that the MPD is usually not dilated in AIP, contradictory to malignant lesions, where the upstream pancreatic duct is dilated.
- *Serology:* Elevated serum IgG levels of subclass IgG4 are useful in diagnosis of AIP;[3] cutoff values of 130–140 mg/dL are considered significant. However, these levels alone are not sensitive or specific enough for making the diagnosis and must be used in conjunction with other diagnostic criteria.
- *Response to therapy:* Steroids are the first-line therapy to use in patients with active AIP. Prednisolone is administered for 1 month at a dose of 0.6–0.8 mg/kg/day (30–40 mg/day) followed by tapering by 5 mg/week, till complete stoppage

of steroids by 3-6 months. Clinical response in the form of improvement in symptoms can be used to guide the rate of steroid taper. Remission with steroids is achieved in majority of cases; however, relapse rated up to 33% has been reported. Maintenance therapy with low-dose steroid for more than a year can be used to reduce the risk of relapse in such cases. Rituximab as monotherapy is useful in those with contraindications to steroids.

REFERENCES

1. Rose NR, Mackay IR (Eds). The Autoimmune Diseases, 4th edition. San Diego, CA: Elsevier Academic Press; 2006.
2. Sah RP, Chari ST, Pannala R, Sugumar A, Clain JE, Levy MJ, et al. Differences in Clinical Profile and Relapse Rate of Type 1 Versus Type 2 Autoimmune Pancreatitis. Gastroenterology. 2010;139:140-8.
3. Chari ST. Diagnosis of autoimmune pancreatitis using its five cardinal features: introducing the Mayo Clinic's HISORt criteria. J Gastroenterol. 2007;42 Suppl 18: 39-41.
4. Shimosegawa T, Chari ST, Frulloni L, Kamisawa T, Kawa S, Mino-Kenudson M, et al.; International Association of Pancreatology. International consensus diagnostic criteria for autoimmune pancreatitis: guidelines of the International Association of Pancreatology. Pancreas. 2011;40(3):352-8.
5. Kamisawa T, Takuma K, Egawa N, Tsuruta K, Sasaki T. Autoimmune pancreatitis and IgG4-related sclerosing disease. Nat Rev Gastroenterol Hepatol. 2010;7(7):401-9.
6. De Pretis N, Frulloni L. Autoimmune Pancreatitis Type 2. Curr Opin Gastroenterol. 2020;36:417-20.
7. Khandelwal A, Shanbhogue AK, Takahashi N, Sandrasegaran K, Prasad SR. Recent advances in the diagnosis and management of autoimmune pancreatitis. AJR Am J Roentgenol. 2014;202(5):1007-21.

CHAPTER 27

Pancreatic Mass Lesion— A Diagnostic Dilemma

VK Gupta

■ INTRODUCTION

Tuberculosis has high prevalence in Asia. Among extrapulmonary tuberculosis, abdominal tuberculosis is seen in approximately 11–16%. Isolated pancreatic tuberculosis is rare and in majority of the cases, it presents as a mass lesion in the head of pancreas. The lesions of tuberculosis affecting other parts of the pancreas are rare. Clinically, it can manifest as obstructive jaundice, chronic pancreatitis, pancreatic abscess, acute pancreatitis, or a pseudocyst. Extrapulmonary tuberculosis is more common in immunodeficient patients. We present a case of pancreatic tuberculosis in an immunocompetent male who presented with features of obstructive jaundice. After confirmation of the diagnosis on cytology of the sample collected on EUS, ATT was given and a major surgical intervention was avoided.

■ CASE REPORT

A 42-year-old male had presented with pain abdomen, fever, anorexia, and weight loss for a duration of 1 month. Clinically, he had icterus and remaining general and systemic examination was noncontributory. Hematological parameters were normal except elevated erythrocyte sedimentation rate (ESR) **(Table 1)**. The liver function test (LFT) was grossly deranged **(Table 2)**. X-ray chest was normal. Ultrasound abdomen found a dilated common bile duct (CBD) in its proximal part with sudden cutoff in the mid CBD, dilatation of intrahepatic biliary radicles (IHBR), and a mass lesion in the head of pancreas. The pancreatic duct was of normal dimension. Magnetic resonance cholangiopancreatography (MRCP) also confirmed the findings of the ultrasound abdomen. Contrast-enhanced computed tomography (CECT) of the abdomen showed a mass lesion in the head of pancreas measuring 4 × 3 cm, causing compression of the CBD in the mid-CBD region **(Figs. 1A and B)**. There were a few scattered lymph nodes in the peripancreatic region. CA 19 9 was also elevated—404 IU **(Table 3)**. To obtain a tissue diagnosis, endoscopic ultrasound- (EUS)-guided fine needle aspiration (FNA) of the mass lesion was done and the aspirate was subjected to cytological examination and gene expert test. The gene expert was positive and the cytology revealed the presence of epithelioid cell granuloma and Langhans giant cells **(Fig. 2)**.

To complete the list of investigations and to relieve the obstruction of the CBD, endoscopic retrograde cholangiopancreatography (ERCP) was performed and the brush cytology sample was collected from the site of CBD obstruction, followed by stenting of the CBD by a 10 Fr 7 cm-long plastic stent. The brush cytology sample did not reveal any

SECTION 6: Diseases of the Pancreas

TABLE 1: Hematological parameters before and after admission.

CBC	At admission	1 month later	2 months later	6 months later
Hb (g/dL)	12.4	12.2	14.1	15.5
TLC	6,400	7.5	5.99	5.63
DLC				
Neutrophils	64	66	63	64.5
Lymphocytes	20	24	26	26.3
Eosinophil	04	03	4.2	3
Monocytes	12	07	6.3	6
Basophils	00		0.5	0.2
Absolute counts				
Neutrophils			3.77	3.63
Lymphocytes			1.56	1.48
Monocytes			0.38	0.34
Eosinophil			25	0.17
Basophils			0.03	0.01
Platelet count (thousand/mm^3)	260	285	148	201
PCV	37	35.8	44.6	47.1
MCV	86	85.0	88.8	89.7
MCH	28.8	28.8	28.1	29.5
MCHC	33.5	33.9	31.6	32.9
RBC	4.3	4.22	5.02	5.25
ESR (Westergren)	65			

(CBC: complete blood count; DLC: differential leukocyte count; ESR: erythrocyte sedimentation rate; Hb: hemoglobin; MCH: mean corpuscular hemoglobin; MCHC: mean corpuscular hemoglobin concentration; MCV: mean corpuscular volume; PCV: packed cell volume; RBC: red blood cells, TLC: total leukocyte count)

TABLE 2: LFT before and after admission.

LFT	At admission	1 month later	2 months later	6 months later
Total bilirubin	7.0	0.76	0.48	0.43
Conjugated bilirubin	5.8			
Unconjugated bilirubin	1.2			
AST	187.0	25	19	18
ALT	344.0	28	10	<10
Alkaline phosphatase	298.0	162	87	84
Total protein	8.5	7.79	8.1	7.56
Albumin, serum	4.2	4.07	4.24	4.15
Globulin	4.3			
A/G ratio	1	1.09	1.1	1.22
GGT, serum		245	68	24

(A/G: albumin/globulin; ALT: alanine aminotransferase; AST: aspartate aminotransferase; GGT: gamma-glutamyl transferase; LFT: liver function test)

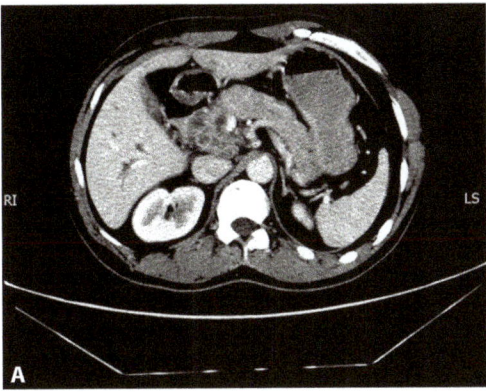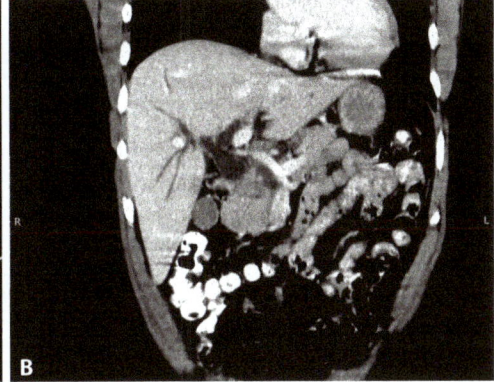

Figs. 1A and B: Contrast-enhanced computed tomography (CECT) abdomen showing pancreatic head mass lesion causing compression of the common bile duct (CBD).

TABLE 3: Cancer antigen (CA) 19-9 value at the time of admission.

CA 19-9	At admission
CA 19-9, serum	400.98

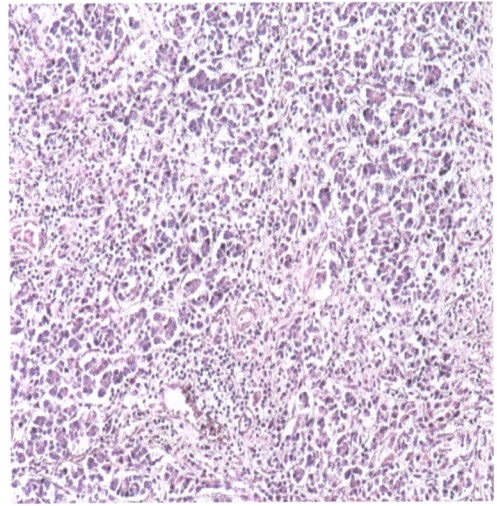

Fig. 2: Microphotograph of the pancreatic fine needle aspirate showing giant cells.

evidence of malignancy. Thus, the diagnosis of pancreatic tuberculosis was established and ATT was started.

He was exhibited ATT for a total duration of 6 months. During this period of treatment, he was regularly followed up with LFTs. He did not have any complications and gradually improved. His symptoms abated within 2–3 weeks.

On completion of ATT, his LFT, CECT abdomen, and CA 19-9 were repeated. All were found to be normal. The biliary stent was removed. He was regularly followed-up for additional 6 months at monthly intervals. As he did not have any evidence of recurrence of disease for 6 months after stopping treatment, his frequency of follow-up was reduced to once in 6 months. Now, he is asymptomatic for more than 3 years after stopping ATT.

■ DISCUSSION

Tuberculosis is the infection caused by mycobacterium tuberculosis. Extrapulmonary tuberculosis accounts for approximately 20% in immunocompetent host and in immunocompromised patients, it can be up to 50%.[1] As per the World Health Organization (WHO), pancreatic tuberculosis accounts for approximately 11–16% of total extrapulmonary tuberculosis. Pancreatic tuberculosis is usually seen in the fourth and fifth decade. Worldwide, the maximum load of tuberculosis and extrapulmonary tuberculosis is from Asia.[2,3] With the advent of the imaging modalities such as CECT and EUS, more and more cases of pancreatic tuberculosis are being diagnosed in both immunocompetent and immunocompromised states. Bhansali et al. did not find any case of pancreatic tuberculosis, in a study of abdominal tuberculosis spanning over 12 years probably because of lack of tools like EUS at that time.[4]

The role of EUS in correctly diagnosing the pancreatic lesions has been highlighted by Sharma et al.[5]

Diagnosis of the pancreatic tuberculosis is a very challenging task as it can present with a variety of symptoms which may be totally nonspecific, such as pain in abdomen, fever, anorexia, weight loss, and sometimes jaundice due to the biliary obstruction. Especially in patients with elevated CA 19-9, pancreatic head mass lesion, and jaundice, the suspicion of pancreatic malignancy is always very strong. Many patients have been subjected to Whipple's surgery, but on examination of the resected specimen of the pancreas and the surrounding lymph nodes, features of tuberculosis are clear and management with antimicrobials for tuberculosis leads to complete recovery. With easy access to EUS, diagnosis of mass lesion in the head of pancreas is made reasonably well and pancreatic tuberculosis mimicking pancreatic malignancy is diagnosed and treated nonsurgically.

To diagnose a case of pancreatic tuberculosis was very difficult and the first case report from Qatar was published as late as 2019 only.[6]

Singh et al. have published a case report of similar case whose diagnosis could be made after Whipple's surgery only, but he recovered fully after the patient received ATT.[7]

Regarding the treatment of the pancreatic tuberculosis, 6-month course of ATT is usually sufficient. Two months of initial intensive therapy with isoniazid, rifampicin, pyrazinamide, and ethambutol is followed by continuation of isoniazid and rifampicin for next 4 months. During the period of treatment, regular follow-up with LFT to look for any evidence of drug-induced hepatotoxicity is very important.

CONCLUSION

Tuberculosis is prevalent all over the world. In western world, immunocompromised hosts have higher prevalence, whereas in Asia, even immunocompetent population gets affected by this disease. Extrapulmonary tuberculosis, especially abdominal tuberculosis, is very frequently being diagnosed with the help of newer diagnostic tools. Pancreatic mass lesion of tuberculosis mimicking malignancy is very common. To avoid any surgery, we must make all efforts to diagnose it conclusively. Standard ATT for 6-month duration is sufficient to treat pancreatic tuberculosis.

REFERENCES

1. Sharma SK, Mohan A. Extrapulmonary tuberculosis. Indian J Med Res. 2004;120(4):316-53.
2. World Health Organization. Global tuberculosis report. Geneva, Switzerland: World Health Organization; 2018.
3. World Health Organization. Global tuberculosis report. Geneva, Switzerland: World Health Organization; 2015.
4. Bhansali SK. Abdominal tuberculosis. Experiences with 300 cases. Am J Gastroenterol. 1977;67(4):324-37.
5. Sharma V, Rana SS, Kumar A, Bhasin DK. Pancreatic tuberculosis. J Gastroenterol Hepatol. 2016;31:310-8.
6. Singh Ali M, Shaukat A, Al-Suwaidi Z, Al-Maslamani M. Tuberculosis of pancreas, the first case reported from Qatar. Int J Mycobacteriol. 2019;8:101.
7. Singh DK, Haider A, Tatke M, Kumar P, Mishra PK. Primary pancreatic tuberculosis masquerading as a pancreatic tumor leading to Whipple's pancreaticoduodenectomy. A case report and review of the literature. JOP. 2009;10(4):451-6.

Section 7

Diseases of the Intestines (Luminal Disorders)

28. **Chronic Constipation**
    Omesh Goyal, Prerna Goyal

29. **Chronic Diarrhea**
    Daya Krishna Jha, Vishal Sharma

30. **Chronic Constipation: Frequently Asked Questions**
    Mayank Jain, Jayanthi Venkataraman

31. **Gallstone Ileus Presenting as Subacute Small Bowel Obstruction**
    Sethubabu, Teja J

32. **Small Bowel Neuroendocrine Tumors**
    Mahiboob Sayyed, Manu Tandan

33. **An Interesting Case of SIBO/Dysbiosis**
    Sanjeev Sachdeva, Ujjwal Sonika

34. **Amoeboma Masquerading as Carcinoma Colon**
    Deepak Lahoti, Shami Kumar, Nitin Bhople, Avesh, Meenakshi Jain

35. **Constipation–Functional Dyspepsia Overlap**
    Uday C Ghoshal, Uzma Mustafa

Chapter 28

Chronic Constipation

Omesh Goyal, Prerna Goyal

■ CASE

A 45-year-old male, with no comorbidities, presented history of chronic constipation (CC) for 10 years. His stool frequency was once in 4-5 days and consistency was hard. He reported mild abdominal discomfort and bloating sensation throughout the day and pain in the anal area during defecation. There was history of occasional bleeding per rectum, bright red in color, and separate from the stools. There was no history of vomiting, weight loss, dyspnea, etc. He reported prolonged sitting on toilet since his twenties. Initially, the patient opted for self-treatment [diet and lifestyle modifications and using some over-the-counter (OTC) laxatives] for 2-3 years. Experiencing no benefit, he consulted local physicians but was unresponsive to the medical treatment. Then the patient was referred to the gastroenterology department of a tertiary care institute for further management.

The patient's detailed medical history, including concomitant drug history and family history were taken. No abnormality was detected on physical examination, except body mass index (BMI) of 27.1 kg/m². Abdominal examination revealed mildly distended abdomen with palpable, nontender lumps (likely fecaliths) in left flank. Per-rectal examination revealed normal anal tone, paradoxical increase in anal sphincter pressure on pushing, and internal hemorrhoids.

Laboratory investigations including complete hemogram, liver, renal and thyroid function tests, random blood sugar, serum calcium, and abdominal ultrasound were normal. Abdominal X-rays (erect/supine) revealed colon loaded with fecal matter, with no significant air–fluid levels. Stool for occult blood was negative. The patient was advised a colonoscopy, which revealed medium-sized internal hemorrhoids and melanosis coli (MC). As there was no secondary cause of constipation, the patient was diagnosed with functional constipation (FC), according to the Rome IV criteria. Further investigations were advised to subcategorize the FC.

Colonic transit time study was performed using 60 radio-opaque markers (ROMs) as per Indian protocol.[1] It revealed retention of 46 ROMs at 36 hours and 32 ROMs at 60 hours (spread throughout the colon), which suggests slow-transit constipation (STC) or functional defecation disorder (FDD). Therefore, high-resolution anorectal manometry (HRARM) was performed using a 12-channel water-perfusion manometry catheter with a balloon at its tip, using standard technique.[2-4] Resting anal pressure was normal, indicating normal IAS. On squeezing, there was adequate increase in anal pressure, indicating normal external anal sphincter (EAS). On attempted defecation (pushing), there was adequate increase in rectal pressure but paradoxical increase in anal pressure, indicating type I

FDD. Rectoanal inhibitory reflex (RAIR) was normal. Rectal sensory testing was normal. Balloon expulsion test (BET) was performed using 50 mL water-filled balloon. The patient was unable to expel the balloon in 1 minute. The combination of anorectal manometry (ARM) findings and BET was diagnostic of anorectal dysfunction (ARD).

The patient was advised biofeedback therapy (BFT) for which he consented. All medications including laxatives were stopped. He received six sessions of BFT under supervision in hospital, in addition to the exercises advised at home. There was remarkable improvement in symptoms and ARM findings.

To conclude, this case highlights a common cause of CC, which failed to improve with routine medical therapy but responded to cause-specific therapy. Therefore, in order to improve overall outcomes, early diagnosis and targeted treatment are essential.

CLINICAL DISCUSSION ON CHRONIC CONSTIPATION

Epidemiology

Constipation is one of the most frequently encountered benign gastrointestinal (GI) disorders.[3-6] Prevalence of CC in the global community studies varies from 11% to 18%;[7] and in Indian studies from 11.6% to 23%.[8-10] In a study on college students in northern India, prevalence of CC was 2.1%.[11] CC has a significant burden on utilization of healthcare resources, including cost of inpatient and outpatient care, laboratory tests, and diagnostic procedures.[12,13]

Definition (Including Stool Frequency and Form)

Constipation has been defined differently at different times. There has been a change from the initial physician-driven stool frequency-based definition of CC to patients' reported symptom cluster-based definition.[3] In essence, symptoms of difficult, infrequent, incomplete defecation of sufficiently long duration, and severe enough to force the patient to seek health care suggest CC.[3,14,15] Patients presenting to the physician, often have their own perception of what constipation means to them. Therefore, it is crucial to enquire in detail about the stool frequency, stool shape, and consistency. Normal stool frequency can vary between three times per day to once every three days due to food and lifestyle variations.[16,17] Bristol stool form scale (BSFS) uses visual images of stool forms and bowel diaries which are reliable methods to characterize bowel habits (**Fig. 1**).[18,19] The BSFS describes seven stool appearance and consistency categories, which correlate with colonic transit time.[20-22] For western population, CC is defined by Bristol stool form (BSF) I–II, while in Indian

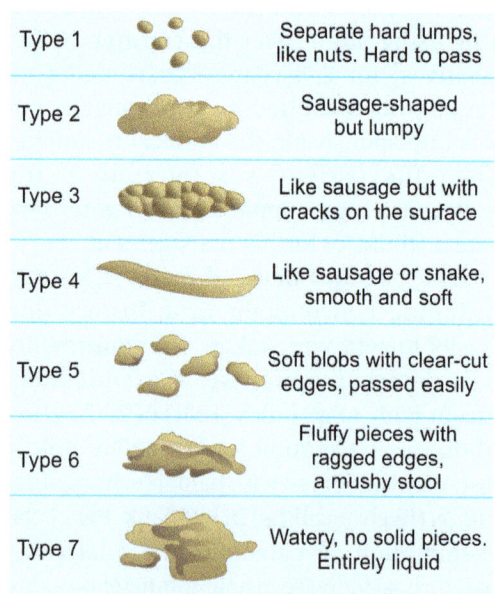

Fig. 1: Bristol stool form scale.

TABLE 1: Common causes of secondary constipation.

Medications	*Analgesics:* NSAIDs and opioids
	Antihypertensives: Diuretics and calcium channel blockers
	Antidepressants
	Antihistamines
	Anti-Parkinsons agents
	Metallic ions
Metabolic disorders	Diabetes, hypothyroidism, and hyperparathyroidism
	Electrolytes imbalance: Hypocalcemia, hypokalemia, and hypomagnesemia
Neuropathy	Autonomic neuropathy
	Hirschsprung's disease
	CNS lesions
	Amyloidosis
Idiopathic and other related conditions	Parkinson's disease
	Paraneoplastic syndromes
	Eating disorders
	Low-fiber/high-protein diet; poor oral intake
	Colonic obstructions: Mass lesions and pseudo-obstruction

(CNS: central nervous system; NSAIDs: nonsteroidal anti-inflammatory drugs)

TABLE 2: Rome IV diagnostic criteria for functional constipation (FC).*

1. Must include two or more of the following:**
   - Straining during more than one fourth (25%) of defecations
   - Lumpy or hard stools (Bristol Stool Form Scale 1–2) more than one fourth (25%) of defecations
   - Sensation of incomplete evacuation more than one fourth (25%) of defecations
   - Sensation of anorectal obstruction/blockage more than one fourth (25%) of defecations
   - Manual maneuvers to facilitate more than one fourth (25%) of defecations (e.g., digital evacuation and support of the pelvic floor)
   - Fewer than three spontaneous bowel movements (SBM) per week
2. Loose stools are rarely present without the use of laxatives
3. Insufficient criteria for irritable bowel syndrome

* Criteria fulfilled for the last 3 months with symptom onset at least 6 months prior to diagnosis
** For research studies, patients meeting the criteria for opioid-induced constipation (OIC) should not be given a diagnosis of FC because it is difficult to distinguish between opioid side effects and other causes of constipation.

patients, addition of type III BSF increases diagnostic sensitivity.[4]

Constipation can be *primary or secondary*. Common causes of secondary constipation are listed in **Table 1**. Primary CC is best defined by Rome IV criteria **(Table 2)**. The Rome IV criteria suggests that all patients with CC without evidence of structural or metabolic abnormalities to explain symptoms and not having significant abdominal pain [not meeting criteria for irritable bowel syndrome with constipation (IBSC)] should be considered under the "umbrella" of FC.[14,21]

In contrast, patients with IBSC have abdominal pain as the predominant symptom along with BSF types 1 or 2, >25% of the times.[14] FC and IBSC may be a part of the spectrum of CC in which patients with severe abdominal pain are on one end and those with no/mild pain are on the other end.[21] The crucial pathophysiological difference between FC and IBSC may lie in different degrees of visceral sensitivities: rectal hyposensitivity (RH) being more common in FC and rectal and colonic hypersensitivity more often seen in patients with IBSC. Most of the hospital-based Indian studies have reported FC to be more common than IBSC among patients with CC.[8,23-25]

Pathogenesis

In epidemiological surveys, several lifestyle factors including inadequate dietary fiber and fluid intake, irregular and inadequate time in the toilet, sedentary life, and consumption of some drugs **(Table 1)** have been reported to contribute to CC.[4,26] However in patients presenting with CC to the clinicians, especially in tertiary care centers, major pathophysiological abnormalities have been found to contribute to constipation in addition to these trivial factors. Pathophysiologically, CC can be divided into three broad categories—STC, normal transit constipation (NTC), and dyssynergic defecation or FDD.[4] FDD is characterized by paradoxical contraction or inadequate relaxation of the pelvic floor muscles during attempted defecation and/or inadequate propulsive forces during attempted defecation. These disorders are frequently associated with symptoms such as excessive straining, feeling of incomplete evacuation, and digital facilitation of bowel movements. It has been suggested that FC might have some organic basis which can alter colonic motility or rectoanal coordination.[27] These include reduced number of enteric neuronal elements including interstitial cells of Cajal, nuclear abnormalities in the ganglia, and reduction of acetylcholinesterase activity.[28,29] Methane-producing gut flora may also be associated with reduced gut motility.[30]

Diagnosis

Diagnosis of CC includes detailed history taking, physical examination, including digital rectal examination (DRE), and investigations to exclude organic causes and explore possible contributing pathophysiological factors, when indicated.[3,31,32] Identifying causes of secondary constipation **(Table 1)** is of utmost importance.[20,33,34] History of alarm symptoms (hematochezia, weight loss, a family history of colorectal cancer (CRC) or inflammatory bowel disease, anemia, positive fecal occult blood tests (FOBT), and onset of constipation at >45 years of age) is crucial. Several studies have demonstrated that some of these alarm features may be reasonably sensitive though not specific to suggest the presence of organic causes of CC.[4,35]

A thoroughly performed DRE in a case of CC can be quite informative. DRE begins with a close inspection of the perianal region, which can reveal excoriations, hemorrhoids, fissures, or masses. An anal contraction in response to a gentle stroke on perianal skin excludes damage to sacral nerve pathways. Palpation with a lubricated index finger in anal canal should include a search for fecal impaction. Resting sphincter tone should be assessed because if it is increased, it may contribute to evacuation difficulties. The anterior wall should be checked for the presence of a rectocele. Placing one hand on the lower abdomen while a finger is inserted into the anal canal, patient should be asked to strain and try to push out the finger; the anal sphincter and puborectalis should relax, and the perineum should descend <3.5 cm.[36] If it does not happen, this indicates FDD.[19,20,22,37,38] Digital assessments of anal tone at rest and during squeezing correlate with the pressures measured by means of manometry.[39,40]

Laboratory investigations (complete blood counts, random blood sugar, renal function tests, calcium levels, and thyroid-stimulating hormone levels) should be done rule out secondary causes of CC, wherever indicated. Performance of colonoscopy in all patients with CC to exclude organic disorders is debatable. While colonoscopy is mandatory in a patient with alarm features, it can also be an important tool in obtaining evidence for the cause of long-standing constipation, especially in a patient with unexplained symptoms, and/or chronic laxative abuse. Colonoscopy is the best modality to rule out mucosal lesions such as rectal ulcers, polyps, inflammatory bowel disease, and CRC.[41]

Fecal occult blood test needs special mention in this context as it is an easily available and cheap test with high sensitivity and specificity to rule out the possibility of CRC.[42,43] FOBT can be immunochemical [fecal immunochemical test (FIT)] or guaiac based. FIT is a preferred test as it does not need any dietary restrictions.[43] In our case, FOBT was negative, but colonoscopic findings revealed presence of hemorrhoids and MC. MC is a noninflammatory, benign, reversible bowel entity in which a brown or black pigment is deposited in the colorectal mucosa. MC is usually caused by the long-term use of anthraquinone laxatives, such as senna, rhubarb, aloe, Rhamnus, and frangula.[44,45] MC can gradually improve over 1 year after stopping the use of laxatives.[46]

Patients with CC (FC or IBSC) who do not respond to reasonable trials of empiric therapy should undergo further evaluation to identify the three overlapping pathophysiological subtypes, i.e., NTC, STC, and FDD.[6,14] The functional diagnostic modalities include ARM, BET, colon transit time (CTT) study, defecography [X-ray or magnetic resonance imaging (MRI)], etc.[3] However because of the lack of widespread availability of these investigations in our country, the workup of a patient with CC often remains inadequate.[47]

Colon transit time is a simple radiological test to assess the colonic transit. The Indian protocol CTT involves giving 20 ROMs filled in two capsules were administered at 0, 12, and 24 hours, and then taking abdominal radiographs obtained at 36 and 60 hours.[1] Retention of ≥30 ROMs at 36 hours (sensitivity 90% and specificity 82%) and ≥14 markers at 60 hours (sensitivity 95% and specificity 100%) was quite accurate to detect slow colon transit and FDD.[1]

Anorectal manometry assesses anorectal pressure changes during rest and simulated defecation of an intrarectal balloon, sphincter tone, and rectoanal reflexes (which evaluate intrinsic and extrinsic innervation and rectal compliance and sensitivity).[21,22,32,35] Although more expensive, HRARM using solid-state probe permits easier calibration and shorter procedure time compared to conventional water-perfused ARM.[48]

In brief, during ARM procedure, the patient is asked to lie in left lateral position and a catheter with balloon at its tip is placed inside the rectum. The basal sphincter pressure (denoting internal anal sphincter activity) and the length of the sphincter zone is estimated. Then, the patient is asked to squeeze and the squeeze sphincter pressure (denoting external sphincter activity) is recorded. Subsequently, the patient is asked to push/bear down so as to simulate the act of defecation. During this period, the maximum intrarectal and the minimum residual anal sphincter pressures are recorded. Defecation index is calculated as the maximum rectal pressure divided by the minimum anal sphincter pressure during attempted defecation. A defecation index value of ≤1.4 is used to indicate FDD. FDD is further classified into four types **(Figs. 2A to D)**.

Rectal sensory testing is performed by inflating an intrarectal balloon with progressively increasing volumes of air (10 mL increments; from 10–400 mL). The patient is asked to report about the first sensation, desire, and urgency to defecate and the maximum tolerable limit while the balloon is being inflated. RH is defined as the maximum tolerable limit >240 mL or at least two of the followings: (1) First sensation at >25 mL,

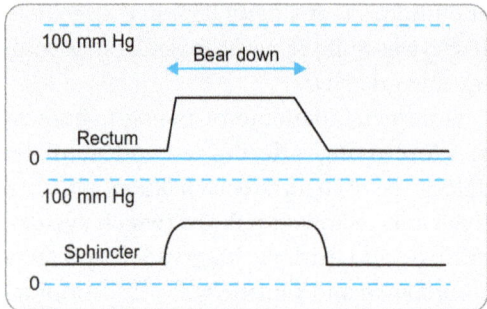
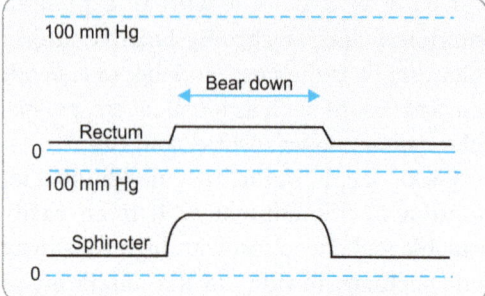
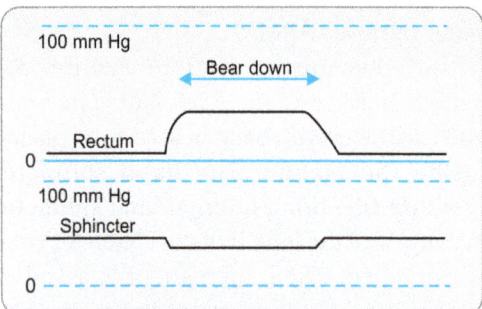
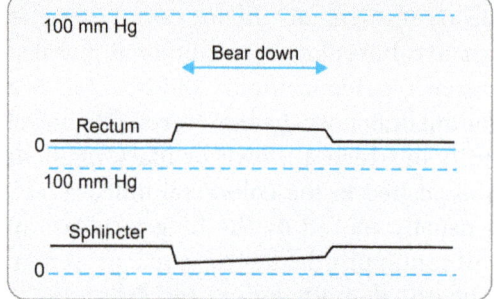

Figs. 2A to D: Classification of dyssynergic defection.

(2) desire to defecate at >150 mL, and (3) urgency to defecate at >200 mL. RAIR is considered present if there is reduction in resting anal sphincter pressure on rectal balloon inflation.

The BET is performed by placing a balloon inside the rectum and filling it with 50 mL warm water. The patient is provided with a stopwatch and is given privacy to expel the balloon in squatting/sitting position. BET is considered abnormal if the patient fails to pass out the balloon in 1 minute.[2]

A standardized protocol of HRARM can diagnose FDD and other neuromuscular and sensory problems and further characterize subtype of FDD. It can, therefore, guide therapists providing corrective BFT.[32,35,49,50]

However, ARM and BET have some limitations. Substantial variations in the procedure methodologies used for BET and ARM exist. Furthermore, success of procedure depends on patient cooperation, procedure may be embarrassing, and test performance may not accurately replicate the actual act of defecation.

If the balloon expulsion or ARM fails to diagnose or exclude a strongly suspected defecatory disorder, a MRI defecography or a fluoroscopic X-ray defecography is recommended.[2] Defecography is a real-time radiology-imaging procedure to visualize how different muscles and organs are moving as the patient defecates, after being given a rectal contrast agent.[51]

The role of MRI in pelvic floor dysfunction is increasing because of its high temporal resolution. MR defecography (MRD) can demonstrate multiplanar information about pelvic floor disturbances during real-time imaging of defecation. Moreover, good temporal resolution, high soft-tissue contrast, lack of radiation exposure, and improved evaluation of triple compartment involvement make it the preferred imaging approach to evaluate patients with pelvic floor dysfunction. MRD can diagnose cystocele, rectocele, and enterocele which can develop due to weakness of the supporting muscles, fasciae, and ligaments.[52] MRD can confirm paradoxical contraction of puborectalis and reveal if puborectalis muscle has become hypertrophic and indenting on the posterior rectal wall.[53]

■ TREATMENT

- *Lifestyle and dietary measures:* These include sufficient fiber intake (20–30 g/day), adequate fluid intake (1.5–2 L/day), physical activity, and avoidance of food and medications that cause constipation.[32,54] When patient does not respond to lifestyle and dietary measures, pharmacotherapy is indicated. These include bulk-forming agents, osmotic laxatives, stimulant laxatives, secretory laxatives, prokinetics, emollients, lubricants, etc.[32]
- *Bulk-forming agents:* They increase the volume and soften stool consistency, thus leading to improved bowel emptying and reduced pain. Most commonly used are psyllium/ispaghula (Plantago ovata) (soluble fiber), bran (insoluble fiber), methylcellulose, and calcium polycarbophil.[55]
- *Osmotic laxatives:* They are non-absorbable molecules and ions which create an intraluminal osmotic gradient that increases electrolyte secretion, resulting in reduced fecal viscosity and increased fecal biomass, with beneficial effects on peristalsis.[32] Examples include polyethylene glycol (PEG), lactulose, sorbitol, mannitol, magnesium citrate, magnesium hydroxide, magnesium sulfate, sodium sulfate, etc. They are comparatively easy to use and inexpensive and can be used as the first-line therapy for CC.[32,56]

  Lactulose is metabolized by colonic bacteria, producing short-chain fatty acids, which are partially absorbed and have a laxative effect.[57,58] Therefore, the dose-response curve of lactulose is nonlinear.[57,58] PEG, however, is neither metabolized or absorbed; therefore, its dose-response curve is linear.[57-59] Osmotic laxatives may be used daily and for long-term. Common side effects of osmotic laxatives include abdominal cramping and bloating, which are dose-dependent.[54] Excessive use of osmotic laxatives can lead to electrolyte imbalance and volume overload in patients with heart and renal failure.[32,60] In addition, lactulose can lead to gas-related side effects (e.g., flatulence).[57]
- *Stimulant laxatives:* In cases not responding adequately to bulk and osmotic laxatives, stimulating laxatives (senna, cascara buckthorn, bisacodyl, sodium picosulfate, and anthraquinone derivatives) may be used. They stimulate peristalsis and thus cause bowel emptying.[32] Most common side effects are abdominal pain, distension, diarrhea, nausea, and vomiting.[21,32,54] In addition to reducing the absorption of water and stimulating intestinal motility, they also increase prostaglandin release. Their main advantage is the rapid mechanism

of action, with evacuation occurring on average within 6–12 hours. Because of their collateral effects (electrolyte disturbances, hypokalemia, and abdominal colic), they should not be used for prolonged periods.

- *Secretory laxatives:* They cause the secretion of chloride into the intestinal lumen. Examples include lubiprostone, linaclotide, and plecanatide.

  Lubiprostone is a bicyclic fatty acid that acts on chloride channels (type 2) on the apical membrane of intestinal cells, which increases chloride secretion and passively draws sodium and water, leading to increased hydration of stool and accelerated peristalsis (without acting on smooth muscles).[59] Lubiprostone is an effective and safe drug (dose 8–24 µg, twice a day).[59,61] Side effects may include nausea, vomiting, and diarrhea.[62]

  Linaclotide is a 14-amino acid peptide that activates guanylate cyclase, located on the luminal membrane of intestinal cells, stimulating the synthesis of cyclic guanosine monophosphate (cGMP), which stimulates the opening of chloride channels.[63] Increased chloride secretion passively leads to water and sodium secretion. Linaclotide dose is 145 µg and the main side effect is diarrhea.[64]

  Plecanatide is a natural analog of uroguanylin, a peptide agonist of the guanylate cyclase-C receptor.[65] Its efficacy and safety profile are similar to those for linaclotide.[65]

- *Prokinetics:* It is a highly selective 5-hydroxytryptamine 4 (5-HT4) agonist that causes accelerated peristalsis and accelerates intestinal transit.[54] Its dose is 2–4 mg, once a day, and main side effects include headache, nausea, and diarrhea.[54,66] Previous drug in the same category, Tegaserod (a nonselective 5-HT4 agonist) has been withdrawn from the market due to cardiac side effects.

- *Methylnaltrexone:* It is a selective µ-opioid receptor antagonist, which acts on peripheral opioid receptors.[67] Thus, it antagonizes the peripheral effect of opioids (e.g., constipation), while it has no effect on the central, analgesic effect.[68] Its dose is 8–12 mg (or 0.15 mg/kg) subcutaneously, on the second day or at 24 hours.[67] It is effective in the treatment of constipation due to the use of opioids.[68] The most common side effects are abdominal pain and flatulence.[68]

- *Enemas or suppositories* may be used in select cases of chronically constipated patients (e.g., those with psychogenic megacolon) or fecal impaction, in which the initial measures (fiber, fluids, and laxatives) were ineffective. Transanal irrigation stimulates the rectum and hydrates the feces, allowing intestinal discharge. The use of these methods should be limited to brief periods and the agents may be composed of sodium phosphate or vegetable oils.

- *Elobixibat (A3309)* is a nonabsorbable molecule that alters the absorption of bile at the terminal ileum, which increases the supply of biliary acids in the proximal colon, with a consequent increase in secretion and colic motility.

- *Probiotics* restore intestinal microbiota and may help in increasing evacuation frequency, improving fecal consistency and diminishing flatulence. The most studied bacteria are Bifidobacterium lactis DN-173 010, Lactobacillus casei Shirota, VSL#3 (a mixture of eight different strains) and *Escherichia coli* (*E. coli*) Nissle 1917.

CHAPTER 28: Chronic Constipation

Flowchart 1: Algorithm for diagnosis and treatment of a patient with chronic constipation (CC).

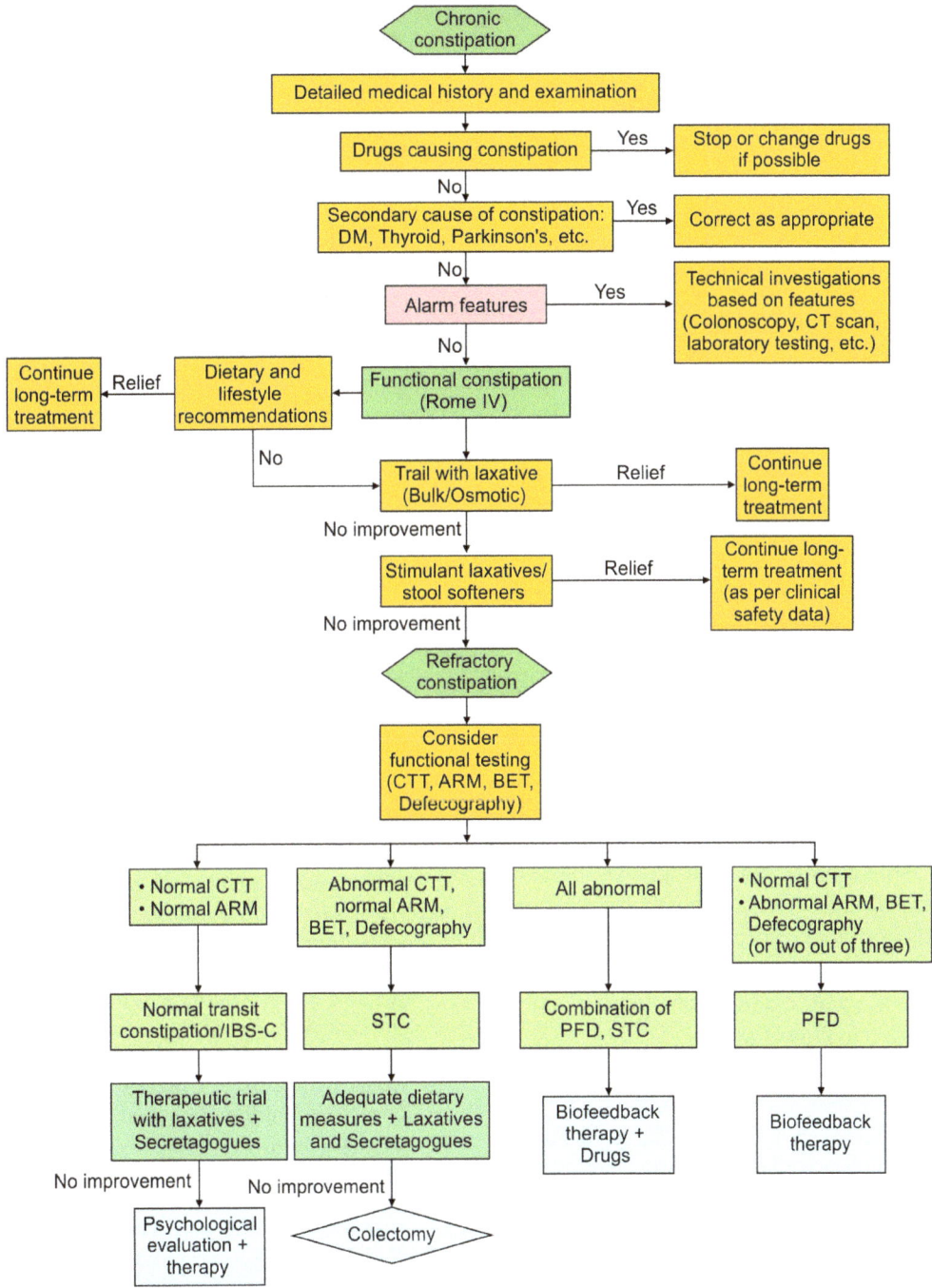

(ARM: anorectal manometry; BET: balloon expulsion test; CT: computed tomography; CTT: colon transit time; DM: diabetes mellitus; IBSC: irritable bowel syndrome with constipation; PFD: pelvic floor disorder; STC: slow-transit constipation)

However, current scientific evidence confirming their benefit in the treatment of CC is lacking.

- *BFT* is a robust recommended treatment for FDD diagnosed by symptoms and ARM. Four-to-six sessions of electromyography or manometry-based BFT carries a 70–80% efficacy rate for FDD compared to standard treatment. Furthermore, it has a sustained response for 12 and 44 months. Standard office-based BFT suffers from limitations—the need for skilled staff, multiple visits, and limited availability at expert centers. Home BFT may be more cost-effective and shows promise for the future.[69]

To conclude, patients with CC not responding to first-line treatment should be classified phenotypically (i.e., FC vs. IBSC) and should be subjected to relevant investigations to reach a pathophysiological diagnosis (FDD/STC/NTC), so that their treatment can be tailored accordingly. Although some treatments are effective for both IBSC and FC, such as prosecretory agents, other treatments are specific to IBSC (e.g., antidepressants, antispasmodics, and cognitive behavior therapy) or FC (e.g., prucalopride), while only BFT would be effective for the subgroup of patients with FDD. Proposed algorithm for diagnosis and treatment of a patient with CC is shown in **Flowchart 1**.

■ REFERENCES

1. Ghoshal UC, Gupta D, Kumar A, Misra A. Colonic transit study by radio-opaque markers to investigate constipation: validation of a new protocol for a population with rapid gut transit. Natl Med J India. 2007;20:225-9.
2. Goyal O, Bansal M, Sood A. Clinical and anorectal manometry profile of patients with functional constipation and constipation-predominant irritable bowel syndrome. Indian J Gastroenterol. 2019;38(3):211-9.
3. Ghoshal UC. Chronic constipation in Rome IV era: The Indian perspective. Indian J Gastroenterol. 2017;36(3):163-73.
4. Ghoshal UC, Sachdeva S, Pratap N, Verma A, Karyampudi A, Misra A, et al. Indian consensus on chronic constipation in adults: A joint position statement of the Indian Motility and Functional Diseases Association and the Indian Society of Gastroenterology. Indian J Gastroenterol. 2018;37(6):526-44.
5. Rubin G, Dale A. Chronic constipation in children. BMJ. 2006;333(7577):1051-5.
6. Rao SS, Patcharatrakul T. Diagnosis and treatment of dyssynergic defecation. J Neurogastroenterol Motil. 2016;22:423-35.
7. Suares NC, Ford AC. Prevalence of, and risk factors for chronic idiopathic constipation in the community: systematic review and meta-analysis. Am J Gastroenterol. 2011;106:1582-91.
8. Jain M, Baijal R. Dyssynergic defecation: demographics, symptoms, colonoscopic findings in north Indian patients. Indian J Gastroenterol. 2017;36:435-7.
9. Makharia GK, Verma AK, Amarchand R, Goswami A, Singh P, Agnihotri A, et al. Prevalence of irritable bowel syndrome: a community based study from northern India. J Neurogastroenterol Motil. 2011;17:82-7.
10. Ghoshal UC, Abraham P, Bhatt C, Choudhuri G, Bhatia SJ, Shenoy KT, et al. Epidemiological and clinical profile of irritable bowel syndrome in India: report of the Indian Society of Gastroenterology Task Force. Indian J Gastroenterol. 2008;27:22-8.
11. Goyal O, Nohria S, Dhaliwal AS, Goyal P, Soni RK, Chhina RS, et al. Prevalence, overlap, and risk factors for Rome IV functional gastrointestinal disorders among college students in northern India. Indian J Gastroenterol. 2021;40(2):144-53.
12. Nellesen D, Yee K, Chawla A, Lewis BE, Carson RT. A systematic review of the economic and humanistic burden of illness in irritable bowel syndrome and chronic constipation. J Manag Care Pharm. 2013;19:755-64.

13. Dennison C, Prasad M, Lloyd A, Bhattacharyya SK, Dhawan R, Coyne K. The health-related quality of life and economic burden of constipation. Pharmacoeconomics. 2005;23:461-76.
14. Lacy BE, Mearin F, Chang L, Chey WD, Lembo AJ, Simren M, et al. Bowel disorders. Gastroenterology. 2016;150:1393-407.
15. Longstreth GF, Thompson WG, Chey WD, Houghton LA, Mearin F, Spiller RC. Functional bowel disorders. Gastroenterology. 2006;130:1480-91.
16. Rutter P. Constipation and diarrhoea. In: Walker R, Whittlesea C (Eds). Clinical Pharmacy and Therapeutics, 5th edition. London: Elsevier; 2012. pp. 209-21.
17. Lembo A, Camilleri M. Chronic Constipation. N Eng J Med. 2003;349(14):1360-8.
18. Rao SS, Rattanakovit K, Patcharatrakul T. Diagnosis and management of chronic constipation in adults. Nat Rev Gastroenterol Hepatol. 2016;13:295-305.
19. Bharucha AE, Pemberton JH, Locke GR 3rd. American Gastroenterological Association technical review on constipation. Gastroenterology. 2013;144:218-38.
20. Serra J, Mascort-Roca J, Marzo-Castillejo M, Delgado Aros S, Ferrándiz Santos J, Rey Diaz Rubio E, et al. Clinical practice guidelines for the management of constipation in adults. Part 1: definition, aetiology, and clinical manifestations. Gastroenterol Hepatol. 2017;40:132-41.
21. Mearin F, Ciriza C, Mínguez M, Rey E, Mascort JJ, Peña E, et al. Clinical Practice Guideline: Irritable bowel syndrome with constipation and functional constipation in the adult. Rev Esp Enferm Dig. 2016;108:332-63.
22. Camilleri M, Ford AC, Mawe GM, Dinning PG, Rao SS, Chey WD, et al. Chronic constipation. Nat Rev Dis Primers. 2017;3:17095.
23. Rooprai R, Bhat N, Sainani R. Prevalence of functional constipation and constipation-predominant irritable bowel syndrome in Indian patients with constipation. Int J Basic Clin Pharmacol. 2017;6:275-85.
24. Ray G. Evaluation of the symptom of constipation in Indian patients. J Clin Diagn Res. 2016;10:OC01-3.
25. Shah N, Baijal R, Kumar P, Gupta D, Kulkarni S, Doshi S, et al. Clinical and investigative assessment of constipation: a study from a referral center in western India. Indian J Gastroenterol. 2014;33:530-6.
26. Ratuapli S, Bharucha AE, Noelting J, Harvey DM, Zinsmeister AR. Phenotypic identification and classification of functional defecatory disorders using high-resolution anorectal manometry. Gastroenterology. 2013;144:314-22.
27. Jain M, Baijal R, Srinivas M, Venkataraman J. Clinical predictors and gender-wise variations in dyssynergic defecation disorders. Indian J Gastroenterol. 2018;37:255-60.
28. Posserud I, Syrous A, Lindstrom L, Tack J, Abrahamsson H, Simren M. Altered rectal perception in irritable bowel syndrome is associated with symptom severity. Gastroenterology. 2007;133:1113-23.
29. Burgell RE, Scott SM. Rectal hyposensitivity. J Neurogastroenterol Motil. 2012;18: 373-84.
30. Miller R, Bartolo DC, Cervero F, Mortensen NJ. Anorectal sampling: a comparison of normal and incontinent patients. Br J Surg. 1988;75:44-7.
31. Bharucha AE, Dorn SD, Lembo A, Pressman A. American Gastroenterological Association medical position statement on constipation. Gastroenterology. 2013;144:211-7.
32. Serra J, Mascort-Roca J, Marzo-Castillejo M, Aros SD, Ferrándiz Santos J, Rey Diaz Rubio E, et al. Clinical practice guidelines for the management of constipation in adults. Part 2: diagnosis and treatment. Gastroenterol Hepatol. 2017;40:303-16.
33. Sharma A, Kurek J, Morgan JC, Wakade C, Rao SSC. Constipation in Parkinson's disease: a nuisance or nuanced answer to the pathophysiological puzzle? Curr Gastroenterol Rep. 2018;20:1.
34. Lee YY, Haque M, Lawenko R, Sharma A. Systemic disorders that affect gastrointestinal motility. Clinical and Basic Neurogastroenterology and Motility. Cambridge, MA: Academic Press; 2020. pp. 601-18.

35. Basilisco G, Coletta M. Chronic constipation: a critical review. Dig Liver Dis. 2013;45:886-93.
36. Talley NJ. How to do and interpret a rectal examination in gastroenterology. Am J Gastroenterol. 2008;103:820-2.
37. Tantiphlachiva K, Rao P, Attaluri A, Rao SS. Digital rectal examination is a useful tool for identifying patients with dyssynergia. Clin Gastroenterol Hepatol. 2010;8:955-60.
38. Rao SSC. Rectal exam: yes, it can and should be done in a busy practice! Am J Gastroenterol. 2018;113:635-8.
39. Tantiphlachiva K, Rao P, Attaluri A, Rao SS. Digital rectal examination is a useful tool for identifying patients with dyssynergia. Clin Gastroenterol Hepatol. 2010;8(11):955-60.
40. Orkin BA, Sinykin SB, Lloyd PC. The digital rectal examination scoring system (DRESS). Dis Colon Rectum. 2010;53(12):1656-60.
41. Rao SS, Go JT. Update on the management of constipation in the elderly: new treatment options. Clin Interv Aging. 2010;5:163-71.
42. Patcharatrakul T, Gonlachanvit S. Outcome of biofeedback therapy in dyssynergic defecation patients with and without irritable bowel syndrome. J Clin Gastroenterol. 2011;45:593-8.
43. Lee JK, Liles EG, Bent S, Levin TR, Corley DA. Accuracy of fecal immunochemical tests for colorectal cancer: systematic review and meta-analysis. Ann Intern Med. 2014;160:171.
44. Van Gorkom BA, Karrenbeld A, van Der Sluis T, Koudstaal J, de Vries EG, Kleibeuker JH. Influence of a highly purified senna extract on colonic epithelium. Digestion. 2000;61:113-20.
45. Mellouki I, Meyiz H. Melanosis coli: a rarity in digestive endoscopy. Pan Afr Med J. 2013;16:86.
46. Rao SSC, Bharucha AE, Chiarioni G, Felt-Bersma R, Knowles C, Malcolm A, et al. Functional anorectal disorders. Gastroenterology. 2016:S0016-5085(16) 00175-X 10.
47. Schmulson M, Corazziari E, Ghoshal UC, Myung SJ, Gerson CD, Quigley EM, et al. A four-country comparison of healthcare systems, implementation of diagnostic criteria, and treatment availability for functional gastrointestinal disorders: a report of the Rome Foundation working team on cross-cultural, multinational research. Neurogastroenterol Motil. 2014;26:1368-85.
48. Kang HR, Lee JE, Lee JS, Lee TH, Hong SJ, Kim JO, et al. Comparison of high-resolution anorectal manometry with water-perfused anorectal manometry. J Neurogastroenterol Motil. 2015;21:126-32.
49. Rao SS, Azpiroz F, Diamant N, Enck P, Tougas G, Wald A. Minimum standards of anorectal manometry. Neurogastroenterol Motil. 2002; 14:553-9.
50. Rao SS. Dyssynergic defecation and biofeedback therapy. Gastroenterol Clin North Am. 2008;37:569-86.
51. Boyadzhyan L, Raman SS, Raz S. Role of static and dynamic MR imaging in surgical pelvic floor dysfunction. Radiographics. 2008;28(4): 949-67.
52. Kalekar T. The Role of Magnetic Resonance Imaging Defecography in the Evaluation of Patients With Chronic Constipation. 2022;41(4):271-7.
53. Nikjooy A, Maroufi N, Ebrahimi Takamjani I, Hadizdeh Kharazi H, Mahjoubi B, Azizi R, et al. MR defecography: a diagnostic test for the evaluation of pelvic floor motion in patients with dyssynergic defecation after biofeedback therapy. Med J Islam Repub Iran. 2015;29:188.
54. Mearin F, Lacy BE, Chang L, Chey WD, Lembo AJ, Simren M, et al. Bowel disorders. Gastroenterology. 2016:S0016-5085(16) 00222-5.
55. Popovic D, Spuran M, Jovanović I. Plantago ovata u terapiji hronične opstipacije-rezultati multicentrične studije. Arch Gastroenterohepatol. 2012;29(1):35-41.
56. Forootan M, Bagheri N, Darvishi M. Chronic constipation: a review of literature. Medicine. 2018;97(20):e10631.
57. Hammer HF, Santa Ana CA, Schiller LR, Fordtran JS. Studies of osmotic diarrhea induced in normal subjects by ingestion of polyethylene glycol and lactulose. J Clin Invest. 1989;84(4):1056-62.

58. Fritz E, Hammer HF, Lipp RW, Hogenauer C, Stauber R, Hammer J. Effects of lactulose and polyethylene glycol on colonic transit. Aliment Pharmacol Ther. 2005;21(3):259-68.
59. Schey R, Rao SS. Lubiprostone for the treatment of adults with constipation and irritable bowel syndrome. Dig Dis Sci. 2011;56(6):1619-25.
60. Hsieh C. Treatment of constipation in older adults. Am Fam Physician. 2005;72(11): 2277-84.
61. Lembo A. Constipation. In: Feldman M, Friedman L, Brandt L (Eds). Sleisenger and Fordtran's gastrointestinal and liver disease, 10th edition. Philadelphia, PA: Elsevier Saunders; 2016. pp. 270-94.
62. Li F, Fu T, Tong WD, Liu BH, Li CX, Gao Y, et al. Lubiprostone is effective in the treatment of chronic idiopathic constipation and irritable bowel syndrome: a systematic review and meta-analysis of randomized controlled trials. Mayo Clin Proc. 2016;91(4):456-68.
63. Corsetti M, Tack J. Linaclotide: a new drug for the treatment of chronic constipation and irritable bowel syndrome with constipation. United European Gastroenterol J. 2013; 1(1):7-20.
64. Bassotti G, Usai-Satta P, Bellini M. Linaclotide for the treatment of chronic constipation. Expert Opin Pharmacother. 2018;19(11):1261-6.
65. Bassotti G, Usai Satta P, Bellini M. Plecanatide for the treatment of chronic idiopathic constipation in adult patients. Expert Rev Clin Pharmacol. 2019;12(11):1019-26.
66. Bassotti G, Usai Satta P, Bellini M. Prucalopride for the treatment of constipation: a view from 2015 and beyond. Expert Rev Gastroenterol Hepatol. 2019;13(3):257-62.
67. Garnock-Jones KP, McKeage K. Methylnaltrexone. Drugs. 2010;70(7):919-28.
68. Thomas J, Karver S, Cooney GA, Chamberlain BH, Watt CK, Slatkin NE, et al. Methylnaltrexone for opioid-induced constipation in advanced illness. N Engl J Med. 2008;358(22):2332-43.
69. Sharma A, Rao SSC, Kearns K, Orleck KD, Waldman SA. Review article: diagnosis, management and patient perspectives of the spectrum of constipation disorders. Aliment Pharmacol Ther. 2021;53(12):1250-67.

Chapter 29

Chronic Diarrhea

Daya Krishna Jha, Vishal Sharma

■ INTRODUCTION

A 27-year-old lady presents with loose stools for 3 months with loss of weight (12 kg) and increasing fatigability.

Question 1: What is chronic diarrhea?
Answer: Diarrhea is a symptom experienced by humans universally. Most patients of diarrhea present with a short-lived episode of infectious origin which usually resolves spontaneously or with antimicrobials.

Chronic diarrhea which is predominantly of noninfectious origin may have various other possible causes.[1] Diarrhea can be defined as alteration of stool frequency, consistency, and volume or weight. Patients commonly define it as change of stool consistency or increased stool frequency; however, researchers have objectified diarrhea using stool weight and volume which is difficult to practice clinically.[2] Bristol Stool Chart is commonly applied clinically as a visual scale for change of stool consistency, where type V and above is considered as diarrhea. Chronic diarrhea is defined as persistent alteration in stool consistency (Bristol type 5 and above) with more than usual frequency of stool lasting >4 weeks.[3] It is important to understand that diarrhea is a symptom and not a disease. Hence, thoughtful application of the basic mechanisms of diarrhea can help facilitating the diagnosis and management.

The diarrhea was insidious in onset but progressive with semisolid to watery stools, no mucus or blood and a stool frequency which has now increased to 8/day. The stool quantity was high and the patient had required two admissions for hypovolemia. The diarrhea was not associated with any abdominal pain. There was no relief with fasting. The stools were watery and explosive but not foul-smelling.

Question 2: What is the clinical classification of chronic diarrhea and how does history suggest the cause of diarrhea?
Answer: Above case description highlights the presentation of watery diarrhea which is a large volume causing hypovolemia, suggestive of small bowel origin. No improvement with fasting suggests osmotic diarrhea.

Chronic diarrhea has vast differential diagnosis underlining the importance of carefully taken history and good physical examination. Chronic diarrhea can be variously described as originating from large bowel or small bowel, caused by maldigestion or malabsorption, based on stool characteristics as watery, fatty, or inflammatory.[4] Understanding the symptom clusters, settings, and impact of illness on patient's life often guides clinicians in differentiating functional from organic diarrhea. Whenever a patient with chronic diarrhea presents, it will be worthwhile to follow a *stepwise approach* in arriving at anticipated diagnosis with limited relevant investigations.

When a patient of chronic diarrhea arrives, following a stepwise approach often helps in deciding the extent and urgency of evaluation. *Firstly*, is it actual diarrhea or fecal incontinence, which can be easily be confirmed by history of soiling of clothes and confirmed on most occasions by digital rectal examination. *Secondly*, is the diarrhea of iatrogenic origin like drug-induced (look for recent changes in drugs), radiation-induced or related to previous surgery. *Thirdly*, is diarrhea chronic lasting >4 weeks. *Fourthly*, is diarrhea of functional origin or organic in nature based on alarm symptoms like nocturnal frequency, fever, weight loss, rectal bleeding, evidence of malnutrition, and dehydration **(Table 1)**.[5] In case of functional diarrhea, it may be associated with pain as in case of irritable bowel syndrome (IBS) or painless in case of functional diarrhea as defined by Rome IV criteria.[6] Some cases of chronic diarrhea which appear to be of functional origin can also be because of small intestinal bacterial overgrowth (SIBO), bile acid diarrhea, or food intolerances. These can be confirmed by therapeutic trials with antibiotics, bile acid sequestrants, or elimination diets.[5]

In cases where diagnosis is not established after initial assessment, further evaluation in the form of basic laboratory tests, stool evaluation, imaging and endoscopy often helps in clinching the diagnosis. Presenting symptoms and basic stool tests helps to categorize the diarrhea as inflammatory, fatty, or watery. Describing diarrhea as small bowel or large bowel can help in deciding the sequence of evaluation among multiple tests available **(Table 2)**. Categorizing patients into one type helps in narrowing the differentials, thus directing the investigation rationally.

TABLE 1: Differentiation between organic and functional diarrhea.

	Organic	*Functional*
Volume	Large	Small
Nocturnal stool	Present in most cases	Absent
Blood	May be present	Absent
Frequency	May be daily or intermittent	Usually Intermittent
Onset	Mostly acute onset	Insidious
Fecal incontinence	May be present	Absent
Weight loss and features of malnutrition	Yes	Absent
Dehydration and hypokalemia	Yes	Absent

TABLE 2: Differentiation between small-bowel and large-bowel diarrhea.

	Small bowel	Large bowel
Volume	Large	Small
Blood	No	Usually present
Rectal symptoms	No	Usually present
Steatorrhea (greasy stool)	May be present	Almost never present
Excessive flatulence (suggest carbohydrate malabsorption)	May be present	No
Foul-smelling stool and pedal edema (Suggest protein malabsorption)	May be present	No
Vitamin deficiency	Yes	No
Pain abdomen	Periumbilical	Hypogastric

Inflammatory diarrhea is suggested by history of small volume, frequent, bloody stools which may be accompanied by mucus or pus, fever, abdominal pain, and tenesmus. Stool evaluation in such patients demonstrates leucocytes, red blood cells (RBCs), and raised leukocyte proteins (fecal calprotectin or lactoferrin).

Fatty stool also known as steatorrhea is indicated by history of greasy or bulky stool which is difficult to flush, oil in stool, weight loss, fat soluble vitamin deficiency, recent onset diabetes, or pain in the abdomen. Floating stool which represents excess gas may be misinterpreted due to excess fat. Steatorrhea can results malabsorption due to mucosal disease (celiac disease) or maldigestion due to either pancreatic exocrine insufficiency (e.g., chronic pancreatitis) or inadequate duodenal bile acid (SIBO, primary biliary cirrhosis). Fatty stool in case of maldigestion (e.g., pancreatic insufficiency) are not watery as the triglycerides are intact on reaching colonic mucosa; however, in case of malabsorption when the breakdown of triglycerides to fatty acids is not affected, fatty acids act as cathartic on colonic mucosa may produce voluminous watery stool.

Watery diarrhea may be caused by intake of poorly absorbed osmotically active substances (osmotic diarrhea) or more commonly, conditions causing secretory diarrhea. These two types of diarrhea can be differentiated on the basis of response to fasting and fecal osmotic gap on most occasions. Osmotic diarrhea typically decreases stool volume in response to fasting, whereas secretory diarrhea continues unchanged **(Table 3)**.

On examination, our patient had pallor with platonychia, the body mass index (BMI) was 17 kg/m^2. The patient had cheilitis and glossitis.

TABLE 3: Differentiation between watery and inflammatory diarrhea.

	Watery	Inflammatory
Stool volume	Large volume	Usually small volume
Blood in stool	No	Yes
Rectal symptoms (tenesmus, mucus or pus)	No	May be present
Abdominal pain	Less common	More common
CRP	Normal	Elevated
Stool • WBC • RBC • Fecal calprotectin	• No • No • Normal	• Yes • Yes • Raised

(CRP: C-reactive protein; RBC: red blood cell; WBC: white blood cell)

Question 3: How do clinical findings help in suggesting an underlying diagnosis?
Answer: Physical findings are more important in estimating the severity and may rarely point toward direct evidence toward etiology of diarrhea. In this case patient had findings of anemia, vitamin insufficiency and low BMI indicative of malabsorption, suggesting mucosal disease.

Findings which may help in suggesting etiology are mentioned in **Table 4**.

Question 4: The hemogram suggested anemia with iron deficiency. What next tests would you advise? Which blood tests should always be considered in evaluation of chronic diarrhea?
Answer: The presence of iron deficiency anemia (IDA) has high sensitivity for small bowel enteropathy, particularly celiac disease. We performed serum iron, serum ferritin, and total iron-binding capacity (TIBC) to confirm IDA. Immunoglobulin A (IgA) anti-tissue transglutaminase (tTG) and total IgA was done for possibility of

TABLE 4: Physical findings suggesting etiology in chronic diarrhea.[5]

Findings	Potential etiology
Orthostasis, hypotension	Dehydration, neuropathy
Muscle wasting, edema	Malnutrition
Hyperpigmentation	Addison disease
Urticaria pigmentosa, dermographism	Mast cell disease
Dermatitis herpetiformis	Celiac disease
Pinch purpura, macroglossia	Amyloidosis
Flushing, right-sided heart murmur, wheeze	Carcinoid syndrome
Thyroid nodule	Hyperthyroidism
Abdominal bruit	Chronic mesenteric ischemia
Arthritis	IBD, Whipple's disease
Lymphadenopathy	HIV infection, lymphoma, cancer
Anal sphincter weakness	Fecal incontinence

(HIV: human immunodeficiency disease; IBD: inflammatory bowel disease)

celiac disease. Evaluation of iron profile confirmed IDA and celiac serology was positive with titers of IgA anti-tTG being high. Patient was subsequently advised for upper gastrointestinal (GI) endoscopy.

To avoid missing serious or common causes for chronic diarrhea, screening investigations should be done to look for malabsorption: full blood count, renal profile, liver function tests, albumin, B12, folate, ferritin, and vitamin D. Testing for C-reactive protein has a high sensitivity for organic disease. Thyroid function tests (to exclude hyperthyroidism) and serological tests for celiac disease (including total IgA levels) form part of a basic screen of investigations. Fecal calprotectin is needed and can help distinguish between inflammatory bowel disease (IBD) and IBS. Values of <50 μg/g make IBD unlikely, but a raised calprotectin can be found in colorectal cancer, infectious gastroenteritis [including tuberculosis (TB)] and with use of nonsteroidal anti-inflammatory drugs.

In cases where there are no pointers indicating etiology of diarrhea may be investigated based on clinical type of diarrhea as discussed subsequently

In cases of *inflammatory diarrhea* basic evaluation may show raised C-reactive protein or erythrocyte sedimentation rate (ESR), decreased serum albumin. Inflammatory diarrhea essentially suggests inflamed and disrupted mucosa which may be caused by IBD (ulcerative colitis or Crohn's disease), infectious etiology (*Entamoeba histolytica*, TB, *Clostridioides difficile*, cytomegalovirus), neoplasia (carcinoma colon, lymphoma), mesenteric ischemia, diverticulitis or radiation colitis rarely. History and evaluation suggestive of inflammatory diarrhea helps guide clinicians towards colonoscopy as the initial evaluation.

In cases with *steatorrhea* fat in stool is routinely identified by Sudan stain and steatorrhea is defined as >7 g of fat per 24 hours in a patient consuming 100 g of fat in diet per day. On identifying fatty diarrhea, evaluation is directed to differentiate malabsorption from maldigestion. Initial evaluation focuses to consider either a structural problem involving small bowel or pancreas. Endoscopy with small bowel biopsy will provide clues for celiac disease and if duodenal aspirates are taken for culture can point toward SIBO. SIBO can also be diagnosed on the basis of (lactulose or glucose) hydrogen breath test. Radiological imaging (CT or endoscopic ultrasonography) may be utilized for structural abnormality involving pancreas, pointing towards pancreatic insufficiency. Additionally imaging can also suggest a cause for cholestatic jaundice, ileal resection, enterocolic fistula, or bowel involvement (as in Crohn's disease) which may present with steatorrhea due to inadequate fat solubilization. Similarly in surgical patients with setting for SIBO a therapeutic trial of gut specific antibiotics may provide best answers in resource limited situations.

In cases with *watery diarrhea* the initial aim is to differentiate osmotic from secretory diarrhea using fecal osmotic gap. Fecal osmotic gap is calculated by subtracting twice the sum of stool sodium and potassium from 290 mOsm/kg, the osmolality of stool in body. Fecal osmotic gap >100 mOsm/kg is characteristic of osmotic diarrhea and gap <50 suggests secretory diarrhea.[7] Osmotic diarrhea is largely due to three reasons: (1) ingestion of osmotic laxatives like magnesium salts, phosphate salts, sulfate salts or polyethylene glycol; (2) ingestion of poorly absorbed sugars like lactose in a lactase deficient individual or sorbitol, which is present in artificial sweeteners; and (3) lastly as a manifestation of generalized malabsorption. Evaluation of patients with osmotic diarrhea is generally straightforward with stool pH <6 indicating intolerance to carbohydrates. Stool ions can be measured in cases with laxative abuse presenting as factitious diarrhea.

Secretory diarrhea has extensive differential diagnosis and may require a wide range of investigation to arrive at accurate diagnosis. Basic mechanism is disruption of epithelial electrolyte transport leading to excess fluids being released from the lumen. Infections are the leading cause of secretory diarrhea and should be evaluated by stool culture, multiplex polymerase chain reaction (PCR) testing and special staining. Immunocompromised status of the patient should be ascertained as chronic infections are more likely to persist in such cases. Endocrine conditions commonly causing diarrhea are diabetic autonomic neuropathy, hyperthyroidism and Addison's disease. Peptide-secreting tumor like carcinoid or gastrinoma are fascinating causes, but rare. Hence, their evaluation should be done in appropriate clinical setting and imaging evidence suggestive of high pretest probability. Bile acid-induced diarrhea (BAD) which can occur due to ileal dysfunction of any cause like post cholecystectomy and congenital defects in bile acid transport or of idiopathic origin. BAD may be responsible for some cases of functional diarrhea and may be part of spectrum of IBS. Bile acid sequestrants can be tried empirically in such cases due to limited availability of diagnostic tests. SIBO should be considered in cases with secretory diarrhea where gut motility is delayed and empirical antibiotics can be initiated. Some cases like neoplastic disorder, mucosal disorders like IBD, and structural lesions such as short-bowel syndrome can be easily arrived at diagnosis after imaging and endoscopic evaluation.

The endoscopy revealed scalloping of duodenal folds and reduced fold height. Histology confirmed subtotal villous atrophy.

Question 5: What are the causes of duodenal scalloping? How to evaluate further?

Answer: Duodenal scalloping is not a specific sign for celiac disease on endoscopy. Conditions that can cause duodenal scalloping include human immunodeficiency virus enteropathy, tropical sprue, giardiasis, eosinophilic enteritis, amyloidosis, and Whipple's disease.[8] In cases where duodenal scalloping is noticed, all patients should have celiac serology done like IgA anti tTG and total IgA. Histology will reveal subtotal or total villous atrophy and increased intraepithelial lymphocytes (IEL >30 cells/hpf) in cases with celiac disease. Other causes of scalloping which can be diagnosed on biopsy include amyloidosis (Congo red staining), eosinophilic enteritis, giardiasis, etc. If negative then patients should be evaluated for alternate causes of duodenal scalloping with human immunodeficiency disease (HIV) serology, duodenal aspirate for giardiasis. If a patient has villous atrophy with features of malabsorption and no specific etiology on evaluation, such cases may be treated as tropical malabsorption.

Question 6: Which patients would need colonoscopy and how to sample for histology?
Answer: Lower GI endoscopy with mucosal biopsy has an important role in inflammatory and secretory diarrhea, with a diagnostic yield of 15–30%. Colonoscopy with routine ileoscopy provides better diagnostic yield than sigmoidoscopy. Biopsy should be taken from multiple segments of the colon even when mucosa appears normal to exclude microscopic colitis or eosinophilic enteritis.[3]

Question 7: What are the common causes of chronic diarrhea in India? Which tests help in making their diagnosis?
Answer: Patients presenting with chronic diarrhea and malabsorption should be considered for common etiology like tropical malabsorption, parasitic infections, intestinal TB, and celiac disease in India.[9] Other etiology include Crohn's disease, immunoproliferative small intestinal disease (IPSID) and acquired immunodeficiency syndrome (AIDS).[10]

Clinical presentation of celiac disease and tropical malabsorption can be similar, however features favoring celiac are: short stature, vomiting/dyspepsia, endoscopic scalloping/attenuation of duodenal folds, histological high-modified Marsh changes, crescendo type of intraepithelial lymphocytosis, surface epithelial denudation, surface mucosal flattening, thickening of subepithelial basement membrane, and celiac seropositivity; while those favoring tropical malabsorption include anemia, abnormal urinary d-xylose test, endoscopic either normal duodenal folds or mild attenuation, histologically decrescendo type of intraepithelial lymphocytosis, low-modified Marsh changes, patchy mucosal changes, and mucosal eosinophilia. Diagnosis of giardiasis can be made on the basis of finding trophozoites in the second part of the duodenum (D2) biopsy or cyst/trophozoites in the spot stool examination. Strongyloidiasis can be diagnosed by the presence of larvae in stool or D2 biopsy. *Isospora*, *Cryptospora*, and *Microspora* are diagnosed by the presence of their respective cysts in any of the three consecutive stool samples stained with special stains like modified Kinyoun's acid-fast stain and Ryan blue stain. Intestinal TB is suggested by endoscopic features and the presence of acid-fast bacilli (AFB) in the biopsy or histopathological features (especially caseating granulomas) or detection of AFB by TB PCR or TB mycobacteria growth indicator tube culture. Crohn's is diagnosed according to European Crohn's and Colitis Organisation (ECCO) criteria, i.e., combination of endoscopic features, histopathology, radiological imaging, and response to treatment. IPSID is a sporadic illness which presents with malabsorption, clubbing and abdominal mass. Endoscopy may show thickened duodenal folds, and biopsy may reveal plasmacytic infiltrate in lamina propria, broadening of villi and atrophic crypts (compare to celiac disease).[11]

Question 8: What are the causes of drug-induced chronic diarrhea?
Answer: Diarrhea is a relatively frequent adverse event, accounting for about 7% of all drug adverse effects. Antimicrobials are responsible for 25% of drug-induced diarrhea.[12] A thorough review must be carried out regarding the previous, recent, or intermittent use of laxatives, antacids, proton-pump inhibitors (PPIs), antibiotics (particularly clindamycin, macrolides, amoxicillin, and quinolones), colchicine, antihypertensive drugs (particularly olmesartan and other angiotensin II receptor blockers, angiotensin-converting enzyme inhibitors, and beta blockers), drugs used in heart disease (digoxin, quinidine, ticlopidine), drugs taken for controlling overweight, obesity, and diabetes mellitus, lithium use, and oncologic therapy, including immunosuppressants, targeted therapy, and immunotherapy.

CASE VIGNETTES: APPLYING THE STEPWISE APPROACH

Case Scenario 1

A 40-year-old female presented with recent onset type 2 diabetes mellitus and 3 month history of diarrhea. She has up to 8 stools a day which is watery, explosive, and nocturnal frequency of 1–2 stools per day. There is no urgency, tenesmus, rectal bleeding, or pain in abdomen. No history of fever or weight loss. She has no history of abdominal surgery, radiation, and was started on oral antidiabetics about 4 months back. Basic laboratory evaluations including blood counts and biochemistry were unremarkable. Stool evaluation showed no pathogens, white blood cells, or occult blood. She underwent a colonoscopy with sigmoid biopsy which was normal. Evaluation for celiac serology was negative.

This patient has chronic diarrhea which has lasted >4 weeks, where there is no history of fecal incontinence. Patient has nocturnal frequency strongly indicating the organic nature of diarrhea. She started on oral antidiabetics, which included metformin and glimepiride about 4 months back. Stool evaluation and history was suggestive of watery diarrhea with absence of features suggestive of inflammatory diarrhea or steatorrhea. Metformin is among the common causes of diarrhea in patients with diabetes mellitus. After stopping metformin, the patient had complete resolution of diarrhea. This case underlies the importance of drug history in cases with chronic diarrhea. Patients with diabetes mellitus (DM) are prescribed drugs like acarbose and metformin which can lead to diarrhea. Celiac disease, microscopic colitis, pancreatic insufficiency, and SIBO are other common causes of diarrhea in patients with diabetes.

Case Scenario 2

A 30-year-old IT professional presented with intermittent diarrhea, abdominal fullness, and increased flatulence for the last 5 years since he has started traveling because of work. He gives a history of mild abdominal cramping pain followed by large-volume watery stool with excessive flatus. He denies a history of nocturnal symptoms, urgency, blood in stool, weight loss, or fecal incontinence. He has been advised multiple short courses of antibiotics thinking of infectious origin diarrhea due to travel with no relief. Physical examination was unremarkable with no rashes, thyromegaly, and hepatomegaly. His routine laboratory evaluation was unrevealing. Stool evaluation done thrice have shown no WBCs, RBCs, pus cells, ova/parasites, and pH of 5.6. Should we investigate such cases or manage as functional bowel disorders?

On applying the stepwise approach. This individual has diarrhea lasting with no fecal incontinence. There is no history to suggest any iatrogenic cause for diarrhea. Has persistent symptoms lasting >4 weeks, establishing chronic diarrhea. Historically patient has no nocturnal symptoms, weight loss, or any alarm symptoms. He has history of pain abdomen with relation to defecation pointing towards a functional cause of diarrhea like IBS. However, his stool evaluation revealed a stool pH of 5.6 which may suggest carbohydrate malabsorption. To differentiate the two disorders a fecal osmotic gap was done which showed a stool sodium of 70 mmol/L and a potassium level of 25 mmol/L. Calculated fecal osmotic gap [290 − 2(75 + 25)] was 90 mmol/L which was suggestive of osmotic diarrhea. Osmotic diarrhea has straightforward differentials, where a stool pH <6 indicates carbohydrate intolerance. A hydrogen breath test done for lactose was suggestive of lactose intolerance. The patient was then advised a lactose-free diet and observed for 3 months, a significant improvement was found in his symptoms.

■ CONCLUSION

Approach to chronic diarrhea involves a stepwise approach and employment of relevant investigation depending on symptom cluster in each patient. Classifying diarrhea as watery, inflammatory, or fatty guides clinicians in reaching etiological diagnosis utilizing suitable investigation. A subset of patients may require empirical therapy in fitting circumstances helping clinch diagnosis.

■ REFERENCES

1. Schiller LR, Pardi DS, Sellin JH. Chronic Diarrhea: Diagnosis and Management. Clin Gastroenterol Hepatol. 2017;15(2):182-193.e3.
2. Mearin F, Lacy BE, Chang L, Chey WD, Lembo AJ, Simren M, et al. Bowel Disorders. Gastroenterology. 2016;S0016-5085(16) 00222-5.
3. Arasaradnam RP, Brown S, Forbes A, Fox MR, Hungin P, Kelman L, et al. Guidelines for the investigation of chronic diarrhoea in adults: British Society of Gastroenterology, 3rd edition. Gut. 2018;67(8):1380-99.
4. Camilleri M, Sellin JH, Barrett KE. Pathophysiology, Evaluation, and Management of Chronic Watery Diarrhea. Gastroenterology. 2017;152(3):515-532.e2.
5. Feldman M, Friedman LS, Brandt LS. Sleisenger & Fordtran's Gastrointestinal and Liver disease: Pathophysiology, Diagnosis, Management, 11th edition. Philadelphia: Elsevier; 2020.
6. Drossman DA, Hasler WL. Rome IV-Functional GI Disorders: Disorders of Gut-Brain Interaction. Gastroenterology. 2016;150(6):1257-61.
7. Shiau YF, Feldman GM, Resnick MA, Coff PM. Stool electrolyte and osmolality measurements in the evaluation of diarrheal disorders. Ann Intern Med. 1985;102(6):773-5.
8. Shah VH, Rotterdam H, Kotler DP, Fasano A, Green PH. All that scallops is not celiac disease. Gastrointest Endosc. 2000;51(6):717-20.
9. Pipaliya N, Ingle M, Rathi C, Poddar P, Pandav N, Sawant P. Spectrum of chronic small bowel diarrhea with malabsorption in Indian subcontinent: is the trend really changing? Intest Res. 2016;14(1):75-82.
10. Ghoshal UC, Mehrotra M, Kumar S, Ghoshal U, Krishnani N, Misra A, et al. Spectrum of malabsorption syndrome among adults & factors differentiating celiac disease & tropical malabsorption. Indian J Med Res. 2012;136(3):451-9.
11. Fine KD, Stone MJ. Alpha-heavy chain disease, Mediterranean lymphoma, and immunoproliferative small intestinal disease: a review of clinicopathological features, pathogenesis, and differential diagnosis. Am J Gastroenterol. 1999;94(5):1139-52.
12. Chassany O, Michaux A, Bergmann JF. Drug-induced diarrhoea. Drug Saf. 2000;22(1):53-72.

Chronic Constipation: Frequently Asked Questions

Mayank Jain, Jayanthi Venkataraman

■ CASE DETAILS

A 32-year-old male, a businessman, presented with constipation for 2 days. The defecation was associated with excessive straining, digital evacuation, and use of pressure over the buttocks. There was no associated abdominal pain, painful defecation, or bleeding per rectum. The patient had taken enemas and over-the-counter laxatives with no significant relief. He had a sedentary lifestyle with low intake of fiber and fluids. Sleep was normal. Duke's anxiety–depressive score was negative. Patient was not on any medication for any particular ailment. There was no history of perianal surgery. There were no alarming features such as weight loss, bleeding, anorexia, or fever. There were no addictions and associated comorbid ailments. There was no family history of gastrointestinal malignancy.

On examination, vitals were normal; body mass index (BMI) was 33.6 kg/m^2. There was no significant pallor and skin texture was normal.

Systemic examination was normal.

Digital rectal examination: Resting and squeeze pressures—normal; on attempted defecation, anal sphincter contraction was present.

Clinical diagnosis: Functional constipation (FC).

Probable pathophysiology: Slow transit constipation in combination with fecal evacuation disorder.

Prescription

Diet: High fiber (20–25 g/day)—fruits and green leafy vegetables and adequate fluids of 1.5–2.0 L/day

Pharmacotherapy: Polyethylene glycol 15 g with water after dinner with prucalopride 2 mg once a day 45 minutes before breakfast.

In absence of clinical response further investigations would include colonic transit study, anorectal manometry (ARM) with or without magnetic resonance (MR) defecography.

In dyssynergia defecation disorders biofeed back therapy is recommended.

■ FREQUENTLY ASKED QUESTIONS

Question 1: How is constipation different in Indians compared to the west?

Answer: In Indians, the average stool frequency is 1–2 per day; stool forms are softer (Bristol 4/5). Thus, patient's perception is most important to determine constipation. Moreover, constipation-associated stools in Indians is often Bristol types I–III compared to types I–II as defined in the west.[1]

Question 2: How does one classify chronic constipation in adults?

Answer: Chronic constipation in adults can be divided into four main categories:
1. *Constipation with alarm symptoms:* Age >45 years, family history of colon cancer, inflammatory bowel disease, gastrointestinal bleed, anemia, weight loss, lump in the abdomen, fever, and significant weight loss.
2. *FC:* This is characterized by two or more of the following for >25% of the defecations:[2]
    - Straining
    - Lumpy or hard stools [Bristol Stool Form Scale (BSFS) 1–2]
    - Sensation of incomplete evacuation
    - Sensation of anorectal obstruction/blockage
    - Manual maneuvers to facilitate (e.g., digital evacuation and support of the pelvic floor)
    - Fewer than three spontaneous bowel movements per week
        - Loose stools are rarely present without the use of laxatives
        - Insufficient criteria for irritable bowel syndrome
    Criteria fulfilled for the last 3 months with symptom onset at least 6 months prior to diagnosis.
3. *Constipation predominant [irritable bowel syndrome with constipation (IBS-C)]:* Irritable bowel syndrome is a disorder of gut brain axis interaction (DGBI) in which recurrent abdominal pain is associated with defecation or a change in bowel habit. Symptom onset should occur at least 6 months before the diagnosis and symptoms should be present during the last 3 months; more than one fourth (25%) of bowel movements with Bristol stool form types 1 or 2 and less than one-fourth (25%) of bowel movements with Bristol stool form types 6 or 7.[2]

TABLE 1: FC/IBS-C subdivided into three categories based on physiological tests.

Category	Features	Physiological test results
Normal transit constipation	Incomplete evacuation +/− abdominal pain	Normal
Slow transit constipation	Infrequent stools <3 per week; hard, pellet-like stools; more common in young women	Delayed colonic transit study
Dyssynergic defecation/FED	Manual evacuation, use of different postures to evacuate, prolonged straining, use of perineal or vaginal pressure	Abnormal balloon expulsion and anorectal manometry

(FC/IBS-C: functional constipation/irritable bowel syndrome with constipation; FDC: fecal evacuation disorder)

FC/IBS-C can be further subdivided into three categories based on physiological tests—normal transit constipation, slow transit constipation, and dyssynergic defecation **(Table 1)**.

4. *Opioid-induced constipation:* Symptoms are similar to FC but associated with introduction or change in dose of opioids.[2]

Question 3: What are the criteria to diagnose dyssynergic defecation?
Answer: In patients with FC and/or IBS-C, there are four types of dyssynergic defecation based on Rao et al criteria.[3]
1. Patients must fulfil the diagnostic criteria for FC and/or IBS-C.
2. Patients must demonstrate dyssynergic pattern (I–IV) i.e. paradoxical increase in anal sphincter pressure (anal contraction), or less than 20% relaxation of the resting anal sphincter pressure, or inadequate propulsive forces observed

with manometry, imaging or electromyographic recordings. These need to be demonstrated during repeated attempts to defecate.
3. Patients must satisfy one or more of the following criteria:
    - Inability to expel an artificial stool (50 mL water-filled balloon) within 1–2 minutes.
    - Inability to evacuate or ≥50% retention of barium during defecography.

Question 4: What are the points in the history that need to be elicited in a patient who says, "I have constipation" **(Box 1)**?

> **BOX 1:** History that needs to be elicited in a patient with constipation.
>
> - Onset and duration
> - Relation to meals and bowel movements
> - Surgical history
> - Addictions—alcohol, tobacco, and smoking
> - Comorbid ailments, e.g., diabetes, neurological diseases, hypothyroidism, and associated FGID
> - Family history of colon cancer, IBD, etc.
> - Drugs, e.g., anticholinergics, antipsychotics, opioids, antihypertensives, antidiabetic, lipid-lowering agents, anticonvulsants, iron, calcium, and aluminum antacids
> - Red flag signs/sympoms—age >45 years, bleeding per rectum, weight loss, abdominal lump, anemia, and fever
> - Dietary history—quantum of fluid, fibre and animal protein itake
> - Lifestyle—exercise, timing of defecation, use of mobile/newspaper while defecating
> - Type of toilet used—Indian/western
> - Maneuvers to facilitate defecation
> - Obstetric history
> - Psychological issues and sleep
>
> (FGID: functional gastrointestinal disorders; IBD: inflammatory bowel disease)

Question 5: What is the Importance of DRE?[4]
Answer: Digital rectal examination is used to determine presence of dyssynergic defecation or to rule out rectal mass. The sensitivity, specificity, and positive and negative predictive value of DRE in the detection of dyssynergia is 69.7%, 81.5%, 82.1%, and 68.75%, respectively. Steps of DRE are given in **Box 2**.

> **BOX 2:** Steps of digital rectal examination.
>
> - Inspection of perineum—skin tags/warts/hemorrhoids/fissure/prolapse
> - Perineal sensation and anocutaneous reflex
> - Digital palpation–resting tone and squeeze
> - Examination while bearing down-push effort of abdominal muscle, relaxation or contraction of anal sphincter, and perineal descent

Question 6: What are the baseline investigations required in our patient?
Answer: These include[1]
- Hemogram
- Fecal occult blood
- T3, T4, and thyroid-stimulating hormone (TSH)
- Blood sugar
- Ultrasonography (USG) abdomen
- Short length colonoscopy/full length dependong on the age, presence of alarm symptoms/family history.

Question 7: What is the initial treatment of constipation?[1]
Answer: Initial treatment should include lifestyle modification and osmotic laxatives. Physicians should recommend adequate dietary fiber intake, drinking plenty of water, regular exercise, and maintaining a healthy sleep pattern. Use of Indian toilet or use of foot stool while using western toilet should be advised. Osmotic laxatives such as lactulose and ispaghula containing nonabsorbable molecules which enhance the water content in the stool, thus softening its consistency and increasing its volume. Stimulant laxatives such as bisacodyl, sodium picosulfate, and senna increase the fluid and electrolyte secretion in the lumen and also enhance the colonic peristalsis. Fiber supplement should be avoided if the

patient is already on high fiber diet and/or has abdominal bloating as a prominent symptom.

Question 8: What are the physiological tests needed in refractory constipation?

Answer:
- *Colonic transit study (Ghoshal protocol):* This test should be done when patient is off enterokinetics/stimulant laxatives for at least 1 week. 20 markers are given at 0, 12, and 24 hours each. Abdominal radiographs are taken at 36 and 60 hours. Retention of more than 30 markers at 36 hours and more than 14 markers at 60 hours is considered abnormal. If markers are distributed along the length of the colon **(Fig. 1)**, patient probably has slow transit; if markers are predominantly in pelvis, this suggests dyssynergic defecation **(Figs. 2 and 3)**.[5]
- ARM **(Fig. 4)** is a sophisticated test to measure pressures at the anorectal region and subclassify dyssynergic pattern into various subtypes. Currently, the London Classification provides a standardized method and nomenclature for description of alterations in anorectal motor and sensory function using office-based investigations.[6]

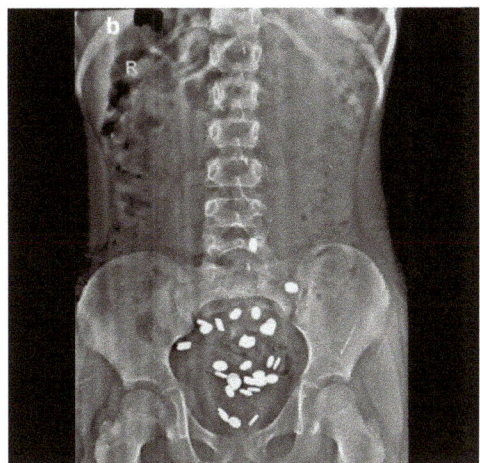

Fig. 2: Markers predominantly in the pelvis.

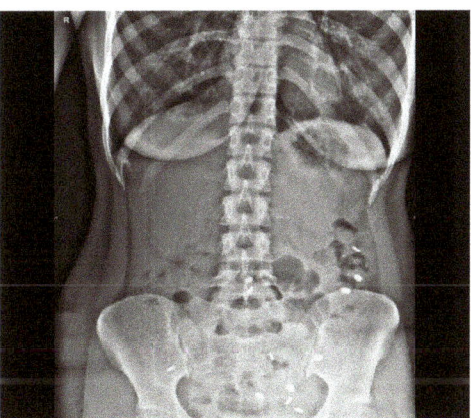

Fig. 3: Patient with FED.

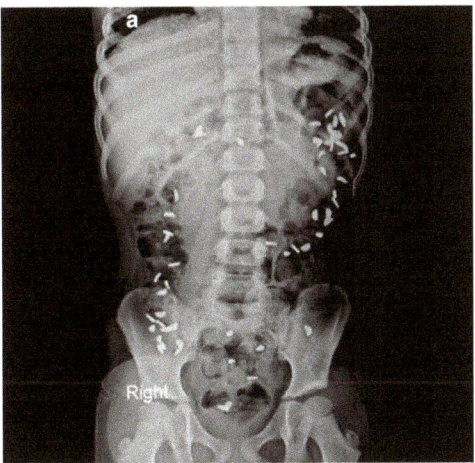

Fig. 1: Markers distributed along the length of colon.

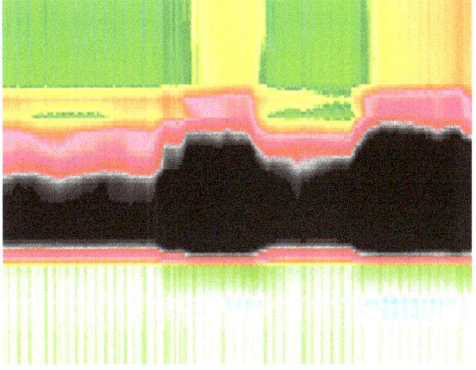

Fig. 4: *ARM:* High squeeze pressure and abnormal push pressure. Inability to expel balloon; RAIR at 80 mL. Diagnosis (FED: fecal evacuation disorder).

Steps of ARM include:[6]
- Stabilization period for 3 minutes to allow anal tone to return to baseline
- Rest: This measures basal anal tone at rest and is recorded over 60 seconds.
- *Short squeeze:* Three squeezes are performed, each of 5 seconds duration, separated by 30 seconds between maneuver recovery intervals.
- Long (endurance) squeeze: This records anal pressure during sustained voluntary effort over 30 seconds.
- *Cough:* This measures rectoanal pressure changes during cough
- *Push:* This measures anal and rectal pressure changes during simulated defecation. Three pushes are performed, each of 15 seconds duration, separated by 30 seconds between maneuver recovery intervals.
- *Rectoanal inhibitory reflex (RAIR):* This measures reflex anal response to rapid rectal distension. Absence of RAIR suggests a possible diagnosis of Hirschsprung's disease.
- Rectal sensory test.
- Balloon expulsion test (BET) or defecography

- *BET:* This is a simple bedside test to rule out dyssynergic defecation. It is safe, cheap, and gives instantaneous information. It may be especially helpful in centers where anorectal manometry is not available. It can be done with the patient lying in left lateral (nonphysiological) or in a sitting posture. A balloon, tied at end of a thin catheter, is placed inside the rectum and is subsequently filled with 50 mL water. The patient is asked to expel it while lying in left lateral position. It can be done during ARM. The time taken to expel the balloon >2 minutes is taken as abnormal.[7]

- *MR/barium defecography:* The study demonstrates presence of rectcoele and abnormal perineal descent. The three tests, the ballooon expulsion, ARM and defecogrsphy are complimentary for diagnosis of obstuction defecation syndrome (ODS). Complementary investigations such as these enhance the diagnostic accuracy on the type of constipation.

Question 9: How can we decide management based on physiological tests **(Table 2)**?
Answer:

TABLE 2: Types of constipation and their treatment options.

Constipation type	Treatment options
Dyssynergic defecation	Biofeedback—significant improvement in symptoms and anorectal manometry parameters
Slow transit constipation	Enterokinetics, e.g., prucalopride
Surgery	• Severe slow transit constipation • Large rectocele • Adult Hirschsprung's disease • Psychological evaluation is must before surgery

Question 10: What is the significance of methane in slow transit constipation of methane and constipation?[8,9]
Answer: High methane-producing bacterial load should be considered in patients with slow transit constipation not responding to stimulant laxatives/enterokinetics. High methane levels inhibit small and large bowel motility. Studies have shown that increased number of Methanobrevibacter smithii in the gut increases the severity of constipation. Rifaximin improves colonic transit and relieves constipation.

Question 11: What are the different drug classes available in India to treat constipation **(Table 3)**?

Answer:

TABLE 3: Drug classes available in India to treat constipation.

Category	Available drugs
Osmotic laxatives	Lactulose, lactitol, polyethylene glycol (PEG), sorbitol
Bulk laxative	Isaphgula husk
Stool softener	Liquid paraffin
Saline laxative	Milk of magnesia
Stimulant laxatives	Bisacodyl and sodium picosulfate
Secretagogues	Linaclotide and lubiprostone
Colonic prokinetic	Prucalopride
Suppository	Bisacodyl and glycerin
Enema	Phosphate and citrate
Newer drugs	Velusetrag and naronapride

CLINICAL PEARLS TO MANAGE SLOW TRANSIT CONSTIPATION

- Always rule out secondary causes of constipation e.g., reduced intake of foods
- Lifestyle improvement includes diet rich in fiber, adequate fluids, relaxant exercises, and adopting the right defecatory posture.
- Screen for dyssynergic defecation
- Stimulant laxatives/enterokinetics—First line
- In absence of response, rule out the possibility of large colonisations of Methanobrevibacter smithii.

CLINICAL PEARLS FOR MANAGING IRRITABLE BOWEL SYNDROME WITH CONSTIPATION

- Stimulant laxatives are not recommended in presence of abdominal pain.
- Ispaghula husk, lactulose, and lactitol are best avoided in bloaters.
- For pain-related IBS, otilonium bromide, mebeverine, drotaverine, or pinaverium bromide are recommended.
- Selective serotonin reuptake inhibitors (SSRI) can be added as they do not worsen the symptoms of constipation; tricyclic antidepressants, even in small dose, are contraindicated.
- Secretagogues such as lubiprostone, linaclotide, and plecanatide can be tried. They, however, are not effective in patients with slow transit.
- Attention must be paid to psychosocial issues with appropriate neuromodulators/psychiatric consultation.

CLINICAL UTILITY OF BIOFEEDBACK THERAPY[10-12]

- Neuromuscular training with visual, audio, or verbal feedback will help improve coordination between contraction of abdominal muscles and relaxation of pelvic floor.
- It improves symptoms and ARM parameters
- The procedure is time-consuming and is often associatd with poor compliance in the Indian setting.
- Biofeeback therapy is an innovative behavioral procedure
- Innovative behavioral therapy intervention (one session of biofeedback at hospital + diaphragmatic breathing exercises and pelvic relaxation exercises at home)—preliminary data—encouraging.
- **Table 4** summarises the diagnostic approach and management of the 4 types of costipation.

CLINICAL PEARLS FOR MANAGING CONSTIPATION IN PREGNANCY

- There are multifactorial factors. These include hormonal effects (progesterone >>estrogen); reduced physical activity and dietary changes; medications, e.g., iron and antiemetics; mechanical; maternal gut microbiome changes; and electrolyte disturbances, thyroid disorders, and diabetes
- Diagnostic tests are best undertaken after delivery.

TABLE 4: Summary of diagnostic AIDS and management.

Constipation subtype	Diagnostic AIDS	Management principles
Functional constipation	• History (Rome IV), DRE physiological tests—CTT, ARM, BET, defecography • Breath tests as per need	• STC—enterokinetics/stimulants, rifaximin if high methane • NTC—secretagogues/laxatives
Dyssynergic defecation	History, DRE, baseline investigations, ARM, balloon expulsion, and defecography	Biofeedback
Constipation with red flags	History, DRE, imaging, colonoscopy, and blood tests	Treat the cause
IBS-C	History—Rome IV (give a positive diagnosis), DRE, and baseline investigations	• Treat pain if significant • Neuromodulators for psychological modifiers • Drugs
Opioid-induced constipation	History, DRE, and baseline tests	Stop or reduce dose, laxatives

(AIDS: acquired immunodeficiency syndrome; ARM: anorectal manometry; BET: balloon expulsion test; CTT: colon transit time; DRE: digital rectal examination; IBS-C: irritable bowel syndrome with constipation; NTC: normal transit constipation; STC: slow transit constipation)

- *Treatment:* Dietary counseling, medications such as lactulose and polyethylene glycol (PEG) are safe during pregnancy.
- *Hemorrhoids and anal fissures:* These are managed conservatively.
- *Thrombosed piles*: If extemely painful, the thrombosed piles are excised and decompressed.

REFERENCES

1. Ghoshal UC, Sachdeva S, Pratap N, Verma A, Karyampudi A, Misra A, et al. Indian consensus on chronic constipation in adults: A joint position statement of the Indian Motility and Functional Diseases Association and the Indian Society of Gastroenterology. Indian J Gastroenterol. 2018;37(6):526-44.
2. Mearin F, Lacy BE, Chang L, Chey WD, Lembo AJ, Simren M, et al. Bowel Disorders. Gastroenterology. 2016:S0016-5085 (16)00222-5.
3. Rao SS, Patcharatrakul T. Diagnosis and Treatment of Dyssynergic Defecation. J Neurogastroenterol Motil. 2016;22(3):423-35.
4. Jain M. Digital rectal examination—a reliable screening tool for dyssynergic defecation. Indian J Gastroenterol. 2018;37:176-7.
5. Ghoshal UC, Gupta D, Kumar A, Misra A. Colonic transit study by radio-opaque markers to investigate constipation: validation of a new protocol for a population with rapid gut transit. Natl Med J India. 2007; 20:225-9.
6. Scott SM, Carrington EV. The London Classification: Improving Characterization and Classification of Anorectal Function with Anorectal Manometry. Curr Gastroenterol Rep. 2020;22(11):55.
7. Lee BE, Kim GH. How to perform and interpret balloon expulsion test. J Neurogastroenterol Motil. 2014;20:407-9.
8. Ghoshal U, Shukla R, Srivastava D, Ghoshal UC. Irritable bowel syndrome, particularly the constipation-predominant form, involves an increase in Methanobrevibacter smithii, which is associated with higher methane production. Gut Liver. 2016;10:932-8.
9. Ghoshal UC, Srivastava D, Misra A. Reduction of breath methane using rifaximin shortens colon transit time and improves constipation: a randomized double-blind placebo controlled trial. Gastroenterology. 2015;148:4 Suppl 1:S308-9.
10. Misra A, Ghoshal UC. Effect of biofeedback therapy on anorectal physiological parameters among patients with fecal evacuation disorder. Indian J Gastroenterol. 2017;36:99-104.
11. Shah N, Baijal R, Kumar P, Gupta D, Kulkarni S, Doshi S, et al. Clinical and investigative assessment of constipation: a study from a referral center in western India. Indian J Gastroenterol. 2014;33:530-6.
12. Jain M, Baijal R. Dyssynergic defecation: demographics, symptoms, colonoscopic findings in north Indian patients. Indian J Gastroenterol. 2017;36:435-7.

Gallstone Ileus Presenting as Subacute Small Bowel Obstruction

Sethubabu, Teja J

INTRODUCTION

Gallstone ileus is an uncommon complication of cholelithiasis, characterized by the mechanical blockage of the gastrointestinal tract caused by the lodgment of one or more gallstones. Although termed "ileus", this obstruction is actually a true mechanical obstruction.[1] Gallstone ileus occurs in 0.15–1.5% of cholelithiasis cases and in <0.1% of all cases of ileus.[1,2] It manifests with nonspecific clinical features, necessitating a heightened suspicion in elderly patients who exhibit signs of small bowel obstruction. The morbidity and mortality rates associated with this condition remain elevated due to the advanced age of affected individuals and the presence of concurrent medical conditions. Previous reports have documented instances of spontaneous resolution following the passage of gallstones measuring <2.5 cm.[3]

CASE REPORT

A 59-year-old female patient presented to our emergency with a 2-day history of pain, initially in right upper quadrant of abdomen that persisted for 4 hours and then subsided, followed by lower abdominal pain with one episode of vomiting, nonbilious, and contained ingested food. Patient had obstipation for 2 days. She had no significant history. Upon admission, her general examination was unremarkable. Vitals were stable with no tachycardia and normal blood pressure and temperature. Abdominal examination revealed mild abdominal distension with tenderness in right and left iliac fossa and hypogastrium. Bowel sounds were not exaggerated and per rectal examination showed no fecal impaction. Initial laboratory parameters showed hemoglobin (Hb) 13g/dL, white blood cells (WBC) 10,860, platelets 1.82 lakhs, urea 66 mg/dL, and creatinine 1.4 mg/dL. Liver function test (LFT) and international normalized ratio (INR) were normal. X-ray erect abdomen was done to confirm the diagnosis of intestinal obstruction which showed multiple air fluid levels, pneumobilia, and Belthazar sign **(Fig. 1)**. Contrast-enhanced computed

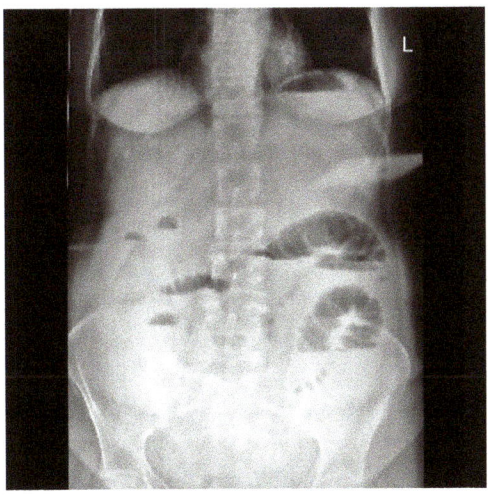

Fig. 1: X-ray erect abdomen showing pneumobilia, multiple air fluid levels, and Belthazar sign.

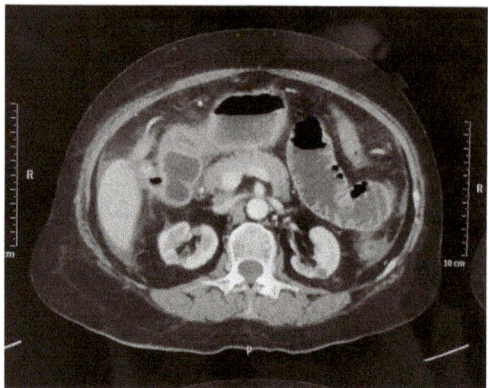

Fig. 2: Pneumobilia, fundus of gallbladder adherent to lateral wall of duodenum without obvious fistulous communication and cholelithiasis.

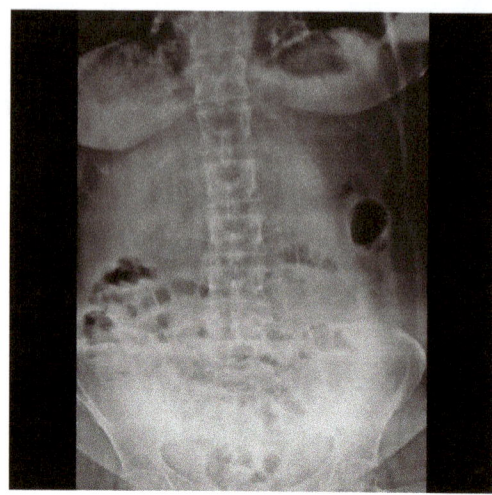

Fig. 4: X-ray erect abdomen showing relief of obstruction with nonspecific dilatation of bowel loops.

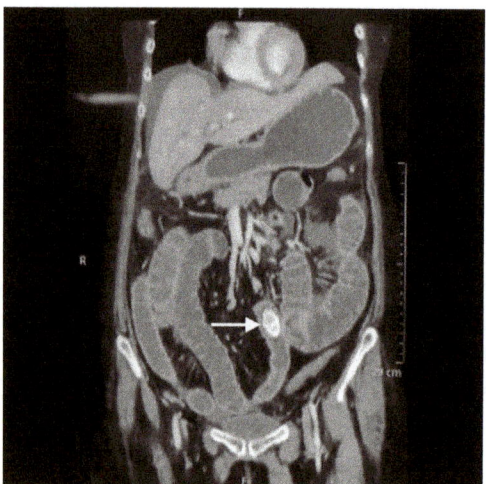

Fig. 3: Multiple dilated jejunal and ileal loops due to large calculus in the mid-ileal loop measuring 26 × 21 mm and collapse of bowel loops distal to obstruction.

tomography (CECT) abdomen was done which revealed pneumobilia, multiple dilated jejunal, and ileal loops due to large calculus in the mid-ileal loop measuring 26 × 21 mm and collapse of bowel loops distal to obstruction and fundus of gallbladder wall adherent to lateral wall of duodenum without obvious direct communication **(Figs. 2 and 3)**. A diagnosis of gallstone ileus was made and the patient was started on conservative management while being planned for surgery. She was monitored for any signs of perforation, sepsis, and worsening intestinal obstruction. On day 3 of admission, the patient's abdominal distension decreased and she passed stool and flatus. Repeat X-ray erect abdomen showed relief of obstruction with nonspecific dilatation of bowel loops **(Fig. 4)**. Patient was started on liquid diet and normal diet. She was asymptomatic and was discharged to follow-up on regular basis for decision regarding cholecystectomy.

■ DISCUSSION

Gallstone ileus, an uncommon complication of cholelithiasis, represents a relatively infrequent cause of mechanical intestinal blockage, accounting for 1–4% of cases.[4-7] As gallstone ileus primarily affects aged more than 65 years, accounting for one fourth of non strangulation intestinal obstruction, there is a heightened risk of morbidity and mortality due to accompanying illnesses, resulting in a mortality rate ranging from 6.7% to 22.7%.[4,7]

The pathogenesis of gallstone ileus stems from acute or chronic cholecystitis, which occurs in conjunction with cholelithiasis. The inflammation and adhesions caused by gallstones facilitate the formation of a cholecystoenteric fistula. The most prevalent type of fistula is the cholecystoduodenal, while the less common types include cholecystocolonic and cholecystduodenocolonic.[4,5] The order for most common sites for impaction is as follows: ileum (50.0-60.5%), jejunum (16.1-26.9%), duodenum (3.5-14.6%), and colon (3.0-4.1%).[4,8] Impacted gallstones are predominantly composed of cholesterol and have an approximate size of 4 cm, falling within the impaction-prone range of ≥2.5 cm.[9]

Diagnosing gallstone ileus presents challenges, but radiological investigations utilizing techniques such as ultrasonography (USG), computed tomography (CT), and plain abdominal radiographs aid in expediting accurate diagnoses in over 50% of cases, reducing preoperative delays.[10] Abdominal radiographs, both erect and supine, serve as the initial imaging modality for intestinal obstruction cases. Rigler et al.[11] described classic radiographic signs, including intestinal obstruction, pneumobilia, the presence of an abnormally located gallstone, and a change in the stone's position on serial exams. The presence of at least two of these signs is considered pathognomonic, with an additional sign described by Belthazar and Schechter,[12] involving the presence of two air–fluid levels in the right upper quadrant. However if the gallstone is not calcified, the findings on plain abdominal films may be nonspecific. Ultrasound evaluates the gallbladder's status, presence of cholelithiasis, choledocholithiasis, and pneumobilia, but visualizing the fistula connecting to the adjacent bowel is usually challenging.

CT imaging provides higher resolution, displays dilated loops, evaluates the bowel wall's condition, and identifies the site and cause of the obstruction. In emergency situations, CECT imaging often reveals Rigler's triad, which encompasses an ectopically calcified gallstone, biliary tree air, and evidence of mechanical bowel obstruction, strongly indicating gallstone-induced intestinal blockage.

The prognosis of gallstone ileus is generally poor and worsens with advancing age. Mortality rates (7.5-15%) and morbidity remain high, primarily due to delayed diagnoses and concurrent conditions such as cardiorespiratory distress, obesity, and diabetes mellitus.[13] The primary goal of treatment is prompt relief of intestinal obstruction to minimize morbidity and mortality. Gallstone ileus typically necessitates emergency surgery to alleviate the blockage. The one-stage procedure involves enterolithotomy, cholecystectomy, and fistula repair, while the two-stage procedure includes enterolithotomy and subsequent biliary surgery. Laparoscopy-guided enterolithotomy has recently emerged as an alternative surgical approach. Nonsurgical treatments comprise endoscopic removal and shock-wave lithotripsy, depending on the specific location. Spontaneous resolution of gallstone ileus following the passage of a gallstone has also been reported.[3] In the current case, the intestinal obstruction spontaneously resolved after the patient passed a gallstone measuring 26 × 21 mm during the observation period.

■ CONCLUSION

Gallstone ileus, despite being a recognized condition, is infrequent given the overall prevalence of gallstones in the general population. The diagnosis is typically confirmed through abdominal CT scans, which identify both the location of the obstruction and the presence of the stone. Surgical intervention represents the primary treatment for gallstone ileus. However considering the potential complications and mortality rates in elderly patients, conservative management may be considered initially for selected cases. The specific site of obstruction, stone size, and the patient's overall condition guide the treatment approach for gallstone ileus. Surgical intervention provides a definitive solution and elective cholecystectomy can help prevent future episodes.

■ REFERENCES

1. Abou-Saif A, Al-Kawas FH. Complications of gallstone disease: Mirizzi syndrome, cholecystocholedochal fistula, and gallstone ileus. Am J Gastroenterol. 2002;97:249-54.
2. Nakao A, Okamoto Y, Sunami M, Fujita T, Tsuji T. The oldest patient with gallstone ileus: report of a case and review of 176 cases in Japan. Kurume Med J. 2008;55:29-33.
3. Farooq A, Memon B, Memon MA. Resolution of gallstone ileus with spontaneous evacuation of gallstone. Emerg Radiol. 2007;14(6):421-3.
4. Clavien PA, Richon J, Burgan S, Rohner A. Gallstone ileus. Br J Surg. 1990;77:737-42.
5. Pavlidis TE, Atmatzidis KS, Papaziogas BT, Papaziogas TB. Management of gallstone ileus. J Hepatobiliary Pancreat Surg. 2003;10:299-302.
6. Raf L, Spangen L. Gallstone ileus. Acta Chir Scand. 1971;137:665-75.
7. Masannat Y, Masannat Y, Shatnawei A. Gallstone ileus: a review. Mt Sinai J Med. 2006;73:1132-4.
8. Reisner RM, Cohen JR. Gallstone ileus: a review of 1,001 reported cases. Am Surg. 1994;60:441-6.
9. Syme RG. Management of gallstone ileus. Can J Surg. 1989;32:61-4.
10. Ayantude AA, Agrawal A. Gallstone ileus: diagnosis and management. World J Surg. 2007;31:1292-7.
11. Rigler LG, Borman CN, Noble JF. Gallstone obstruction: pathogenesis and roentgen manifestations. JAMA. 1941;117:1753-60.
12. Balthazar EJ, Schechter LS. Air in gall bladder: a frequent finding in gallstone ileus. Am J Roentgenol. 1978;131:219-22.
13. Rodriguez Hermosa JI, Codina Cazador A, Girones Vila J, Roig Garcia J, Figa Francesch M, Acero FD. Gallstone ileus: results of analysis of a series of 40 patients. Gastroenterol Hepatol. 2001;24:489-94.

Small Bowel Neuroendocrine Tumors

Mahiboob Sayyed, Manu Tandan

■ INTRODUCTION

Neuroendocrine tumors (NETs) are heterogeneous group of malignancies arising from neural crest-derived cells and can occur throughout the body. These tumors may secrete various hormones depending on their organ of origin, leading to several hormone-mediated effects. Initially, the term Karzinoid (carcinoma-like) was coined by Siegfried Oberndorfer. With the advent of immunohistochemistry and molecular biology which revealed the heterogeneous nature of this disease, the term was later changed to NET. Small bowel NETs (SBNETs) arise from enterochromaffin cells of the lining epithelium of digestive tract which secretes majority of body's serotonin.[1]

Neuroendocrine tumors are classified depending on the site of origin as foregut, midgut, or hindgut. Based on the histology, it can be classified as well differentiated or poorly differentiated. **Figure 1** shows the incidence of NET increasing yearly [all sited from the Surveillance, Epidemiology, and End Results (SEER) database].

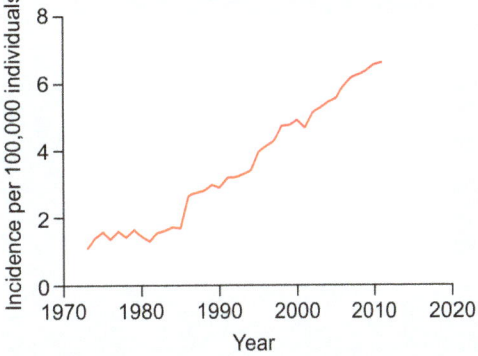

Fig. 1: Age-adjusted yearly incidence of neuroendocrine tumor from all sited from SEER database.[2]

■ CASE

A 60-year-old gentleman presented with history of recurrent episodes of abdominal pain associated with vomiting and abdominal distension. The symptoms were relieved after placement of Ryles tube and after keeping him nil orally for few days, signifying subacute intestinal obstruction. Clinically, he was well built, alert, and oriented. He did not have pallor, icterus, clubbing, pedal edema, or palpable lymphadenopathy. Mild abdominal tenderness could be elicited at the periumbilical region. His routine blood work is shown in **Table 1**.

Ultrasonography (USG) abdomen showed small mesenteric nodule. Further evaluation was done with contrast-enhanced computed tomography (CECT) abdomen which revealed round-to-oval, irregularly marginated, speculated soft tissue, density measuring 44 × 33 mm in the mesentery with desmoplastic reaction along with subtle retraction of ileal loops (**Fig. 2**). The diagnostic possibility of NET was considered

TABLE 1: Routine blood parameters.	
Blood test	Parameters
Hb	13.6 mg/dL
TLC	17,000 cells/mm³
Platelets	4.33 lakhs
Creatinine	0.16 mg/dL
Bilirubin	0.7 mg/dL
ALP	128 U/L
Albumin	3.4 g/dL

(ALP: alkaline phosphatase; Hb: hemoglobin; TLC: total leukocyte count)

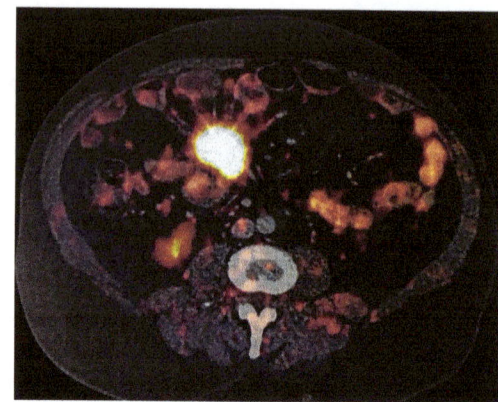

Fig. 3: DOTATATE-PET showing intense fluorodeoxyglucose (FDG) avid, large, irregular, enhancing soft tissue density lesion in the mesentery.

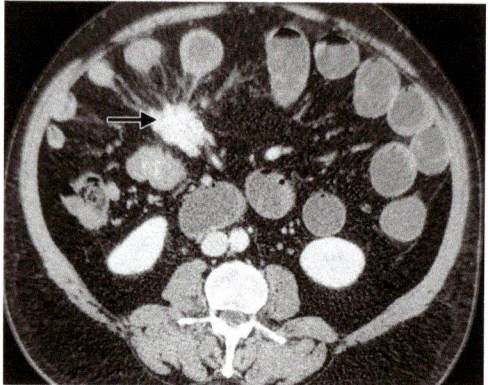

Fig. 2: Contrast-enhanced computed tomography (CECT) abdomen showing round-to-oval, irregularly marginated, speculated, soft tissue density in the mesentery with desmoplastic reaction.

based on the characteristic enhancement pattern. Serum chromogranin level was however normal. ⁶⁸Gallium (⁶⁸Ga) DOTATATE positron emission tomography–computed tomography (PET-CT) showed two foci of intense tracer avid (SUV max 14) arterial phase enhancing asymmetrical nodular wall thickening, involving mid- and distal-ileal loops, respectively **(Fig. 3)**. Another intense fluorodeoxyglucose (FDG) avid (SUV max 48), large, irregular, enhancing soft tissue density lesion (38 × 26 × 29 mm) was seen in the mesentery with significant desmoplastic reaction and tethering of adjacent ileal loops. DOTATATE picture confirmed the diagnosis of ileal NET with involvement of mesenteric lymph nodes. Intraoperative findings revealed cramped and edematous segment of small bowel with a 5 × 5 cm lesion in this segment. Mesentery was fibrotic with mesenteric deposits and severe desmoplastic reaction. Small bowel resection and anastomosis was done. Grossly, tumor on external surface showed dense adhesions with formation of mass in mesentery. On cut section, two yellowish white nodules were seen. Histopathology revealed monomorphic population of round cells with round-to-oval nuclei with salt and pepper chromatin and granular cytoplasm. The cells were arranged in solid nests **(Fig. 4)**. The mitotic figures were 1–2/high power field (HPF). The postoperative recovery was uneventful.

■ DISCUSSION

Although considered rare, SBNETs are increasing in incidence and prevalence, mostly due to increased detection and improved survival.[2]

The clinical presentation of SBNETs varies from mechanical obstruction of surrounding structures by tumor or symptoms arising as a result of secretion of active substances by the tumor. The classic clinical triad of carcinoid syndrome including diarrhea, wheezing, and right-sided valvular heart disease is seen less commonly. This syndrome results from secretion of bioactive amines such as serotonin, histamines, prostaglandin, and tachykinins from the tumor. Recent survey of patients with SBNET showed that 36% reported pain as their initial presenting symptom, 26% as flushing, and 24% reported diarrhea as their first symptom.[3]

Other less common symptoms are pellagra-like skin lesions, telangiectasia, peripheral edema, and arthritis. Some patients can present with asymptomatic mass detected on imaging done for other reason. Sometimes patient can also present with intestinal obstruction needing surgery. Up to 50% of patients with SBNETs can develop fibrosis of mesenteric lymph nodes, potentially causing tethering and kinking of the mesentery, leading to obstruction, pain, and mesenteric ischemia.[4]

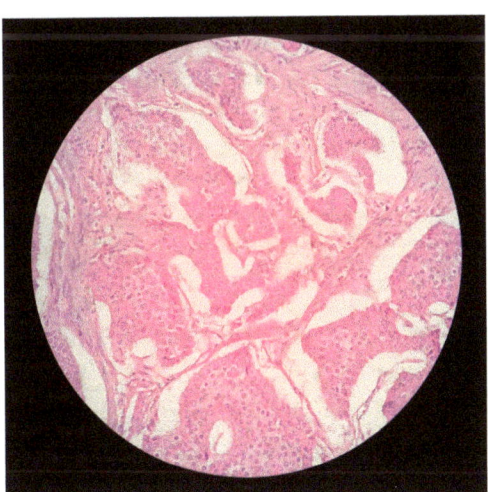

Fig. 4: Cellular tumor composed of monomorphic population of round cells arranged in solid nests having round-to-oval nuclei with salt and pepper chromatin and granular cytoplasm.

■ DIAGNOSIS

The diagnostic strategy in these cases is largely dictated by the clinical presentation. In patients presenting with the classic triad of carcinoid syndrome, biochemical testing is helpful to diagnose the disease. Biochemical testing includes 24-hour urinary 5-hydroxyindoleacetic acid (5-HIAA) (sensitivity 85% and specificity 90%) and serum chromogranin (sensitivity 71% and specificity 50%).[5,6] Serum chromogranin A (CgA) is useful for monitoring the disease progression and its recurrence. Several foods (avocados, pineapples, bananas, kiwi fruit, and walnuts) can increase urinary HIAA and should be avoided before measuring the levels. Similarly, serum chromogranin levels can be spuriously elevated in patients taking proton pump inhibitors (PPIs). Pancreastatin is a post-translational cleavage fragment of CgA that is more specific and sensitive than CgA in detecting progression and predicting survival.[7] Moreover, its level is unaffected by PPI use.

Imaging

Imaging with ^{68}Ga DOTA PET is helpful in localizing the lesion. Imaging may identify the site of primary tumor, involvement of nodes, and presence of metastatic disease, which will aid in surgical planning and provide a baseline for monitoring of disease progression.

Broadly, imaging modalities can be divided into anatomic and functional **(Box 1)**.

BOX 1: Imaging modalities.

Anatomic:
- USG
- CECT/MRI

Functional:
- DOTATATE
- OctreoScan

(CECT: contrast-enhanced computed tomography; MRI: magnetic resonance imaging; USG: ultrasonography)

Contrast-enhanced computed tomography is often used as the initial diagnostic imaging because of the widespread availability and noninvasive nature. Small bowel NETs cause desmoplastic reaction in mesenteric lymph nodes, resulting in spiculations with stellate pattern on imaging.[8] Small bowel NETs and metastases are hypervascular, imparting them the characteristic enhancement on arterial phase.[8] Magnetic resonance imaging (MRI) has greater sensitivity for detecting liver metastasis which appear hypointense on T1-weighted and hyperintense on T2-weighted MRI images. ^{68}Ga DOTA PET-CT (DOTATATE, DOTATOC, or DOTANOC) is increasingly being utilized for confirming the lesions seen on cross-sectional imaging and determining the extent of the disease throughout the body. Ga^{63} DOTATATE reveals the location of the lesions by uptake of somatostatin analogs (SSA) through cell-surface receptors and has a diagnostic sensitivity and specificity of 96% and 100%, respectively.[9]

Histopathology

Small bowel NETs tend to have a nested architecture with centrally placed, oval nuclei with a "salt-and-pepper" appearance on hematoxylin and eosin staining. Immunohistochemistry staining for synaptophysin and chromogranin is usually performed to confirm the diagnosis.[10]

Classification

Tumor differentiation (well vs. poorly differentiated) and grading of tumor (G1, G2, and G3) as shown in **Table 2** is important in providing prognostic information.[11]

■ TREATMENT

Medical

Medical treatment is indicated in patients with:
- Unresectable or residual disease remaining following surgery
- Hormonal symptoms refractory to surgery
- Comorbidities or disease burden (particularly in the liver) preclude surgical treatment.

Somatostatin analogs are the mainstay for the medical treatment of hormonal symptoms of NETs. NETs express high levels of somatostatin receptors. Activation of these by synthetic somatostatin peptide mimetics decreases signaling in cell proliferation pathways while reducing hormone secretion. The PROMID study provided level-I evidence of SSA's ability to

TABLE 2: Classification and grading criteria for neuroendocrine neoplasm of gastrointestinal and hepatopancreatobiliary organs.[11]

Terminology	Differentiation	Grade	Mitosis rate (mitosis/2 mm³)	Ki67 index
NET, G1	Well differentiated	Low	<2	<3%
NET, G2	Well differentiated	Intermediate	2–20	3–20%
NET, G3	Well differentiated	High	>20	>20%
NEC small cell type	Poorly differentiated	High	>20	>20%
NEC large cell type	Poorly differentiated	High	>20	>20%
MiNEN	Well or poorly differentiated	Variable	Variable	Variable%

(NEC: neuroendocrine carcinoma; NET: neuroendocrine tumor; MiNEN: mixed neuroendocrine neoplasm)

slow midgut NET growth.[12] The CLARINET trial showed the effect of another SSA, lanreotide, on progression-free survival in advanced pancreatic, midgut, and hindgut NETs with Ki-67 of <10%.[13]

Other Medical Therapies

Everolimus is a mTOR (mammalian target of rapamycin) inhibitor which suppresses tumor cell survival, angiogenesis, and growth. In the RADIANT-3 trial, everolimus improved progression-free survival in pancreatic NETs; however, its role in small bowel NETs needs further evaluation.[14]

Peptide receptor radionuclide therapy (PRRT) is a form of systemic radiotherapy that allows the administration of targeted radionuclides (^{90}Y-DOTATOC and ^{177}Lu-DOTATATE) into tumor cells that express a large quantity of somatostatin receptors. By conjugating radioisotope to an SSA, concentration of the drug can be increased selectively in tumor cells, where after binding to the receptor, the isotope is internalized. The randomized, phase III trial (NETTER-1), demonstrated its efficacy in both progression-free survival and overall survival.[15]

Telotristat is a tryptophan hydroxylase inhibitor, an enzyme governing the rate-limiting step in serotonin synthesis. By inhibiting this enzyme, telotristat reduces serotonin production, which can reduce symptoms associated with carcinoid syndrome such as diarrhea. In a randomized trial, telotristat effectively controlled diarrhea in patients in whom bowel movements were not adequately controlled by SSA.[16]

Chemotherapy is reserved for high-grade tumors and in those with aggressive growth. Capecitabine/temozolomide-based chemotherapy is an option in such cases.

Surgery

Surgical treatment is the mainstay for definitive diagnosis and treatment of small bowel NETs. In addition, surgery is required to manage the obstructive complications of NETs.

■ REFERENCES

1. Bellono NW, Bayrer JR, Leitch DB, Castro J, Zhang C, O'Donnell TA, et al. Enterochromaffin cells are gut chemosensors that couple to sensory neural pathways. Cell. 2017;170(1):185.
2. Dasari A, Shen C, Halperin D, Zhao B, Zhou S, Xu Y, et al. Trends in the Incidence, Prevalence, and Survival Outcomes in Patients With Neuroendocrine Tumors in the United States. JAMA Oncol. 2017;3(10):1335.
3. Basuroy R, Bouvier C, Ramage JK, Sissons M, Srirajaskanthan R. Delays and routes to diagnosis of neuroendocrine tumours. BMC Cancer. 2018;18(1):1122.
4. Druce MR, Bharwani N, Akker SA, Drake WM, Rockall A, Grossman AB. Intra-abdominal fibrosis in a recent cohort of patients with neuroendocrine ('carcinoid') tumours of the small bowel. QJM. 2010;103(3):177-85.
5. Carling R, Degg T, Allen K, Bax N, Barth J. Evaluation of whole blood serotonin and plasma and urine 5-hydroxyindole acetic acid in diagnosis of carcinoid disease. Ann Clin Biochem. 2002;39(Pt 6):577-82.
6. Vezzosi D, Walter T, Laplanche A, Raoul JL, Dromain C, Ruszniewski P, et al. Chromogranin A measurement in metastatic well-differentiated gastroenteropancreatic neuroendocrine carcinoma: screening for false positives and a prospective follow-up study. Int J Biol Markers. 2011;26(2):94-101.
7. Woltering EA, Voros BA, Beyer DT, Thiagarajan R, Ramirez RA, Mamikunian G, et al. Plasma Pancreastatin Predicts the Outcome of Surgical Cytoreduction in Neuroendocrine Tumors of the Small Bowel. Pancreas. 2019;48(3):356-62.
8. Horton KM, Kamel I, Hofmann L, Fishman EK. Carcinoid tumors of the small bowel:

9. Yang J, Kan Y, Ge BH, Yuan L, Li C, Zhao W. Diagnostic role of Gallium-68 DOTATOC and Gallium-68 DOTATATE PET in patients with neuroendocrine tumors: a meta-analysis. Acta Radiol. 2014;55(4):389-98.
10. Bellizzi AM. Immunohistochemistry in the diagnosis and classification of neuroendocrine neoplasms: what can brown do for you? Hum Pathol. 2020;96:8.
11. Nagtegaal ID, Odze RD, Klimstra D, Paradis V, Rugge M, Schirmacher P, et al. The 2019 WHO classification of tumours of the digestive system. Histopathology. 2020;76(2):182-8.
12. Rinke A, Müller HH, Schade-Brittinger C, Klose KJ, Barth P, Wied M, et al. Placebo-controlled, double-blind, prospective, randomized study on the effect of octreotide LAR in the control of tumor growth in patients with metastatic neuroendocrine midgut tumors: a report from the PROMID Study Group. J Clin Oncol. 2009;27(28):4656-63.
13. Caplin ME, Pavel M, Ćwikła JB, Phan AT, Raderer M, Sedláčková E, et al. Lanreotide in metastatic enteropancreatic neuroendocrine tumors. N Engl J Med. 2014;371(3):224-33.
14. Yao JC, Shah MH, Ito T, Bohas CL, Wolin EM, Cutsem E Van, et al. Everolimus for Advanced Pancreatic Neuroendocrine Tumors. N Engl J Med. 2011;364(6):514.
15. Strosberg J, El-Haddad G, Wolin E, Hendifar A, Yao J, Chasen B, et al. Phase 3 Trial of 177Lu-Dotatate for Midgut Neuroendocrine Tumors. N Engl J Med. 2017;376(2):125.
16. Kulke MH, Hörsch D, Caplin ME, Anthony LB, Bergsland E, Öberg K, et al. Telotristat Ethyl, a Tryptophan Hydroxylase Inhibitor for the Treatment of Carcinoid Syndrome. J Clin Oncol. 2017;35(1):14-23.

a multitechnique imaging approach. AJR Am J Roentgenol. 2004;182(3):559-67.

CHAPTER 33

An Interesting Case of SIBO/Dysbiosis

Sanjeev Sachdeva, Ujjwal Sonika

■ INTRODUCTION

The human gastrointestinal tract is populated by large population of diverse microorganisms, jointly known as gut microbiota.[1] The composition and density of microbiota in proximal gut differs significantly from that in the colon.[2] Gut microbial dysbiosis, which is defined as alteration in quantum, composition, or function of gut microbes, can contribute to various gastrointestinal and extraintestinal disorders.[3] The small intestine usually has no or few coliform bacteria and overall quantity of microbes is limited. Small intestinal bacterial overgrowth (SIBO) is characterized by presence of excessive number of microbes in the small bowel and etiopathogenesis of this entity is multifactorial **(Table 1)**.[1] SIBO is an evolving area of research worldwide and there are very few clinical guidelines available for management of this intriguing disorder.[1,4] Recently published Asian–Pacific consensus[1] defined SIBO as the growth of bacteria ≥10^5 colony-forming unit (CFU) or

TABLE 1: Causes of small intestinal bacterial overgrowth (SIBO).

Structural abnormalities	Motility disorders	Biochemical abnormalities	GI and systemic diseases
• Postoperative adhesions • Small bowel diverticula • Small bowel stricture and fistulas • Blind-loop syndrome • Incompetent ileocecal valve • Inflammatory bowel disease, particularly Crohn's disease	• Chronic intestinal pseudo-obstruction • Drugs (e.g., opiates) • Irritable bowel syndrome and other functional bowel disorders • HIV-associated autonomic neuropathy • Parkinsonism and amyloidosis	• Hypochlorhydria (e.g., atrophic gastritis and proton pump inhibitors therapy) • Biliary diseases and cholecystectomy	• Connective tissue diseases (e.g., scleroderma) • Diabetic autonomic neuropathy and hypothyroidism • Tropical sprue, celiac disease, and other causes of malabsorption syndrome • Chronic pancreatitis • Common variable immunodeficiency • Cirrhosis of liver • Nonalcoholic fatty liver disease • Obesity and its surgical treatment

(GI: gastrointestinal; HIV: human immunodeficiency virus)

≥10³ CFU/mL (particularly if coliforms are present) on a quantitative culture of upper gut aspirate.[2,4-12] Microbiological spectrum of SIBO may vary depending on underlying pathophysiology.[1,13-16]

Although quantitative upper gut aspirate culture is the existing gold standard for diagnosing SIBO, it is invasive, expensive, complex, and limited by the fact that only 30% of gut bacteria can be cultured.[1] As a result in clinical practice, hydrogen-methane breath testing has gained popularity over culture due to its ease and noninvasive nature. Among breath tests, glucose hydrogen breath test (GHBT) is preferred over lactulose hydrogen breath test (LHBT) due to better sensitivity and specificity as per a recent meta-analysis.[17] The role of more recent diagnostic methods such as culturomics, metabolomics, D-xylose, and ^{13}C-based breath testing requires further assessment.[1]

Several microbes have been proposed to produce methane in human gut and these include few Bacteroides and Clostridium, but the bulk of methane production is credited to the Archaea Methanobrevibacter smithii[18] which creates this product from hydrogen and carbon dioxide. Methane produced in the gut is mainly excreted in flatus, but about one fifth is excreted in the breath.[19] >30% of healthy adult human subjects are predominant methane producers.[20] As individuals with high breath methane may also have elevated methanogen microbes in stools, a recent guideline coined a new term "intestinal methanogen overgrowth (IMO)".[4] A recent consensus proposed that methane-producing microbes slow gut transit and cause constipation. The North American Consensus proposed a cutoff for high breath methane levels to be ≥10 parts per million (ppm).[12]

Experimental and clinical data show that methane hampers gut motility and hence, methane concentration may inversely correlate with stool frequency and Bristol Stool Form Score (BSFS).[21-24] Ghoshal et al.[22] reported greater number of Methanobrevibacter smithii in stool samples of patients with irritable bowel syndrome (IBS), especially constipation-predominant IBS (IBS-C) compared to healthy controls and found an inverse correlation between the copy number of Methanobrevibacter smithii and the stool frequency. Chatterjee et al. showed that severity of constipation was related to degree of methane production.[23] Also, few recent studies showed improvement in gut transit as well as constipation with administration of oral antibiotics directed at gut methanogens.[25-28] A meta-analysis showed association of breath methane with constipation and delayed gut transit.[29] In addition, two recent meta-analyses reported an association of methane positivity on breath testing with IBS-C.[30,31]

So, based on this interesting concept of role of methane-positive SIBO in gut dysmotility, we present an interesting case of refractory chronic constipation, wherein excess methane was associated with slow colonic transit and gut-specific antibiotic therapy targeted at methanogens resulted in dramatic improvement in patients' symptoms, stool form, and stool frequency.

CASE REPORT

A 24-year-old male presented to us with complaints of constipation for the last 8 years without any significant change in severity. He complained of passing hard, lumpy, pellet-like stools (Bristol type 1) **(Fig. 1)**,[32] reduced frequency (<3/week) and urge for defecation, feeling of bloating, and incomplete evacuation. But there was no history of digital evacuation of stools or rectal prolapse. Over 8 years, he had used different laxatives as well as rectal suppositories and enemas with little benefit. There was no history of alarm symptoms such as gastrointestinal bleeding, anorexia, weight loss, fever, lump abdomen, or symptoms suggestive of anemia. He had no addictions. There was no history of diabetes, hypothyroidism, tuberculosis, or other comorbidities. However, he had family history of colon cancer-related death of his grandfather. His general physical and systemic examination including abdominal examination were normal. Digital rectal examination was also normal.

A provisional clinical diagnosis of functional constipation (as per Rome IV criteria)[33] **(Fig. 2)** was made and relevant investigations were carried out in view of refractory chronic constipation and also family history of colon cancer. Differential diagnosis of functional constipation includes IBS-C and secondary causes of constipation among which drug-induced constipation needs a special mention. Three subtypes of functional constipation include: (1) normal transit constipation (NTC), (2) slow transit constipation (STC), and (3) fecal evacuation disorder (FED). Clinical features of reduced stool frequency and hard, pellet-like stool in our case pointed toward possibility of STC.

Laboratory findings revealed hemoglobin as 13.6 g/dL, fasting blood sugar 91 mg/dL, glycated hemoglobin (HbA1c) 5.2%, serum

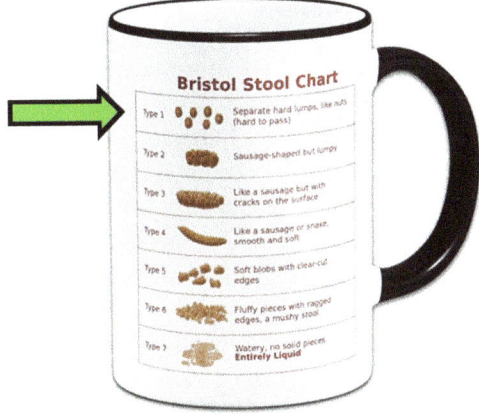

Fig. 1: Bristol Stool Form Score at presentation.

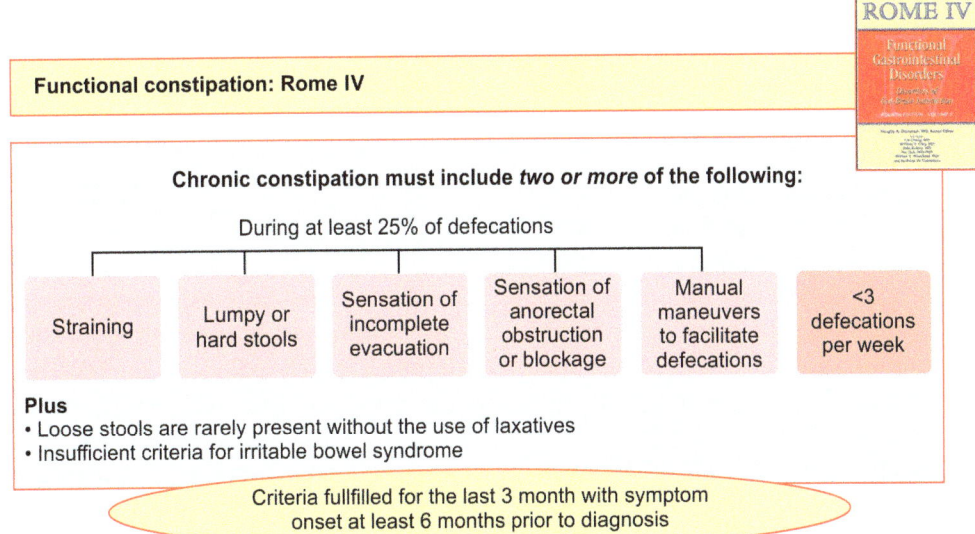

Fig. 2: Rome IV criteria for diagnosis of functional constipation.

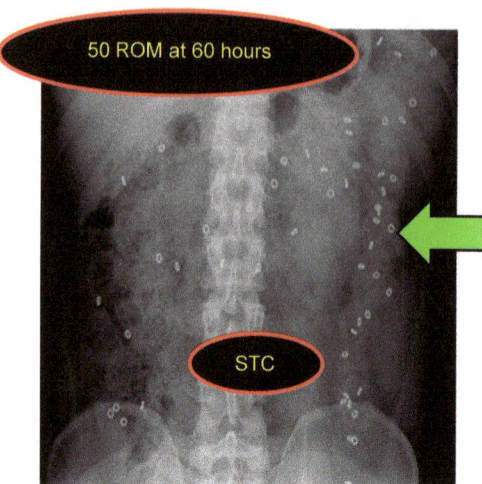

Fig 3: ROM-based CTT study. (CTT: colonic transit time; ROM: radio-opaque marker; STC: slow transit constipation)

thyroid-stimulating hormone (TSH) 2.1 mIU/L, serum creatinine 0.8 mg/dL, and serum albumin 4.1 g/dL. Fecal occult blood test was negative. Colonoscopic study was normal. Radio-opaque marker- (ROM)- based colonic transit time (CTT) study using Ghoshal's protocol[34] showed 50 ROMs at 60 hours (normal <14). Distribution of the markers was throughout the colon suggesting diagnosis of STC **(Fig. 3)**. Anorectal manometry, balloon expulsion test, and magnetic resonance imaging (MRI) defecography were all normal.

With diagnosis of functional constipation (STC-type) refractory to first-line laxatives (such as fiber, milk of magnesia, lactulose, and polyethylene glycol) and oral lubiprostone (a secretagogue), the patient was started on tablet prucalopride (an enterokinetic agent) 2 mg once daily, and in addition advised to follow lifestyle interventions (such as intake of adequate fluid and natural fiber, using Indian style toilet, and a lot of daily physical activity). After 6 weeks, he had no major improvement in constipation. At this time, we added tablet bisacodyl (stimulant laxative) 10 mg once daily. The patient stopped bisacodyl on his own after 4 weeks due to side effects of crampy abdominal pain, and moreover no significant relief in constipation.

At this point, we decided to do test for his breath methane as this is one of the correctable causes of STC. GHBT was performed using a standard protocol[35] (QuinTron Breathtracker™ Digital Microlyzer, Quin Tron Inc., Milwaukee, WI, USA). After ingestion of glucose, there was persistent rise of breath hydrogen >12 ppm above the fasting value, suggesting SIBO, and there was also high breath methane excretion (>35 ppm) both in fasting state and after ingestion of glucose, suggesting methane-positive SIBO **(Fig. 4)**.

In view of presence of SIBO and excessive breath methane, the patient was treated with tablet rifaximin 550 mg thrice daily for 2 weeks to eradicate methane-positive SIBO. On this treatment, his symptoms of constipation improved remarkably with stool frequency increasing to one per day and BSFS improving to 3–4 without laxatives or enemas. He remained fine at follow-up period at 3 months without recurrence of symptoms. Repeat colonic transit study at 3 months showed only 13 markers at 60 hours (which is considered normal). Repeat GHBT at 3 months did not show SIBO and showed normal hydrogen and methane **(Fig. 5)**.

■ DISCUSSION

This patient had slow transit type of functional constipation as evidenced by clinical symptoms as well as findings on ROM-based colonic transit study. His symptoms were refractory to first-line laxatives (such as fiber, milk of magnesia, lactulose, and polyethylene glycol), oral lubiprostone (a secretagogue), and even rectal suppositories and enemas. His anorectal manometry, balloon

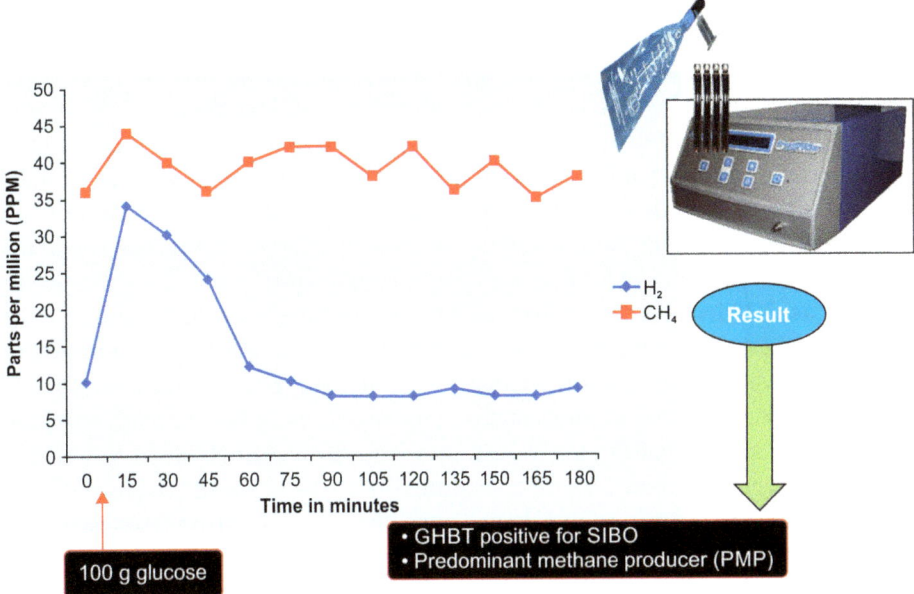

Fig. 4: Glucose hydrogen breath test (GHBT) at presentation, showing presence of small intestinal bacterial overgrowth (SIBO) and predominant methane production.

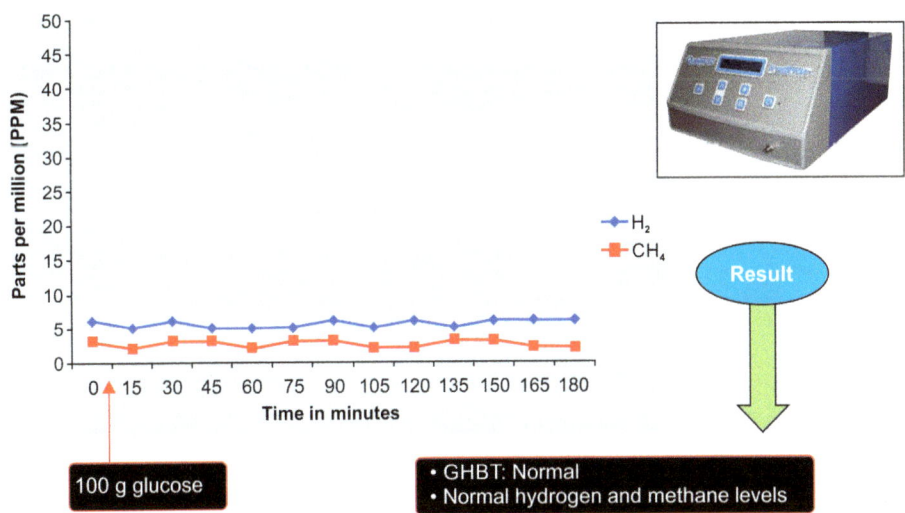

Fig. 5: Glucose hydrogen breath test (GHBT) at 3 months follow-up, showing absence of small intestinal bacterial overgrowth (SIBO) and normal breath hydrogen and methane.

expulsion test, and MRI defecography were all normal, hence ruling out FED. Clinical history, normal basic laboratory tests, and normal colonoscopy essentially ruled out any possible secondary cause of refractory chronic constipation. Empirical treatment with prucalopride (an enterokinetic agent), bisacodyl (stimulant laxative), and lifestyle interventions (such as intake of adequate fluid and natural fiber, using Indian style toilet, and lot of daily physical activity) also did not help this patient. His GHBT clinched the issue as it showed methane-positive SIBO which responded dramatically to oral antibiotic therapy with rifaximin. On follow-up, there was sustained improvement of symptoms, and follow-up colonic transit study as well as GHBT was normal. So this proves the hypothesis that methane-positive SIBO can slow down gut transit and reducing gut methane production by antibiotics such as rifaximin can restore gut motility and result in improvement in constipation.

About 30–62% of healthy people have methane-producing microflora in their gut.[36] Both in vitro and in vivo studies indicate that excessive methane production can inhibit gastrointestinal motility and hence, its concentration may inversely correlate with stool form and frequency.[21-23,37] It has been shown that greater the area under the curve for breath methane, the greater the reduction in gut motility, and hence greater the severity of constipation.[1] The mechanism of delayed gut transit due to excessive methane may be related to alteration in intestinal motility and decrease in gut serotonin production.[25]

Several recent meta-analysis have reported association of breath methane with constipation and delayed gut transit.[29-31] Recently published Indian consensus on chronic constipation categorically emphasized the role of gut methane in pathogenesis of chronic constipation and

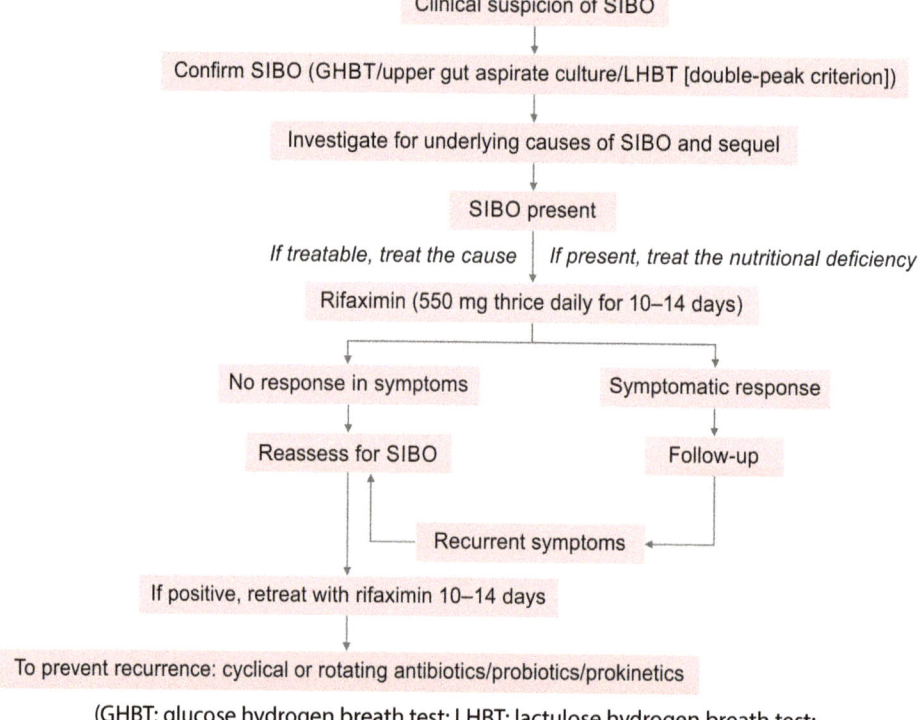

Flowchart 1: Algorithm for management of SIBO as per Asian–Pacific consensus on SIBO.

(GHBT: glucose hydrogen breath test; LHBT: lactulose hydrogen breath test; SIBO: small intestinal bacterial overgrowth)

advised on testing of breath methane in those with STC.[38] The role of methane-associated SIBO has therapeutic implications. Various antibiotics used for management of methane-related SIBO include rifaximin, neomycin, or combination of these two drugs. Three randomized controlled trials, one from India and two from the United States of America (USA), reported that reduction of methane production by treatment with oral antibiotics leads to improvement in constipation.[26-28] The study from India also showed that reduction in breath methane by oral antibiotic therapy was associated with acceleration of colonic transit.[27] Larger multicentric studies on the issue of methane-associated SIBO are eagerly needed. SIBO (of any type) has been reported to recur following successful treatment with antibiotics.[39,40] Predictors of recurrence of SIBO include elderly age, long-term treatment with proton pump inhibitors (PPIs), persistence of predisposing condition, and prior abdominal surgery. Recently published Asian–Pacific consensus on SIBO emphasized on the role of methane in pathogenesis of SIBO, especially those presenting clinically with slow transit type constipation and hence recommended antibiotic therapy to tackle excess methane production, and advised an algorithm for management of SIBO[1] **(Flowchart 1)**.

In conclusion, the current case report suggests that excess methane production must be evaluated in patients with STC, especially those refractory to stimulant laxative and colokinetic medications. Treatment of excess methane production by oral antibiotic therapy can lead to reduction in gut methane which translates into improved gut transit and relief in symptoms of constipation. Further studies on this enigmatic issue are expected in near future.

REFERENCES

1. Ghoshal UC, Sachdeva S, Ghoshal U, Misra A, Puri AS, Pratap N, et al. Asian-Pacific consensus on small intestinal bacterial overgrowth in gastrointestinal disorders: an initiative of the Indian Neurogastroenterology and Motility Association. Indian J Gastroenterol. 2022;41(5):483-507.
2. Ghoshal UC, Ghoshal U. Small intestinal bacterial overgrowth and other intestinal disorders. Gastroenterol Clin North Am. 2017;46:103-20.
3. Lynch SV, Pedersen O. The human intestinal micro-biome in health and disease. N Engl J Med. 2016;375(24):2369-79.
4. Pimentel M, Saad RJ, Long MD, Rao SSC. ACG clinical guideline: Small intestinal bacterial overgrowth. Am J Gastroenterol. 2020;115:165-78.
5. Khoshini R, Dai SC, Lezcano S, Pimentel M. A systematic review of diagnostic tests for small intestinal bacterial overgrowth. Dig Dis Sci. 2008;53:1443-54.
6. Toskes PP. Bacterial overgrowth of the gastrointestinal tract. Adv Intern Med. 1993;38:387-407.
7. Ghoshal UC, Srivastava D, Misra A, Ghoshal U. A proof-of-concept study showing antibiotics to be more effective in irritable bowel syndrome with than without small-intestinal bacterial overgrowth: a randomized, double-blind, placebo-controlled trial. Eur J Gastroenterol Hepatol. 2016;28:281-9.
8. Ghoshal UC, Srivastava D, Ghoshal U, Misra A. Breath tests in the diagnosis of small intestinal bacterial overgrowth in patients with irritable bowel syndrome in comparison with quantitative upper gut aspirate culture. Eur J Gastroenterol Hepatol. 2014;26:753-60.
9. Posserud I, Stotzer PO, Björnsson ES, Abrahamsson H, Simrén M. Small intestinal bacterial overgrowth in patients with irritable bowel syndrome. Gut. 2007;56:802-8.
10. Erdogan A, Rao SS, Gulley D, Jacobs C, Lee YY, Badger C. Small intestinal bacterial overgrowth: duodenal aspiration vs. glucose breath test. Neurogastroenterol Motil. 2015;27:481-9.

11. Ghoshal UC, Baba CS, Ghoshal U, Alexander G, Misra A, Saraswat VA, et al. Low-grade small intestinal bacterial overgrowth is common in patients with nonalcoholic steatohepatitis on quantitative jejunal aspirate culture. Indian J Gastroenterol. 2017;36:390-9.
12. Rezaie A, Buresi M, Lembo A, Lin H, McCallum R, Rao S, et al. Hydrogen and methane-based breath testing in gastrointestinal disorders: the North American Consensus. Am J Gastroenterol. 2017;112:775-84.
13. Bohm M, Siwiec RM, Wo JM. Diagnosis and management of small intestinal bacterial overgrowth. Nutr Clin Pract. 2013;28:289-99.
14. Husebye E, Skar V, Hoverstad T, Melby K. Fasting hypochlorhydria with Gram-positive gastric flora is highly prevalent in healthy old people. Gut. 1992;33:1331-7.
15. Fried M, Siegrist H, Frei R, Froehlich F, Duroux P, Thorens J, et al. Duodenal bacterial overgrowth during treatment in outpatients with omeprazole. Gut. 1994;35:23-6.
16. Ghoshal U, Ghoshal UC, Ranjan P, Naik SR, Ayyagari A. Spectrum and antibiotic sensitivity of bacteria contaminating the upper gut in patients with malabsorption syndrome from the tropics. BMC Gastroenterol. 2003;3:9.
17. Losurdo G, Leandro G, Ierardi E, Perri F, Barone M, Principi M, et al. Breath tests for the non-invasive diagnosis of small intestinal bacterial overgrowth: A systematic review with meta-analysis. J Neurogastroenterol Motil. 2020;26:16-28.
18. Eckburg PB, Bik EM, Bernstein CN, Purdom E, Dethlefsen L, Sargent M, et al. Diversity of the human intestinal microbial flora. Science. 2005;308(5728):1635.
19. Sahakian AB, Jee SR, Pimentel M. Methane and the gastrointestinal tract. Dig Dis Sci. 2010;55(8):2135-43.
20. Levitt MD, Furne JK, Kuskowski M, Ruddy J. Stability of human methanogenic flora over 35 years and a review of insights obtained from breath methane measurements. Clin Gastroenterol Hepatol. 2006;4(2):123-9.
21. Pimentel M, Lin HC, Enayati P, van den Burg B, Lee HR, Chen JH, et al. Methane, a gas produced by enteric bacteria, slows intestinal transit and augments small intestinal contractile activity. Am J Physiol Gastrointest Liver Physiol. 2006;290:G1089-95.
22. Ghoshal U, Shukla R, Srivastava D, Ghoshal UC. Irritable bowel syndrome, particularly the constipation-predominant form, involves an increase in Methanobrevibacter smithii, which is associated with higher methane production. Gut Liver. 2016;10:932-8.
23. Chatterjee S, Park S, Low K, Kong Y, Pimentel M. The degree of breath methane production in IBS correlates with the severity of constipation. Am J Gastroenterol. 2007;102:837-41.
24. Lee KM, Paik CN, Chung WC, Yang JM, Choi MG. Breath methane positivity is more common and higher in patients with objectively proven delayed transit constipation. Eur J Gastroenterol Hepatol. 2013;25:726-32.
25. Ghoshal UC, Srivastava D, Verma A, Misra A. Slow transit constipation associated with excess methane production and its improvement following rifaximin therapy: a case report. J Neurogastroenterol Motil. 2011; 17(2):185-8.
26. Pimentel M, Chang C, Chua KS, Mirocha J, DiBaise J, Rao S, et al. Antibiotic treatment of constipation-predominant irritable bowel syndrome. Dig Dis Sci. 2014;59:1278-85.
27. Ghoshal UC, Srivastava D, Misra A. A randomized double-blind placebo-controlled trial showing rifaximin to improve constipation by reducing methane production and accelerating colon transit: a pilot study. Indian J Gastroenterol. 2018;37: 416-23.
28. Low K, Hwang L, Hua J, Zhu A, Morales W, Pimentel M. A combination of rifaximin and neomycin is most effective in treating irritable bowel syndrome patients with methane on lactulose breath test. J Clin Gastroenterol. 2010;44:547-50.
29. Kunkel D, Basseri RJ, Makhani MD, Chong K, Chang C, Pimentel M. Methane on breath testing is associated with constipation: a systematic review and meta-analysis. Dig Dis Sci. 2011;56:1612-8.

30. Gandhi A, Shah A, Jones MP, Koloski N, Talley NJ, Morrison M, et al. Methane positive small intestinal bacterial overgrowth in inflammatory bowel disease and irritable bowel syndrome: a systematic review and meta-analysis. Gut Microbes. 2021;13:1933313.
31. Shah A, Talley NJ, Jones M, Kendall BJ, Koloski N, Walker MM, et al. Small intestinal bacterial overgrowth in irritable bowel syndrome: a systematic review and meta-analysis of case-control studies. Am J Gastroenterol. 2020;115:190-201.
32. Lewis SJ, Heaton KW. Stool form scale as a useful guide to intestinal transit time. Scand J Gastroenterol. 1997;32:920-4.
33. Mearin F, Lacy BE, Chang L, Chey WD, Lembo AJ, Simren M, et al. Bowel Disorders. Gastroenterology. 2016:S0016-5085(16)00222-5.
34. Ghoshal UC, Gupta D, Kumar A, Misra A. Colonic transit study by radio-opaque markers to investigate constipation: validation of a new protocol for a population with rapid gut transit. Natl Med J India. 2007;20(5):225-9.
35. Sachdeva S, Rawat AK, Reddy RS, Puri AS. Small intestinal bacterial overgrowth (SIBO) in irritable bowel syndrome: frequency and predictors. J Gastroenterol Hepatol. 2011;26 Suppl 3:135-8.
36. Attaluri A, Jackson M, Valestin J, Rao SS. Methanogenic flora is associated with altered colonic transit but not stool characteristics in constipation without IBS. Am J Gastroenterol. 2010;105:1407-11.
37. Jahng J, Jung IS, Choi EJ, Conklin JL, Park H. The effects of methane and hydrogen gases produced by enteric bacteria on ileal motility and colonic transit time. Neurogastroenterol Motil. 2012;24(185-90):e192.
38. Ghoshal UC, Sachdeva S, Pratap N, Verma A, Karyampudi A, Misra A, et al. Indian consensus on chronic constipation in adults: a joint position statement of the Indian Motility and Functional Diseases Association and the Indian Society of Gastroenterology. Indian J Gastroenterol. 2018;37(6):526-44.
39. Lauritano EC, Gabrielli M, Scarpellini E, Lupascu A, Novi M, Sottili S, et al. Small intestinal bacterial overgrowth recurrence after antibiotic therapy. Am J Gastroenterol. 2008;103:2031-5.
40. Sangam A, Dalal A, Arivarasan K. Recurrence of small intestinal bacterial overgrowth after successful antibiotic therapy in patients with irritable bowel syndrome: frequency and predictors. J Neurogastroenterol Motil. 2015;21:S3.

34

Amoeboma Masquerading as Carcinoma Colon

Deepak Lahoti, Shami Kumar, Nitin Bhople, Avesh, Meenakshi Jain

■ INTRODUCTION

The term amoeboma was introduced by Ochner and DeBakey in 1939[1] and it refers to a rare complication of amoebic colitis which may masquerade as colonic malignancy. Amoeboma is a tumor-like mass involving the whole thickness of the bowel wall and is a rare manifestation of amoebiasis. It may mimic Crohn's disease, carcinoma of the colon, non-Hodgkin's lymphoma, tuberculosis, fungal infection, acquired immunodeficiency syndrome (AIDS) associated lymphoma, and Kaposi's sarcoma on colonoscopy. Many case reports[2] describe amoeboma diagnosed only in the surgical specimen after surgery to treat malignancy. Hence, it is extremely important to consider the possibility of amoeboma in any patient presenting with a right iliac fossa mass, tumor-like lesion on colonoscopy, or as a differential of lower gastrointestinal bleed, although its incidence seems to be declining.

■ CASE REPORT

Case 1

A 72-year-old female, known case of diabetes mellitus and atrial fibrillation on anticoagulants, was admitted in intensive care unit (ICU) with severe symptomatic anemia with congestive cardiac failure with right lower limb cellulitis and urinary tract infection (UTI). Her per abdominal examination was unremarkable. Her initial laboratory investigations showed hemoglobin (Hb) 6.8 g/dL, total leukocyte count (TLC) 9,100/mm^3, platelet count 3.86 lakhs/mm^3, albumin 3.2 g/dL, and creatinine 1.11 mg/dL and liver function test (LFT) was grossly normal. Cardiac enzymes were within normal range. The patient was managed with blood transfusions, intravenous antibiotics, diuretics, anticoagulant, oxygen therapy, and other supportive care. However during hospitalization in ICU, patient had an episode of maroon color bleeding per rectum. Her Hb dropped from 9.5 to 7.9 g/dL. Anticoagulant therapy was withheld. Colonoscopy done showed large ulceroproliferative mass lesion in transverse colon with active ooze with no significant obliteration of bowel lumen **(Fig. 1A)**. Multiple biopsies were taken. Endotherapy was done to achieve hemostasis. Possibility of carcinoma colon was kept. Contrast-enhanced computed tomography (CECT) whole abdomen showed focal area of circumferential mural thickening in the mid-transverse colon and hepatic flexure with surrounding streakiness and tiny lymph nodes in this region. No ascites was reported. Histopathology report showed focal ulceration of mucosa with trophozoite stage of amoeba and granulation tissue **(Fig. 1B)**. No granuloma/neoplasia was seen. Amoebic serology immunoglobulin G (IgG) was

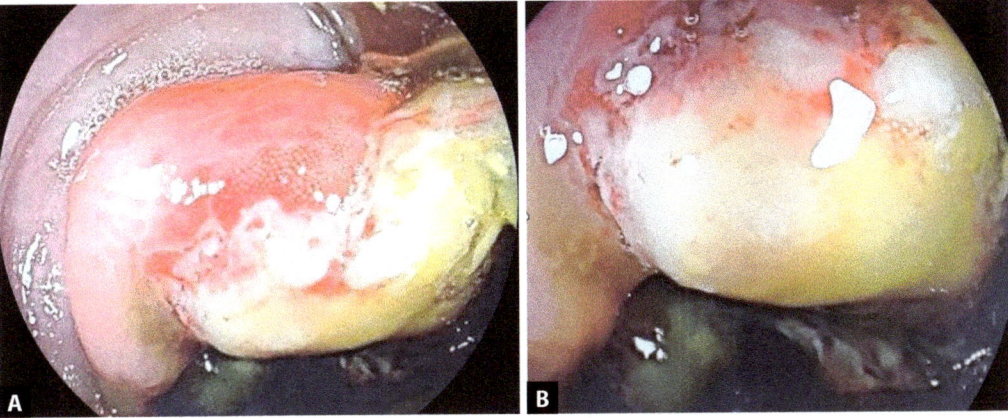

Figs. 1A and B: Colonoscopy showed large ulceroproliferative mass in transverse colon.

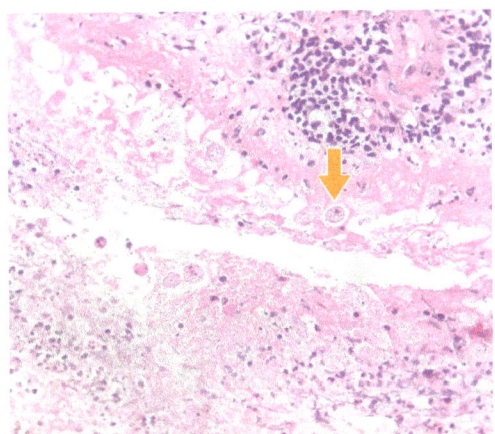

Fig. 2: Focal aggregations of amoeba trophozoites (orange arrow) were demonstrated by Hematoxylin and Eosin (H&E) stain.

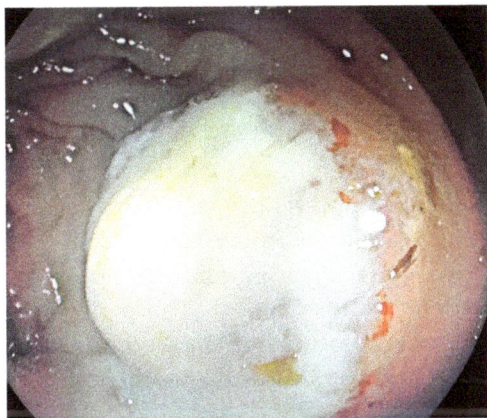

Fig. 3: Colonoscopy showed large ulceroproliferative lesions seen in descending colon.

29.87 IU **(Fig. 2)**. Diagnosis of amoeboma was made and she was started on intravenous metronidazole. Her bleeding stopped and Hb stabilized. She gradually improved and was then discharged on oral metronidazole for total of 14 days.

Case 2

A 54-year-old female, known case of diabetes mellitus and hypothyroidism, had history of pain left side abdomen for around 15 days, associated with constipation and anorexia. There was no history of bleeding per rectum, vomiting, dysuria, or fever. The patient was evaluated outside. Complete blood count (CBC) showed Hb 9.7 g/dL, TLC 9.5×10^3/mm^3, and creatinine 0.86 mg/dL. CECT abdomen was suggestive of focal thickening at splenic flexure of colon and cecum, possibly neoplastic. The patient presented to us for further management. Colonoscopy showed large ulceroproliferative lesions seen in transverse and descending colon with overlying slough **(Fig. 3)**. Scope could not

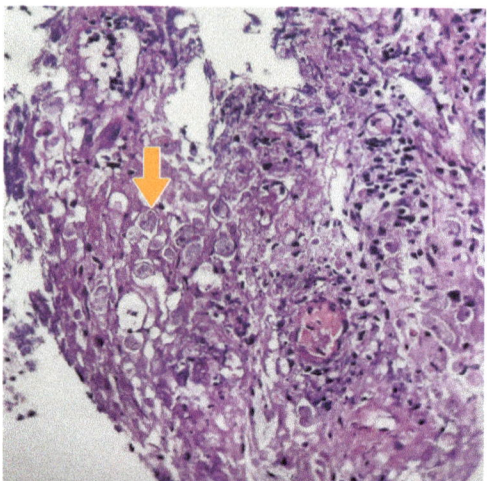

Fig. 4: Focal aggregations of amoeba trophozoites (orange arrow) seen in the background of acute on chronic inflammatory smear seen on Hematoxylin and Eosin (H&E) stain.

be negotiated further. Biopsies were taken; histopathology report showed exudates; acute on chronic inflammatory cells with trophozoite stage of amoeba suggested amoebic colitis **(Fig. 4)**. The patient was started on oral metronidazole and is now symptomatically responding to therapy.

■ DISCUSSION

Intestinal amoebiasis is caused by the protozoan *Entamoeba histolytica* (*E. histolytica*). Amoebiasis is largely a disease of resource-limited countries and *E. histolytica* is endemic in India, Africa, and parts of Central and South America, where almost half the population is infected.[3,4] The parasite exists in two forms, a cyst stage (the infective form), and a trophozoite stage (the form that causes invasive disease).

Sometimes, longstanding intestinal amoebiasis develop chronic inflammatory exophytic masses because the necrotic tissue is replaced by an extensive inflammatory reaction and pseudotumor formation known as amoebomas, mimicking as colonic carcinoma. In our two cases, clinical picture suggested high suspicion of carcinoma too.

Amoebomas are found, in decreasing order of frequency, in the cecum, ascending colon, rectosigmoid, transverse colon, and descending colon.[5] They are usually solitary with variable size and may measure up to 15 cm in diameter, mostly seen in men.

There are few isolated case reports; exact incidence of this disease is unknown. It should be suspected when a patient from an endemic area presents with pain or mass in right side of abdomen with fever, bloody diarrhea, or bleeding per rectum.[3] In our case, patient (case 1) was admitted in hospital with unrelated complaints and developed lower gastrointestinal bleeding in ICU. The findings on colonoscopy, as mentioned earlier, were strongly suggestive of a colonic malignancy in both of our patients. Sometimes colonic amoeboma with amoebic liver abscess may be misdiagnosed as a metastatic colonic malignancy.[6,7] A high index of suspicion is thus essential when dealing with colonic masses and liver lesions, especially in the endemic areas to avoid unnecessary surgeries. Most of the time, amoeboma is diagnosed postoperatively in surgical specimen.[7]

The treatment of amoeboma, if diagnosed correctly by imaging and colonoscopic biopsy, is mainly conservative. Treatment options include 5–10 days of oral metronidazole, followed by diloxanide furoate or paromomycin to eradicate carrier state. If the lesion has not regressed after full medical treatment, colonic resection may be done, particularly if possibility of malignancy cannot be ruled out.[3]

To conclude, colonic amoeboma is a rare complication of invasive amoebiasis, mimics carcinoma of the colon on computed tomography (CT) scan as well as colonoscopy findings. Infection is known to occur in non-endemic areas among individuals who have never traveled abroad.[8] With globalization and widespread traveling, this entity is expected to pose diagnostic challenges for clinicians in nonendemic areas as well.

Awareness about this entity is important especially among surgeons and gastroenterologists so as to avoid unnecessary surgery at first place.

REFERENCES

1. Ochner A, DeBakey M. Surgical consideration of amoebiasis. Surg Gynecol Obstet. 1939;69: 392-402.
2. Shirley DT, Farr L, Watanabe K, Moonah S. A Review of the Global Burden, New Diagnostics, and Current Therapeutics for Amebiasis. Open Forum Infect Dis. 2018; 5:ofy161.
3. Datta PK, Lal P, Bakshi SD. Surgery in the tropics. In: Williams NS, Bulstrode CJK, Ronan O'Connell P (Eds). Bailey and Love's Short Practice of Surgery, 26th edition. London: CRC Press; 2013. pp. 68-92.
4. Sicklick JK, D'Angelica M, Fong Y. The Liver. In: Beauchamp, Evers, Mattox (Eds). Sabiston Textbook of Surgery, 19th edition. Saunders Elsevier; 2012. pp. 1411-75.
5. Li E, Stanley SL Jr. Protozoa. Amoebiasis. Gastroenterol Clin North Am. 1996;25: 471-92.
6. Sharma D, Patel LK, Vaidya VV. Amoeboma of ascending colon with multiple amebic liver abscesses. J Assoc Physicians India. 2001;49:579-80.
7. Simsek H, Elsurer R, Sokmensuer C, Balaban YH, Tatar G. Ameboma mimicking carcinoma of the caecum: case report. Gastrointest Endosc. 2004;59(3):453-4.
8. Salit IE, Khairnar K, Gough K, Pillai DR. A possible cluster of sexually transmitted Entamoeba histolytica: genetic analysis of a highly virulent strain. Clin Infect Dis. 2009;49:346.

Constipation–Functional Dyspepsia Overlap

Uday C Ghoshal, Uzma Mustafa

■ INTRODUCTION

We discuss here a case of a 42-year-old female who presented to the outpatient clinic, with a two-year history of hypogastric pain and discomfort, which occurred daily, and got relieved after bowel movement. She also experienced constipation (predominant stool type Bristol 1–2), frequency 2–3 times/week, with straining, feeling of incomplete evacuation, and repeated ineffective attempts but no manual evacuation. She presented with epigastric fullness, which increased postprandially almost daily, and reported experiencing anorexia, nausea, and occasional vomiting. She suffered from marked abdominal bloating that increased towards evening. Symptom severity limited her daily life activity and she suffered from anxiety and disturbed sleep. She had no alarm symptom. She was a vegetarian. She consulted multiple doctors both of modern medicine, homoeopathy and Ayurveda, but had no relief. An upper gastrointestinal (GI) endoscopy done elsewhere was normal. Tests for *Helicobacter pylori* were negative. Full colonoscopy and ultrasonography (USG) abdomen were normal. Her clinical diagnosis was an overlap of functional dyspepsia (FD) and irritable bowel syndrome with constipation (IBS-C). A colon transit study using radio-opaque markers revealed slow transit. A lactulose hydrogen breath showed high breath methane.

The patient was treated with prucalopride 2 mg once daily and a stimulant laxative (bisacodyl) 10 mg at bedtime. She was advised to avoid high FODMAP (fermentable oligosaccharides, disaccharides, monosaccharides, and polyols) foods. Although she tried to follow the diet, she found it difficult to adhere. Her symptoms improved but only partially, with 3–4 spontaneous bowel movements (Bristol stool type 3) per week. Her symptoms of nausea and vomiting resolved and dyspepsia improved. However, her prior complaint of incomplete bowel movement, straining, abdominal bloating, and flatulence persisted. The patient was not satisfied and requested something more to be done to relieve her symptoms. The patient was continued on prucalopride and bisacodyl. Additionally, rifaximin 550 mg thrice daily was added for 10 days to her treatment regime. Thereafter, her symptoms improved remarkably. A repeat lactulose hydrogen breath showed reduction in breath methane. A repeat colon transit study indicated improvement. The patient has been currently on follow-up for last 2 months and is doing well.

■ DISCUSSION

The above-mentioned case discussed FD-IBS-C overlap. The diagnosis was based on

CHAPTER 35: Constipation–Functional Dyspepsia Overlap

BOX 1: Rome IV criteria for irritable bowel syndrome.

Recurrent abdominal pain, at least 1 day per week in the last 3 months, associated with two or more of the following:
- Related to defecation
- Associated with a change in frequency of stool
- Associated with a change in form (appearance) of stool

Onset at least 6 months ago

BOX 2: Subtyping for irritable bowel syndrome (IBS).

- IBS-C: More than one fourth (25%) of bowel movements with Bristol Stool Scale types 1–2 and less than one fourth (25%) with types 6–7 in the past 2 weeks
- IBS-D: More than one fourth (25%) of bowel movements with Bristol Stool Scale types 6–7 and less than one fourth (25%) with types 1–2 in the past 2 weeks
- IBS-M: More than one fourth (25%) of bowel movements with Bristol Stool Scale types 1–2 and more than one fourth (25%) with types 6–7 in the past 2 weeks
- IBS-U: Patients meet diagnostic criteria for IBS but their bowel habits cannot be accurately categorized in any of the above subtypes

(IBS-C: IBS with constipation; IBS-D: IBS with diarrhea; IBS-M: IBS mixed type; IBS-U: IBS unclassified)

BOX 3: Rome IV criteria for functional dyspepsia.

1. *One or more of the following:*
   - Bothersome postprandial fullness
   - Bothersome early satiation
   - Bothersome epigastric pain
   - Bothersome epigastric burning

   And
2. No evidence of structural disease (including at upper endoscopy) that is likely to explain the symptoms.

   Must fulfill criteria for PDS and/or EPS for the last 3 months with symptom onset at least 6 months ago.

   Heartburn is not a dyspeptic symptom but may often coexist.

   Symptoms that are relieved by evacuation of feces or gas should generally not be considered as part of dyspepsia.

(EPS: epigastric pain syndrome; PDS: postprandial distress syndrome)

Rome IV criteria for IBS and its subtyping (**Boxes 1 and 2**) and FD (**Box 3**).

It is known that FD is a highly prevalent GI disorder with quite a number of patients who are dissatisfied with the treatments.[1] Although FD may occur exclusively, studies suggest that it may overlap with other GI disorders affecting different part of the digestive system, such as overlap with gastroesophageal reflux disease (GERD), epigastric pain syndrome (EPS), postprandial distress syndrome (PDS), and constipation.[2] The presence of motor or functional abnormalities in one region of the GI tract increases the likelihood of abnormalities in others. Prior studies have demonstrated a noteworthy overlap between dyspepsia and constipation symptoms.[3-5] Such relationships suggest that in lieu of an exclusive pathophysiology, an inclusive one may explain symptoms in multiple areas of the GI tract. A multicentric pan-Asian study of disorders of gut brain interaction (DGBI) identified a symptom cluster, comprising constipation symptoms associated with upper abdominal discomfort.[6] When compared to the IBS with diarrhea (IBS-D), the IBS-C patients have been reported to suffer from more severe upper GI symptoms, particularly early satiety and postprandial fullness.[3,7]

The FD–constipation overlap may be attributed to several factors that may explain the coexistence of the two disorders. It is imperative to understand the pathophysiology of the overlap to decide on the treatment plan.

Constipation-induced cologastric brake may result in FD symptoms: The colonic motility is a normal physiological phenomenon which is characterized by rhythmic contractions that propel triturated food content and waste along the large bowel. The cologastric brake inhibits gastric emptying if there is lack of expulsion of the colonic content (the fecal matter), which is an essential, neurally and hormonally mediated physiological mechanism, thereby controlling the transit time and absorption of nutrients. Any abnormality in the colonic motility pattern can lead to upper GI symptoms and bowel movement irregularities. An experimental investigation aimed at assessing the anomaly of the cologastric brake revealed that deliberate suppression of defecation led to delayed gastric emptying in healthy volunteers. This observation implied a potential connection between the cologastric brake and the development of upper abdominal symptoms among patients experiencing constipation.[8,9] A study indicated that some patients with slow transit constipation presented with delayed gastric emptying, which subsequently normalized after subtotal colectomy.[10] Another study found that electrogastrographic parameters improved after colectomy in patients with chronic constipation.[11] A separate investigation observed that isovolumetric rectal distensions delayed upper gut transit.[12] Research conducted on children who presented with FD–constipation overlap revealed a correlation with delayed gastric emptying and symptoms were alleviated following treatment with osmotic laxatives.[13]

FD–constipation overlap share impaired GI motility: The GI motility impairment associated with FD may have delayed gastric emptying, while with constipation, it is slow colonic transit. Both the motor abnormalities may coexist in patients experiencing FD–constipation overlap. An empirical study observed slower gastric emptying in patients experiencing severe constipation than in IBS-D.[14] IBS patients without overlapping FD exhibit normal gastric emptying of solids. However, constipation-predominant IBS patients who experienced concurrent dyspepsia presented with delayed gastric emptying of solids and overlapping postprandial fullness and nausea.[15]

Constipation-induced distension of transverse colon may lead to overlap of symptom perception for FD–constipation: Colonic distension might occur due to factors affecting GI motility and function, such as bloating, constipation, intraluminal content accumulation, and GI motility disorders. An investigation aimed at assessing the anomaly caused by distension of colon revealed that balloon inflation in transverse colon during colonoscopy-induced symptoms in upper abdomen.[16] Observational studies using magnetic resonance imaging investigations suggest that dilated transverse colon could hold more colonic content in IBS-C patients than other colon segments and was responsible for bloating severity in IBS-C patients.[17]

Elevated methane levels driven by gut microbiota dysbiosis: Imbalance in gut microbiota composition, i.e., dysbiosis, leads to elevated levels of methane in gut.[18-21] Gut microbiota dysbiosis may contribute to functional constipation and IBS-C.[22] Gut microbiota imbalance may alter serotonin transporter (SERT) expression, leading to chronic constipation.[23] Reportedly, the SERT genotype has also been associated with PDS.[24] The microbiota–gut–brain axis may have a role in co-occurrence of symptoms related to digestion and gut function.[25]

The complex pathophysiology of FD–constipation overlap calls for a holistic treatment approach, which may include combinations of fecal evacuants, pan-GI prokinetics, and medications to reduce elevated methane levels in gut.

Fecal evacuants to relieve constipation-induced dyspeptic symptoms: Improvement in bowel emptying is linked with improvement in gastric emptying. Many studies have observed this relationship, including one wherein subtotal colectomy enhanced postoperative gastric emptying.[10] Similarly, attainment of normal bowel movements through pharmaceutical interventions and fecal disimpaction led to resolution of the dyspeptic symptoms.[26]

Pan-GI prokinetics for holistic amelioration of FD-constipation overlap symptoms: The pathophysiology of FD-constipation overlap indicates pan-GI hypomotility. The use of pan-GI prokinetic emerges as a holistic treatment option. For instance, prucalopride relieved gastroparesis symptoms such as postprandial fullness, early satiety, nausea, vomiting, and bloating, as well as expedited gastric emptying.[27] The Asia-Pacific guidelines for management of FD-constipation overlap suggests that in event of nonavailability of pan-GI prokinetic, a combination of gastrokinetic with stimulant laxative may help.[2]

Addressing methane levels in the gut: Elevated methane levels in gut are associated with symptoms of constipation and dyspepsia.[18-21] Treating small intestinal bacterial overgrowth (SIBO) with rifaximin reduced methane levels and improved constipation.[28] A high level of breath-methane during fructose challenge test was a response-predictor to low-FODMAP diet among patients.[29] The Asia-Pacific guidelines for management of FD-constipation overlap suggests that restricting high fiber diet, which are abundant in FODMAPs, may help in reducing gut-methane levels.[2,30]

In our case study, the initial treatment with prucalopride and bisacodyl did not give satisfactory relief to the patient. Understandably, the overlap of FD with constipation led to more severe disease burden, compromised quality of life, and poor treatment outcomes. Thus, the principle of treatment pivoted upon improving symptoms of dyspepsia and gastric emptying by emptying the colon, improving the motility, and following low-fiber diet to reduce methane production and improve constipation.

Being vegetarian from northern India, the patient found it difficult to follow a low-FODMAP diet. This can be explained by the regional heterogeneity in dietary pattern and food consumption pattern.[31] In northern India, the challenges to adherence to low-FODMAP diet include high prevalence of vegetarianism, cultural preference of wheat over rice, intake of high volumes of lactose containing milk, prevalence of lactose malabsorption, and generous use of high FODMAP additives such as onion and garlic.[31]

Evidently, this case highlights that there is an overlap of symptom perception in FD and constipation and it is challenging to clearly distinguish and treat the two conditions. Taken together, the putative pathophysiology of FD-constipation overlap pivots on cologastric brake, transverse colon distension, impaired GI motility, and elevated methane levels driven by gut microbiota dysbiosis. Grossly, the treatment lines include pan-GI prokinetic, stimulants, laxatives, antibiotics, and low-fiber diet. It is important that patients experiencing FD-constipation overlap consult healthcare professionals for thorough evaluation, accurate diagnosis, and personalized treatment plan.

REFERENCES

1. Xiong L, Gong X, Siah KTH, Pratap N, Ghoshal UC, Abdullah M, et al. Rome foundation Asian working team report: Real world treatment experience of Asian patients with functional bowel disorders. J Gastroenterol Hepatol. 2017;32(8):1450-6.
2. Gwee KA, Lee YY, Suzuki H, Ghoshal UC, Holtmann G, Bai T, et al. Asia-Pacific guidelines for managing functional dyspepsia overlapping with other gastrointestinal symptoms. J Gastroenterol Hepatol. 2023;38(2):197-209.
3. Talley NJ, Dennis EH, Schettler-Duncan VA, Lacy BE, Olden KW, Crowell MD. Overlapping Upper and Lower Gastrointestinal Symptoms in Irritable Bowel Syndrome Patients with Constipation or Diarrhea. Am J Gastroenterol. 2003;98(11):2454-9.
4. Ford AC, Marwaha A, Lim A, Moayyedi P. Systematic Review and Meta-analysis of the Prevalence of Irritable Bowel Syndrome in Individuals With Dyspepsia. Clin Gastroenterol Hepatol. 2010;8(5):401-9.
5. Matsuzaki J, Suzuki H, Asakura K, Fukushima Y, Inadomi JM, Takebayashi T, et al. Classification of functional dyspepsia based on concomitant bowel symptoms. Neurogastroenterol Motil. 2012;23(4):325-e164.
6. Tien K, Siah H, Gong X, Yang XJ, Whitehead WE, Chen M, et al. Rome Foundation-Asian working team report: Asian functional gastrointestinal disorder symptom clusters. Gut. 2017:1-8.
7. Gwee KA, Lu CL, Ghoshal UC. Epidemiology of irritable bowel syndrome in Asia: Something old, something new, something borrowed. J Gastroenterol Hepatol. 2009;24(10):1601-7.
8. Tjeerdsma HC, Smout AJPM, Akkermans LMA. Voluntary suppression of defecation delays gastric emptying. Dig Dis Sci. 1993;38(5):832-6.
9. Parkman HP, Sharkey E, Mccallum RW, Hasler WL, Kenneth L, Sarosiek I, et al. Constipation in patients with symptoms of gastroparesis: Analysis of Symptoms and Gastrointestinal Transit. Clin Gastroenterol Hepatol. 2022;20(3):546-58.
10. Hemingway DM, Finlay IG. Effect of colectomy on gastric emptying in idiopathic slow-transit constipation. Br J Surg. 2000;87(9):1193-6.
11. Homma S, Hasegawa J, Maruta T, Watanabe N, Matsuo H, Tamiya Y, et al. Isopower maps of the electrogastrogram (EGG) after total gastrectomy or total colectomy. Neurogastroenterol Motil. 2002;11(6):441-8.
12. Coremans G, Geypens B, Vos R, Tack J, Margaritis V, Ghoos Y, et al. Influence of continuous isobaric rectal distension on gastric emptying and small bowel transit in young healthy women. Neurogastroenterol Motil. 2004;16(1):107-11.
13. Boccia G, Buonavolontà R, Coccorullo P, Manguso F, Fuiano L, Staiano A. Dyspeptic Symptoms in Children: The Result of a Constipation-Induced Cologastric Brake? Clin Gastroenterol Hepatol. 2008;6(5):556-60.
14. Nielsen OH, Gjørup T, Christensen FN. Gastric emptying rate and small bowel transit time in patients with irritable bowel syndrome determined with 99mTc-labeled pellets and scintigraphy. Dig Dis Sci. 1986;31(12):1287-91.
15. Stanghellini V, Tosetti C, Barbara G, De Giorgio R, Cogliandro L, Cogliandro R, et al. Dyspeptic symptoms and gastric emptying in the irritable bowel syndrome. Am J Gastroenterol. 2002;97(11):2738-43.
16. Swarbrick ET, Bat L, Hegarty JE, Williams CB, Dawson AM. Site of Pain From the Irritable Bowel. Lancet. 1980;316(8192):443-6.
17. Lam C, Chaddock G, Laurea LM, Costigan C, Cox E, Hoad C, et al. Distinct Abnormalities of Small Bowel and Regional Colonic Volumes in Subtypes of Irritable Bowel Syndrome Revealed by MRI. Am J Gastroenterol. 2017;112(2):346-55.
18. Algera JP, Colomier E, Melchior C, Hreinsson JP, Midenfjord I, Clevers E, et al. Associations between postprandial symptoms, hydrogen and methane production, and transit time in irritable bowel syndrome. Neurogastroenterol Motil. 2023;35(2):1-12.

19. Kunkel D, Basseri RJ, Makhani MD, Chong K, Chang C, Pimentel M. Methane on breath testing is associated with constipation: a systematic review and meta-analysis. Dig Dis Sci. 2011;56(6):1612-8.
20. Chatterjee S, Park S, Low K, Kong Y, Pimentel M. The degree of breath methane production in IBS correlates with the severity of constipation. Am J Gastroenterol. 2007;102(4):837-41.
21. Triantafyllou K, Chang C, Pimentel M. Methanogens, methane and gastrointestinal motility. J Neurogastroenterol Motil. 2014;20(1):31-40.
22. Ohkusa T, Koido S, Nishikawa Y, Sato N. Gut microbiota and chronic constipation: a review and update. Front Med. 2019;6:1-9.
23. Cao H, Liu X, An Y, Zhou G, Liu Y, Xu M, et al. Dysbiosis contributes to chronic constipation development via regulation of serotonin transporter in the intestine. Sci Rep. 2017;7(1):1-12.
24. Oshima T, Toyoshima F, Nakajima S, Fukui H, Watari J, Miwa H. Genetic factors for functional dyspepsia. J Gastroenterol Hepatol. 2011;26(Suppl 3):83-7.
25. De Palma G, Collins SM, Bercik P. The microbiota-gut-brain axis in functional gastrointestinal disorders. Gut Microbes. 2014;5(3):419-29.
26. Fernandes VPI, Lima MCL, Camargo EE, Collares EF, Bustorff-Silva JM, Lomazi EA. Gastric emptying of water in children with severe functional fecal retention. Brazilian J Med Biol Res. 2013;46(3):293-8.
27. Carbone F, Van Den Houte K, Clevers E, Andrews CN, Papathanasopoulos A, Holvoet L, et al. Prucalopride in Gastroparesis: a Randomized Placebo-Controlled Crossover Study. Am J Gastroenterol. 2019;114(8):1265-74.
28. Ghoshal UC, Srivastava D, Misra A. A randomized double-blind placebo-controlled trial showing rifaximin to improve constipation by reducing methane production and accelerating colon transit: A pilot study. Indian J Gastroenterol. 2018;37(5):416-23.
29. Wilder-Smith CH, Olesen SS, Materna A, Drewes AM. Predictors of response to a low-FODMAP diet in patients with functional gastrointestinal disorders and lactose or fructose intolerance. Aliment Pharmacol Ther. 2017;45(8):1094-106.
30. Gwee KA, Ghoshal UC, Chen M. Irritable bowel syndrome in Asia: Pathogenesis, natural history, epidemiology, and management. J Gastroenterol Hepatol. 2018;33(1):99-110.
31. Mustafa U, Ghoshal UC. The challenges of implementing low fermentable oligo-, di-, monosaccharides and polyol diet in India: An analysis of available data. Indian J Gastroenterol. 2022;41(1):104-13.

Index

Page numbers followed by *b* refer to box, *f* refer to figure, *fc* refer to flowchart, and *t* refer to table

A

Abdomen
  contrast-enhanced computed tomography of 150, 168*f*, 177*f*, 214*f*
  ultrasound of 82*f*, 172*f*
Abdominal compartment syndrome 26
Abnormal push pressure 205*f*
Abscess 7,9
  aspirate 9
  hepatic 8
  multiloculated 10
  multiple 10
Achalasia 23*f*, 37, 53
  cardia 24, 52*f*
  diagnosis of 24
  types 21
Acid reflux 43
  composite score analysis 41
Acid-fast bacilli 199
Acinar cell injury 166
Acquired immunodeficiency syndrome 66, 199, 208, 228
Acute pancreatitis 165
  diagnosis of 165
  etiology of 166*t*
  grades of severity of 167
  management of 165
  pathogenesis of 166*t*
Adefovir 131, 132
Advised biofeedback therapy 182
Alagille syndrome 112
Alanine
  aminotransferase 6, 81, 92, 106, 141, 176
  transaminase 4, 14, 100, 101, 130, 147, 150
  level, serum 135
Albumin 4, 28, 29, 176
Alcohol 166
Aldafermin 88

Alkaline phosphatase 4, 6, 81, 92, 100, 101, 112, 117, 122, 130, 141, 150, 156, 214
  serum 135
Allergic vasculitis 37
American College of Gastroenterology guidelines 65
American Society of Gastrointestinal Endoscopy 141, 142
Amoebiasis 13, 230
  intestinal 230
Amoeboma 228
Amylase, serum 141
Amyloidosis 183, 199, 219
Anaerobes 9
Anal fissures 208
Anal sphincter
  external 181
  pressure 181
  weakness 197
Anchovy paste 9
Anemia 14, 184, 199
Angiodysplasia 62, 65
Angioectasia 64*f*, 65, 67*f*
Angiotensin-converting enzyme levels 116
Anorectal dysfunction, diagnostic of 182
Anorectal manometry 185, 189, 202, 208
  combination of 182
  high-resolution 181
Anorexia 221
Antacids 200
Antiangiogenic drugs, use of 69
Antibiotic
  oral 10
  prophylactic 168
  therapy 9, 113
Antibodies, anti-mitochondrial 113
Anticoagulants 65
Antidepressants 183

Antiemetics 207
Anti-Epstein-Barr virus 35
Antihistamines 183
  first-generation 117
Antihypertensive drugs 200
Anti-liver kidney microsomal antibody 125, 135
Antineutrophil cytoplasmic antibodies 156
Antinuclear antibody 106, 117, 125, 135
Antioxidants 88
Anti-Parkinson's agents 183
Anti-reflux
  mucosal ablation 42, 44
  mucosectomy 42, 44
  surgery 45
Anti-smooth muscle antibody 117, 125, 135
Antithrombotic drugs 66
Aortoenteric fistula 58, 66
Appetite, loss of 99
Argon plasma coagulation 60, 65, 67*f*, 70
Arterial oxygen, partial pressure of 167
Artesunate-based regimens 16
Arthritis 197, 215
Ascites 105, 130, 131
  development of 107
  diuretic resistant 28
Asian Pacific Association for Study of Liver 93, 106-108
Aspartate aminotransferase 6, 81, 92, 106, 141, 176
  elevation of 14
Aspartate transaminase 4, 100, 101, 112, 130, 147, 150
  serum 135
Aspirin 65
Atherosclerosis 150
Atlanta classification, revised 167*t*, 169*t*
Autoimmune markers 125, 135

Index

Autoimmune pancreatitis 160, 160*t*, 172, 173
   diagnosis of 172
Autonomic neuropathy, human immunodeficiency virus-associated 219
Azathioprine 156, 166
Azotemia, prerenal 26, 27

B

Bacilli, gram-negative 8
Balloon
   expulsion test 182, 186, 189, 206, 208
   inflation 234
   occluded retrograde transvenous obliteration 72
Barium
   esophagogram 51
   studies, accuracy of 51
   swallow 18, 19
Basophils 176
B-cell acute lymphoblastic leukemia 130
Belthazar sign 209*f*
Bevacizumab 69
Bezafibrate 118
Bile
   acid sequestrants 118
   duct
      benign 147
      disease, immunoglobulin G4-related 159
      injury 115
   pigments 100*f*
Biliary diseases 219
Biliary tract, diseases of 139
Bilirubin 4, 72
Biofeedback therapy, clinical utility of 207
Biopsy 149, 158, 160
   esophageal 18
   multiple 228
Bisacodyl 235
Bleeding 62, 130
   active 60
   complications 136
   drug-induced 65
   manifestations 117
   per rectum 202
   recurrent 61
   ulcers 61
   variceal 131
   vessel, delineation of 68
Bloating 235
   abdominal 232
   sensation 181
Blood
   active oozing of 151*f*
   clots 58
   parameters 214*t*
   pressure 105, 143
      systolic 59, 167
   sugar 204
      random 6, 184
   test 214
   urea nitrogen 27, 93
Blue rubber bleb nevus syndrome 66
Body mass index 33, 105, 125, 181
Bowel loops, nonspecific dilatation of 210*f*
Breath tests 220
Bridge therapy 110
Bristol stool 232
   chart 194
   form scale 182, 182*f*, 220, 221*f*
Bronchoalveolar lavage 35
Brucella 13
   melitensis 15
Brucellosis 15
Bruit, abdominal 197
Bulk forming agents 187

C

Calcium
   levels 184
   polycarbophil 187
Calculus obstructing cystic duct 146
Calprotectin, fecal 196
Camellia sinensis 123
Cameron lesions 58
Canalicular membrane 13, 114
Cancer
   antigen 177*t*
   pancreatic 148, 149*fc*
Candida 33, 37
   albicans 37
   cell wall of 35
   colonization 37
   esophagitis 33, 36
      diagnosis of 37
      perplexing cases of 33
   infections 36
   proliferates 37
   pseudohyphae of 34
   septate hyphae of 36
Capecitabine 217
Capsule endoscopy 71
Carbohydrate malabsorption 201
Carcinoma
   ampullary 147
   hepatocellular 83, 84*f*
   neuroendocrine 216
   periampullary 147
Cardiac failure, congestive 228
Cardiovascular disease 83
Cartridge-based nucleic acid amplification test 35
Cavity, oral 37
Cefoperazone sulbactam 10
Ceftriaxone 9, 10
Celiac disease 66, 196, 199, 219
Cells 4
Cenicriviroc 88
Central nervous system 49, 183
Cerebral failure 109
Cerebrovascular accident 49
Cetirizine 115
Charcot's triad 143
Chemokine receptor antagonist 88
Chemotherapy 149, 217
Chest
   examination 57
   percussion of 33
   roentogram 135
Chicago classification 21
Cholangiocarcinoma 117, 147, 159
Cholangiohepatitis 147
Cholangiopancreatography, endoscopic retrograde 9, 142, 144*f*, 149, 170, 175
Cholangitis 13, 156
   acute 143
   moderate acute 143
   primary biliary 115
Cholecystectomy 211, 219
Cholecystitis, acute calculus 143
Choledocholithiasis 141, 211
Cholelithiasis 210*f*
   presence of 211
Cholestasis 100*f*, 115, 136
   causes of 117
   drug-induced 112, 115*t*
   intrahepatic 112, 116, 117
   pathogenesis of 113
   pregnancy-generated 115
   progressive familial intrahepatic 112, 116
   severe 116

Index

Cholestastic features 116
Cholestatic disorders 112, 117, 118
  prototypical immune-mediated 115
Cholestatic hepatic injury 113
Cholestyramine 113, 118
Chronic constipation 181, 182, 189*fc*, 202
  pathogenesis of 224
Chronic diarrhea 194, 195, 197*t*, 201
  causes of 199
  clinical classification of 194
Ciprofloxacin 10
Circulatory failure 109
Cirrhosis 28, 62, 132, 132*t*, 219
  absence of 83
  atrophic 132
  compensated 131
  cryptogenic 83
  decompensated 105
  diagnosis of 132
  Laennec subclassification of 132*t*
  potential reversibility of 132
  primary biliary 196
  reversal of 130, 132
Cirrhotic nodules 130*f*
Clavulanate 10
Clostridioides difficile 197
Clots, maintenance of 60
Coagulation failure 109
Coil-assisted retrograde transvenous obliteration 73
Colitis
  amoebic 228
  ulcerative 197
Colon 211
  carcinoma of 197, 228
  length of 205*f*
  transit time 181, 189, 208, 222*f*
Colonic transit study 202, 205
Colonoscopy 181, 228, 229, 229*f*, 234
Colorectal cancer, family history of 184
Common bile duct 4, 142, 154, 175
  carcinoma of 146
  compression of 177*f*
  dilated 141, 142*f*, 172
  stones 144*f*
Complete blood count 176, 184, 229
Compression, extrinsic 49
Computed tomography 35*f*, 64, 85, 158*f*, 161*f*, 189
  scan 147
Connective tissue
  diseases 37, 219
  disorders 116
Constipation 107, 183, 189, 203, 204*b*, 207, 207*t*, 208, 232-234
  causes of 183
  chronic 181, 182, 189*fc*, 202
  functional 181, 183*t*, 203, 208
  normal transit 107, 184, 221
  opioid-induced 183, 208
  secondary 183*t*
  slow-transit 181, 189, 206-208, 221, 222*f*
  subtype 208
  types of 206, 206*t*
Contraceptives, oral 125
Contrast-enhanced computed tomography 150, 168*f*, 175, 177*f*, 213, 214*f*, 215, 216, 228
Coronavirus disease 2019 (COVID-19)
  global pandemic of 37
  history of 33
Corticosteroids 124
Courvoisier's law 146
C reactive protein 6, 108, 196
  elevated 33
  raised 154
Creatinine 4
Crescentic endoscopic mucosal resection 44
Crohn's disease 37, 66, 197, 198, 219, 228
Cryptospora 199
Cyclic guanosine monophosphate, synthesis of 188
Cyclosporine 115
Cystic artery 152*f*
  pseudoaneurysm 151*f*
  spontaneous rupture of 150
Cystic duct 157*f*
Cystic fibrosis 116
Cytomegalovirus 37, 102, 106, 108, 197
  esophagitis 37
Cytopenias 16

D

Dapagliflozin 88
Dehydration 195
Dehydrogenase, serum lactate 92
Dengue
  fever 14
  hemorrhagic fever 13
Diabetes mellitus 146, 183, 189, 229
Diabetic autonomic neuropathy 219
Dialysis, slow low-efficiency 29
Diaphragmatic irritation 7
Diarrhea 194, 217, 233
  bile acid-induced 198
  chronic 194, 195, 197*t*, 201
  drug-induced chronic 200
  functional 195*t*
  inflammatory 196, 196*t*, 197
  large-bowel 195*t*
  organic 195*t*
  osmotic 196
  secondary 198
  small bowel 195*t*
  watery 196, 196*t*, 198
Diethylenetriamine pentaacetate scan 113
Dieulafoy's lesion 58, 62, 65, 66
Differential leukocyte count 4, 176
Digital rectal examination 107, 202, 204*b*
Digital subtraction angiography 152*f*
Diloxanide furoate 10
Diphenhydramine 117
Diplopia 48
Direct endoscopy necrosectomy 169*f*
Disaccharides 232
Disseminated intravascular coagulation 14
Distal esophageal
  ring 19
  spasm 21, 53
Distress, respiratory 130
Double duct sign 147
Double pigtail stent placement 168*f*
Double-balloon enteroscope 67, 70
Dubin–Johnson syndrome 116
Ductal obstruction 166
Ductopenia 115

Ductular reaction 100*f*
Duke's anxiety-depressive
  score 202
Duodenal bile acid,
  inadequate 196
Duodenal papilla, prominent 156*f*
Duodenoscopy 156*f*
Duodenum 156*f*, 211
  part of 199
Dysarthria 48
Dyspepsia, functional 232, 233*b*
Dysphagia 18, 19, 36, 47, 48
  acute 50
  benign etiology of 50*t*
  causes of 49*t*
  differential diagnosis of 20*t*
  esophageal 18, 47- 49, 49*t*
  evaluation of 52*f*
  malignant 50, 50*t*
  management of 47
  mechanical 49, 50*t*
  structural 49
  transfer 18
  transit 18
Dyspnea 181
Dyssynergia defecation
  classification of 186*f*
  disorders 202, 206

E

Eating disorders 183
Edema
  pedal 130
  peripheral 215
Efruxifermin 88
Ehlers–Danlos syndrome 66
Electrohydraulic laser 144
Electrolyte disturbances 207
Elobixibat 188
Emollients 187
Empagliflozin 88
Encephalopathy, hepatic 14,
  105, 131
Endoscopic therapy 42, 43, 59,
  61, 62
Endoscopic ultrasound 141, 142*f*,
  170, 172
  guided glue injection 73
Endoscopy 18, 40, 43, 51, 59
End-stage liver disease 62, 131
  model for 73, 93, 102, 128
Enemas 188, 222
Entamoeba histolytica 197, 230
Entecavir 131, 132

Enteritis, nonspecific 66
Enterocolic fistula 198
Enterokinetic agent 223
Enterolithotomy 211
  laparoscopy-guided 211
Enteroscopy 65
  antegrade 65
  deep 71
Enzyme 217
Eosinophil 114*f*, 176
Eosinophilic infiltration 36*f*
Epidemiology 122, 182
Epigastric pain syndrome 233
Epinephrine
  administration 62
  injection 61
Epstein–Barr virus 13, 102, 108
Erdheim–Chester disease 156
Ertapenem 10
Erythrocyte sedimentation
  rate 176, 197
Escherichia coli 8, 188
Esophageal acid exposure 43
Esophageal candidiasis, Kodsi's
  grading of 37*t*
Esophageal manometry, high-
  resolution 18, 23*f*,
  40, 42
Esophageal motility disorders 21
Esophageal mucosa 36*f*
  pseudotracheabization
    of 51*f*
Esophageal pressure 23*f*
  dynamics 53
Esophageal strictures 24
Esophageal varices 74
Esophageal web 19
Esophagitis 58
  eosinophilic 37, 50, 51*f*
  radiation-induced 37
Esophagogastric junction 50, 51
  disorder of 21
Esophagogastroduodenoscopy
  21, 33
Esophagus
  diseases of 31
  distal 61
  hypercontractile 21, 53
Estrogen 69, 115
Ethanolamine 61
European Association for Study
  of Liver-Chronic Liver
  Failure Consortium 107
European Crohn's and Colitis
  Organisation 199

European Society of
  Gastrointestinal
  Endoscopy 66, 141, 142
Exclusion criteria 156, 156*t*
Extended-spectrum beta-
  lactamases 10
Extracorporeal albumin dialysis
  110
Extracorporeal shock wave
  lithotripsy 144

F

Farnesoid X receptor agonists 88,
  90, 118
Fat
  macrovesicular 102
  planes, loss of 149
Fatty liver 82*f*
  disease 85
    nonalcoholic 81, 83, 85,
      219
Fecal evacuation disorder 203,
  205*f*, 221
Fecal immunochemical test 185
Fecal microbiota
  transplantation 110
Fecal occult blood test 185, 205
Fenofibrate 118
Fever 6, 11, 13, 57, 130, 221
  causes of 13
  enteric 15
  persistent 14
  prodrome of 99
Fibrates 118
Fibroblast growth factor
  analogs 88
Fibrosis 132, 132*t*, 173
  4 score 85, 130
  advanced 83, 132
  pericellular 102
  progression 84
Fistula repair 211
Fluid
  collection, acute
    peripancreatic 169
  therapy 167
Fluoroscopic contrast studies 51
Forrest classification 61, 61*t*
Fresh frozen plasma 135
Functional constipation 181,
  183*t*, 203, 208
  diagnosis of 221*f*, 222
  subtypes of 221
  transit type of 222

Functional defecation disorder 181
Functional dyspepsia 232, 233*b*
   overlap of 232
Functional luminal imaging probe 23, 24
Fundal gastric varices 74
Fungal infection 13, 228
Fungi 8

G

Gallbladder 6, 157*f*
   adherent, fundus of 210*f*
   carcinoma of 146
   diseases of 139
   empyema of 146
   malignancy of 117
   status 211
   swelling 146
Gallstone 166
   ileus 209, 210, 211
      prognosis of 211
      stems, pathogenesis of 211
   pancreatitis 170
Gamma-aminobutyric acid B agonist 96
Gamma-glutamyl
   transferase 81, 147, 176
   transpeptidase 92, 100, 101, 112, 135
Gastric
   antral vascular ectasia 58, 62
   cardia 61
   outlet obstruction 37
   peroral endoscopic pyloromyotomy 44
   varices 73
      isolated 73
      Saad-Caldwell classification of 74*f*
      Sarin's classification of 73*f*
      treatment of 73
   vein 74*f*
Gastritis, atrophic 219
Gastroduodenal erosions 58
Gastroesophageal reflux disease 40, 42*t*, 43, 44*fc*, 233
   subtypes of 43
Gastroesophageal varices 72
Gastrointestinal
   bleeding 55, 64, 71, 92, 105, 125, 221
   diseases 219
      immunoglobulin G4-related 153

disorders
   benign 182
   functional 204
hematemesis 57
hemorrhage, incidence of 15
malignancy 202
mesenchymal tumor 50
organs, neuroendocrine neoplasm of 216*t*
tumors
   benign 62
   malignant 62
Gastropathy, portal 59
Gastrorenal shunt 73, 74*f*
Gestational disorders 112
Ghoshal protocol 205
Giant cells 177*f*
Giardiasis, diagnosis of 199
Glandular structures 157
Glasgow alcoholic hepatitis score 93
Glasgow-Blatchford score 58*t*
Glimepiride 115
Globulin 176
Globus sensation 18
Glomerulonephritis 27
   acute 26
   fibrillary 27
   membranoproliferative 27
Glomerulopathy, immunotactoid 27
Glomerulosclerosis, focal segmental 27
Glucocorticoids 160
Glucose hydrogen breath test 220, 223*f*, 224
Glycyrrhizin 124
Granular cytoplasm 214, 215*f*
Granulocyte
   colony-stimulating factor 95
   epithelial lesions, presence of 173
   monocyte stimulating factors 110
Gut brain axis interaction, disorder of 203
Gut microbiota
   dysbiosis 234
   imbalance 234

H

Haptoglobin levels 92
Headache 3
Heart burn, functional 42, 43*t*

Helicobacter pylori 57, 232
Heller's myotomy, laparoscopic 24
Hematobilia 66
Hematochezia 58
Hematoxylin and eosin stain 229*f*, 230*f*
Hemobilia 58, 150, 152
Hemochromatosis 108, 131
Hemoclip 60
   application 68
Hemodiafiltration techniques 110
Hemodialysis 29
Hemoglobin 4, 64, 70, 100, 101, 147, 176, 204, 214, 228
   C, sickle 134
   S polymerase, oral inhibitor of 137
   glycated 4
Hemolysis 16, 136
Hemophagocytosis, feature of 14
Hemorrhage
   nonvariceal
      gastrointestinal 62
      recent 61
   variceal 105
Hemorrhoids 208
   internal 181
Hemostasis 60, 61
   noncontact thermal technique of 60
Hemosuccus
   entericus 66
   pancreaticus 58
Hepatic crisis, acute sickle 134
Hepatic duct 155*f*, 157*f*
   common 155*f*
Hepatic fibrosis, noninvasive detection of 85
Hepatic inflammation, noninvasive detection of 86
Hepatic steatosis, noninvasive detection of 85
Hepatitis 115
   A 13
      virus 4, 106, 113, 135
   acute viral 112
   alcoholic 92, 93*t*
   autoimmune 108, 125, 126*f*, 128, 131, 136
   B E antigen 130
   B
      chronic 85, 131, 132*t*
      core antigen 108, 135

surface antigen 4, 99, 106,
    108, 113, 125, 130, 135
  virus 108, 125, 135
C
  chronic 85
  virus 4, 106
  chronic viral 131
  E virus 4, 99, 106, 107, 113, 135
  coinfection 4
  severe alcoholic 92, 96, 99, 102
  viruses 35
Hepatopancreatobiliary organs,
    neuroendocrine
    neoplasm of 216t
Hepatopathy, sickle 134
Hepatorenal syndrome 26, 28, 95
  management of 28
  pathophysiology of 27
  types of 28
Herb-induced liver injury 121
  classification 122
Herpes
  simplex
    esophagitis 37
    virus 13, 106, 108
  virus 37
Hiatus hernia 41f
High-resolution impedance
    manometry 23
Hirschsprung's disease 183
  diagnosis of 206
Hormonal therapy 69
Human gastrointestinal tract 219
Human immunodeficiency virus
    4, 106, 112, 219
  disease 197, 199
  infection 36, 51
Hydroxyurea 137
Hydroxyzine 117
Hyperbilirubinemia 3
  conjugated 116
Hypercalcemia 166
Hyperemesis gravidarum 115
Hyperparathyroidism 183
Hypertension 64, 146
  portal 99
Hypertriglyceridemia 166
Hypocalcemia 183
Hypochlorhydria 219
Hypodensity, peripheral 151f
Hypoglycemia 14
Hypokalemia 183, 195
Hypomagnesemia 183
Hypothyroidism 125, 146, 183,
    219, 221, 229
Hypoxia 14

I

Ileum 211
Imipenem cilastatin 10
Immunoglobulin G4-related
    disease 153, 155f,
    159, 161fc
  diagnosis of 158
  spectrum of 153f
Immunoglobulin
  A nephropathy 27
  hepatitis A virus 107, 125
  M 3, 4, 99, 106, 113
  hepatitis E virus 125
Infections 112
  evidence of 94
  nonhepatotropic 14
  parasitic 37
  viral 116
Inflammatory bowel disease 184,
    197, 204, 219
Infliximab 115
Injury 81
Intense fluorodeoxyglucose
    214, 214f
Intensive care unit 26, 34, 127, 228
International Club of Ascites
    Diagnostic Criteria 28
International normalized ratio 4,
    14, 72, 93, 100, 101, 106,
    122, 130
Intestinal blockage, gallstone-
    induced 211
Intestinal methanogen
    overgrowth 220
Intestinal obstruction needing
    surgery 215
Intestinal pseudo-obstruction,
    chronic 219
Intestine, diseases of 179
Intrabolus pressure 21
Intrahepatic biliary radicle
    dilatation 3, 4
Intrahepatic cholestasis 112, 116,
    117
  benign recurrent 112
  causes of 112t
  etiology of 114
  recurrent benign 112, 116
Intraluminal liquid 21
Intramuscular long-acting
    ocreotide 68
Iron 207
  deficiency anemia, presence
    of 196

Irritable bowel syndrome 107,
    183, 189, 195, 203, 207,
    219, 220, 232, 233b
Ischemia 166
  mesenteric 197
Isoenzymes, multiple 117
Isoniazid 115
Isospora 199

J

Jaundice 7, 13-15, 122, 130, 135,
    150
  causes of 13, 148
  cholestatic 198
    pattern of 116
  development of 107
  favors 93
  febrile 13
Jejunum 211
  proximal part of 65

K

Kaposi's sarcoma 228
Karzinoid 213
Kayser-Fleischer ring
  absence of 135
  assessment 108
Kidney
  disease
    chronic 28, 85
    improving global outcomes
      guidelines 26
  failure 14, 108
  injury, acute 26-28
Kinyoun's acid-fast stain,
    modified 199
Kiyosue and Saad-Caldwell
    classification
    systems 73
Klebsiella pneumoniae 8, 36

L

Lactoferrin 196
Lactulose 187
  hydrogen breath test 220, 224
Lamivudine 131, 132
Laxatives 235
  intermittent use of 200
  secondary 187, 188
Lenalidomide 69
Leptospira interrogans 15
Leptospirosis 13, 15

Lesions
  large ulceroproliferative 229
  local structural 49
  malignant 156
  onflammatory 65
Leukocyte proteins, raised 196
Levofloxacin 10
Lille score 103
Linaclotide 188, 207
Lipoprotein
  high-density 81
  low-density 81
Lithotripsy, mechanical 144
Liver
  abscess 7, 8*f*, 10*t*, 11
    amoebic 7, 10
    clinical features of 7
    pyogenic 10
    treatment of 9
  biopsy 85, 99, 100*f*, 130*f*, 136
    percutaneous 136
    transjugular 102, 128
  cholestatic disorders of 112
  cirrhosis 72, 84*f*, 219
  disease 79, 125
    alcohol-associated 85
    chronic 26, 107, 125
    decompensated chronic 92
    end-stage 62, 131
    metabolic 125
    severity 127
  enzyme 156
    elevation 83
  failure 108
    acute 13, 28, 134
    acute-on-chronic 28, 92, 101, 105-107, 110*f*, 125, 126*f*, 128
    chronic 106, 108
    manifestations of 107
  fatty 82*f*
  fibrosis 84*f*
    test 85
  function
    abnormalities 154
    test 14, 33, 99, 141, 142, 175, 176, 209, 228
  inflammation 81
  injury
    drug-induced 107, 108, 121
    herb-induced 121
  kidney microsomal antibody 113
  parenchyma 8*f*
  stiffness measurement 130
  support therapies 110
  surface 8*f*
  transplantation 109, 127, 134
Lower esophageal sphincter 21, 23*f*, 41*f*, 47, 50, 52*f*
  relaxation, failure of 23*f*
Lubiprostone 188, 207, 222
Lumen-apposing metal stent 168*f*
Luminal disorders 179
Lump abdomen 221
Lymphadenopathy 33, 197
Lymphocytes 176
  intraepithelial 199
Lymphohistiocytosis, hemophagocytic 16
Lymphoplasmacytic infiltration 159*f*, 172, 173

M

Macrophage activation syndrome 13
Maddrey's discriminant function 93, 102
Magnesium
  citrate 187
  hydroxide 187
  sulfate 187
Magnetic resonance
  cholangiopancreatography 113, 142, 155*f*, 157*f*, 175
  elastography 86
  imaging 7, 85, 148, 161*f*, 170, 215, 216
  pancreatography 170
Malabsorption syndrome, causes of 219
Malaria 13
  double antigen 35
  hepatopathy 14
  cerebral 14
Malformation, arteriovenous 59, 62, 65
Malignancy 13, 58, 117, 166
Malignant atrophic papulosis 66
Mallory-Denk bodies 100*f*, 102
Mallory-Weiss
  syndrome 58
  tears 59, 61
    hallmarks of 61
Mannitol 187
Manometry, esophageal 21, 41*f*, 51
Marshall organ failure score, modified 167*t*
Mass
  formation of 214
  large ulceroproliferative 229*f*
Masson trichrome stain 130*f*
Mean arterial pressure 28
Mean corpuscular
  hemoglobin 176
    concentration 176
  volume 176
Mechanical dysphagia 49, 50*t*
  causes of 50*t*
Meckel's diverticulum 66
Melanosis coli 181
Melena 57, 58
Meropenem 10
Mesenteric deposits 214
Metabolic disorders 183
Metallic ions 183
Methanobrevibacter smithii 206, 220
Methicillin-resistant Staphylococcus aureus 10
Methylcellulose 187
Methylnaltrexone 188
Methylprednisolone 33
Metolazone 115
Metronidazole 9, 10
Microbiota-gut-brain axis 234
Microscopic agglutination test 15
Microspora 199
Midodrine 27, 29
Mitosis rate 216
Molecular adsorbent recirculating system 29, 110
Molecular patterns, pathogen-associated 96
Monocytes 176
Monosaccharides 232
Monotherapy 174
Motor dysphagia 49, 50, 50*t*
  causes of 50*t*
Motor end plate 49
Mucocele 146
Mucosal disease 196
Mucous membrane 13
  detachment of 34
Multiorgan
  dysfunction, sepsis-induced 15
  failure 134
Multiphase computed tomography 72, 99
Multiple air fluid levels 209*f*
Multiple bile plugs 114*f*

Multiplex polymerase chain
    reaction testing 198
Muscular dystrophies 49
Myasthenia gravis 49
Mycobacterium avium complex
    infection 116
Myotomy 52f

N

N-acetyl cysteine 95
Nasopharyngeal swab 35
Nausea 3
Necrotic collection, acute 169
Nephritis, interstitial 27
Nephropathy, membranous 27
Nervous system, peripheral 49
Neural crest-derived cells 213
Neuroendocrine
    neoplasm, mixed 216
    tumors, small bowel 213
Neuromuscular disease 49
Neuropathy 183
    autonomic 183
    peripheral 69
Neutrophil 114f, 176
    gelatinase-associated
        lipocalin 27
Neutrophilic infiltration 102
Nevirapine 115
N-methyl-D-aspartate 96
Nocturnal stool 195
Nodules, small 132
Nonacid reflex 43
Nonalcoholic fatty liver disease
    81, 83, 85, 219
    management of 86
    pharmacotherapy of 87
    spectrum of 84f
Noncontrast computed
    tomography 113
Nonerosive reflux disease 42
Non-Hodgkin's lymphoma 228
Nonsteroidal anti-inflammatory
    drugs 26, 65, 66, 115, 183
Nucleoside
    analogs 131
    inhibitor 132
Nucleotide analogs 131
Nutrition 109
Nutritional therapy 94

O

Obeticholic acid 90

Obscure gastrointestinal bleeding
    etiology of 66t
    evaluation of 70fc
Obstructive jaundice 146, 148
    clinical diagnosis of 156
    immunoglobulin
        G4-related 153
Oddi dysfunction sphincter 166
Odynophagia 18, 36
Oligosaccharides,
        fermentable 232
Oral prednisolone therapy 100t
Organ failure 108, 110f
    assessment, sequential 105
    progressive 108
    score 108
Organ system 167
Oropharyngeal dysphagia 18, 48,
        49, 49t
    features 18
Oropharynx, surgical resection
        of 49
Osler-Weber-Rendu syndrome 66
Osmotic laxatives 187, 207
Osteomalacia 117
Oxaloacetic transaminase 3

P

Packed red blood cell
        transfusion 150
Pain
    abdominal 6, 57, 105, 154, 195,
        196, 201
    retrosternal 36
Pancreas 6, 117, 147, 160
    carcinoma of head of 146, 147
    diseases of 163
    divisum 166
Pancreatic duct 157f, 170, 172
    stricture 147
Pancreatic fluid collections,
        management of 170fc
Pancreatic mass lesion 175, 177f
Pancreatitis 158f
    acute 165
    alcohol-related 169
    autoimmune 160, 160t,
        172, 173
    chronic 146, 196, 219
    idiopathic duct-centric 160
    immunoglobulin 4-related
        160
    mild 168
    severity of 167t

Pancreatoduodenectomy 148
Pancreatography, endoscopic
        retrograde 170
Panesophageal pressurization 23f
Papilla 151f
Paraneoplastic syndromes 183
Parasites 8
Paratyphi 13
Parenchymal disease 28
Parkinson's disease 183
Paromomycin 10
Pegbelfermin 88
Pelvic floor disorder 189
Pelvis 205f
Pentoxifylline 94
Peptic ulcer
    bleeding, treatment of 60
    disease 58
Peptide receptor radionuclide
        therapy 217
Percutaneous transhepatic biliary
        drainage 149
Peripancreatic fluid
        collections 168
    nomenclature of 169t
Peripheral smear 92
Peristalsis, disorder of 21
Per-oral endoscopic myotomy
        24, 52f
Peroxisome proliferator-activated
        receptor agonists 88
Pharyngeal pouch 19
Phenobarbital 118
Phlebectasia 65
Pioglitazone 89
Piperacillin tazobactam 10
Plantago ovata 187
Plasma
    coagulation 60
    exchange 95, 106, 110
    use of 94
Platelet
    count 4, 100, 101, 150, 176
    transfusions 16
Plecanatide 188, 207
Plug-assisted retrograde
        transvenous
        obliteration 72
Plummer-Vinson syndrome
        49, 66
Pneumobilia 209f, 210f, 211
Polidocanol 61
Polyethylene glycol 187, 202
Polygonum multiflorum 123
Polyols 232

Polyposis
 familial adenomatous 66
 syndromes 66
  inherited 66
Portal vein 4, 74*f*
Portosystemic pressure
  gradient 75
Positron emission tomography-
  computed tomography
  214
Postcorrosive lower esophageal
  stricture 52*f*
Post-percutaneous transluminal
  coronary angioplasty 64
Postprandial distress
  syndrome 233
Postprocedure reflux 24
Prednisolone 94, 154, 156, 173
Pregnancy 207
 intrahepatic cholestasis
  of 112, 116
Pressure-flow analysis 23
Probiotics restore intestinal
  microbiota 188
Procalcitonin 108
 levels, normal 102
Progesterone 69
Prokinetics 60, 187, 188
Protein 4
Prothrombin time 3, 4, 93, 106
 elevated 136
Proton pump inhibitors 24, 37,
  43, 43*t*, 44, 60, 200, 225
 standard dose of 40
  therapy 219
Prucalopride 223, 235
Pseudocyst 169, 175
Pseudoxanthoma elasticum 66
Psoralea corylifolia 123
Pyrrolizidine alkaloids 123

Q

Quincke's triad 150
Quinine 16
Quintron breathtracker™ digital
  microlyzer 222

R

Radiation exposure 85
Radiofrequency ablation 62
Radio-opaque marker 181, 222,
  222*f*, 232
Radiotherapy, systemic 217

Rectal pressure 185
Rectal sensory test 185, 206
Rectoanal inhibitory
  reflex 182, 206
Rectocele, large 206
Red blood cell 135, 176, 196
Reflux disease 37
Refractory gastroesophageal
  reflux disease 40, 43*t*
 symptoms of 40
Renal diseases, histological types
  of 27
Renal function tests 184
Renal thrombotic
  microangiopathy 27
Renal vein 74*f*
Respiratory failure 109
Reticulonodular opacities,
  bilateral 35*f*
Reverse transcription-polymerase
  chain reaction 35
Reynold's pentad 14
Rigor 3
Rituximab 174
Rockall score, pre-endoscopic 59*t*
Roundworms 8
Ryle's tube, placement of 213

S

Salmonella typhi 13
Salt and pepper chromatin 215*f*,
  216
Saroglitazar 88
Satellitosis 100*f*
Schatzki's ring 19, 50
Scleroderma 219
Sclerosants 60, 61
Sclerosing cholangitis 115, 155*f*,
  157, 159
 immunoglobulin 4-related
  159
 primary 115
Sclerotherapy, endoscopic 57, 59
Selective serotonin reuptake
  inhibitor 44, 207
Semaglutide 88
Senecio scandens 123
Sensorium, altered 130
Sepsis 14, 108, 116
 bacterial 13
Serology, viral 125
Serotonin
 norepinephrine reuptake
  inhibitor 44

synthesis 217
 transporter expression 234
Serum ascites albumin
  gradient 99, 130
Serum chromogranin 215
 A 215
 level 214
Shock
 absence of 28
 wave lithotripsy 211
Sickle cell
 anemia 134
 disease 134
 hepatopathy 134
  spectrum of 136
 intrahepatic
  cholestasis 134, 137
Single-organ kidney failure 109
Skin lesions 33
Small bowel
 bleed, endoscopic treatment
  of 65
 resection 214
 vascular lesions 66
Small intestinal bacterial
  overgrowth 195, 223*f*,
  224, 235
 causes of 219*t*
Small intestinal disease,
  immunoproliferative
  199
Smooth muscle antibodies 106
Sodium glucose cotransporter 2
  inhibitors 88, 89
Sodium sulfate 187
Soft tissue density lesion 214
Somatostatin analogs 68, 216
 uptake of 216
Sore throat 130
Splenic embolization,
  partial 73, 75
Splenic vein 74*f*
Staphylococcus aureus 8
Steatohepatitis 85
 nonalcoholic 72, 84, 84*f*, 87*b*,
  88*t*, 125
Steatorrhea 118, 196, 197
Steatosis, macrovesicular 100*f*
Stenosis, aortic 62
Steroids 94, 166
 anabolic 115
 androgenic 118
 therapy 101*t*, 173
 treatment 103
 use of 102

Stevens-Johnson syndrome 37
Stimulant laxatives 187, 207, 223
Stone, double impaction of 146
Stool
 blood in 196
 softener 207
 volume 196
Storiform fibrosis 157, 159*f*, 172
Streptococcus pyogenes 8
Stretta procedure 43
Subacute small bowel obstruction 209
Subepithelial basement membrane, thickening of 199
Superior mesenteric vein 74*f*
Superselective transcatheter embolization 68
Surgery 217
 biliary 211
Swallowing, physiology of 47
Synthetic anabolic androgenic steroids 113
Systemic inflammation, pancreatic manifestation of 173
Systemic inflammatory response syndrome 166
Systemic lupus erythematosus 49

T

Tachycardia 64, 105, 209
Tachypnea 105, 166
Tamoxifen 115
Telangiectasia 75, 215
 hereditary hemorrhagic 69
 inherited hemorrhagic 62
Telbivudine 131
Telotristat 217
 reduces serotonin production 217
Temozolomide 217
Tenofovir 131, 132
Thalidomide 68, 69
Thermal
 ablation 61
 coagulation 60
Thiazides 166
Thorax, computed tomography of 24, 35*f*
Thyroid
 disease 125
 disorders 207

hormone receptor beta 88
 nodule 197
 stimulating hormone 184, 204, 222
Ticarcillin 10
Tinidazole 10
Tirzepatide 88
Tortuous splenic vein 72
Total leukocyte count 4, 6, 72, 100, 101, 176, 214
 raised 3
Total parenteral nutrition 116
Total villous atrophy 199
Tranexamic acid 70
Transjugular intrahepatic portosystemic shunt procedure 29, 73
Transoral incisionless fundoplication 43
Transverse colon 229*f*, 234
Trauma 166
Treitz ligament 67
Triglycerides 16
Trophozoites, amoebic 9
 focal aggregations of 229*f*, 230*f*
Tropical sprue 219
Tryptophan hydroxylase inhibitor 217
Tuberculosis 13, 116, 175, 177, 221, 228
 extrapulmonary 175
Tubular necrosis, acute 26, 27
Tumors 148
 cellular 215*f*
 grading of 216
 mucinous 166
 necrosis factor alpha 94
 neuroendocrine 213, 213*f*, 216
 small intestinal 66
Typhoid fever 13, 15

U

Ulcers 64*f*
 deep esophageal 35*f*
 duodenal 59
 esophageal 37
 mucosal 34*f*
 gastric 59
 small intestinal 66
Ultrasound 142
 abdominal 81, 141, 147

Upper esophageal sphincter 47
 disorder of 49
Upper gastrointestinal
 bleeding, nonvariceal 57
 endoscopy 59, 99
 hemorrhage 150
Urea 4
Urinary bladder pressure 26
Urinary D-xylose test, abnormal 199
Urinary tract infection 228
Ursodeoxycholic acid 96, 113, 117, 124

V

Vague abdominal pain 117
Vanishing bile duct syndrome 115
Vascular endothelial growth factor 68
Vater ampulla 147
Vena cava, inferior 74*f*
Video capsule endoscopy 65, 70
Videofluoroscopy 19
Virus
 anti-hepatitis
  C 125
  E 3
 hepatotropic 107
 non-hepatitis B 83
Vitamin 87, 88
 deficiency 195
 fat-soluble 117
Vomiting 3, 181, 235
von Willebrand factor disease 69
Voxelotor 137

W

Water-filled balloon 182
Watermelon stomach 62
Weight loss 81, 86, 148, 156, 181, 221
Whipple's procedure 148, 153
White blood cell 93, 196, 209
Wilson's disease 108, 125, 131

X

Xerosis 117
X-rays, abdominal 181

Z

Zenker's diverticulum 19, 47

EU GSPR Authorised Reprsentative
Logos Europe, 9 rue Nicolas Poussin
1700, La Rochelle, France
Phone: +33 (0) 6 67 93 73 78
E-mail: contact@logoseurope.eu

www.ingramcontent.com/pod-product-compliance
Ingram Content Group UK Ltd.
Pitfield, Milton Keynes, MK11 3LW, UK
UKHW050429150426
5217IPUK00019B/1303